SERIOUS STRENGTH TRAINING

CONTENTS

Part III   The Six Phases of Training

PREFACE

Strength training and bodybuilding are a religion, an obsession, for the many people whose purpose is to build and sculpt their bodies into a state of muscular, symmetrical perfection. It is the only sport dedicated solely to the aesthetics of the human body. The roots of strength training and bodybuilding lie in Greek and Roman antiquity. These civilizations used physical activity as a means of striving for a perfect balance between body and mind. Sculptures from these ancient societies reflect their perceptions of the perfect human form—large, strong, well-defined muscles, all in perfect proportion, or balance.

Today, however, some bodybuilders at the professional level seem to have abandoned the ideal of the perfect human body for the novelty of a freaky body part. They seem to favor mass over symmetry, bulk over chiseled lines, bloat over definition, and quantity over quality. While mass is important, we must realize that its value does not exceed the value of symmetrical lines, well-proportioned limbs, and deeply striated muscles. To attain the ultimate body, one must never lose sight of the balance that shapes the perfect form. To achieve this level of development requires dedication, patience, and—most important—a solid understanding of the body, training principles, exercise prescription, nutrition, and planning. This book introduces a revolutionary approach to strength training and bodybuilding that will bring the body to its perfect state, naturally, with *Periodization*. Read on to see how this book can help you build the ultimate physique!

Get Bigger and Stronger!

Dr. Tudor O. Bompa developed Periodization in Romania in 1963. The Eastern Bloc countries used his unique system for years, as they achieved virtual domination of the athletic world. The system has also been published worldwide in many journals and magazines. Bompa is the author of several books, including *Theory and Methodology of Training: The Key to Athletic Performance* (1983, 1985, 1990, and 1994) and *Periodization of Strength: The New Wave in Strength Training* (1993). In 1988, he applied his concept of Periodization to the sport of bodybuilding, and his Periodization of Bodybuilding system has been published in *Ironman* magazine as the "Ironman Training System" from 1991 to present.

Periodization for serious strength training and bodybuilding is a method of organizing training to achieve optimum gains in mass, strength, and definition, without encountering the pitfalls of overtraining, stagnation, and injury. Different training phases such as *anatomical adaptation, hypertrophy, maximum strength, muscle definition,* and *transition* are manipulated according to individual training goals. This approach ensures that an athlete will peak at appropriate times and can build or maintain a splendid physique year-round. Whether you are just beginning to train or are a seasoned pro, this book has the training plan you need, complete with detailed daily training programs.

Get Massive and Ripped!

For the first time, a nutritional and supplement program has been designed to correspond with each different phase of training.

The body's needs change as training changes, so we must take nutrition and supplementation into account and not leave it to chance. The Metabolic Diet, coupled with the Periodization of supplementation, gives athletes the tools needed to reach optimal levels of strength, mass, and definition.

Dr. Mauro Di Pasquale was a world-class athlete for over 15 years, winning the world championship in powerlifting in 1976 and the World Games in 1981. Today he balances a busy career as a licensed physician in Ontario, Canada, with his demanding schedule as a consultant and researcher.

Get Smart!

Cutting-edge research, conducted by kinesiologist and former NWA (National Wrestling Alliance) lightweight wrestler Lorenzo Cornacchia, gives you the last word on the best exercises for strength, mass, and shape. Scientific studies, using state-of-the-art EMG (electromyography) equipment, target the exercises that cause the greatest stimulation in the muscles and identify those exercises that can be potentially harmful. Part II, Maximum Stimulation Exercises, ranks exercises in order of their effectiveness and provides pictures for each movement, to ensure proper execution.

Get Started!

For those who have been using the Periodization training system over the past few years, it has meant better results—increased muscle size, tone, and definition—without the ever-present pain, strain, and exhaustion typical of other programs. For those about to begin using these techniques, don't look back. Training will never be the same again!

ACKNOWLEDGMENTS

Because our goal throughout this project has been to provide the most up-to-date and useful strength training and bodybuilding information, we called on the expert assistance of several noted colleagues. We are grateful to the following people for their expert contributions to the completion of this book:

Lenny Visconti, BPhe, BSc(PT), CAFC

Bill McIlroy, PhD

Cassandra Volpe, PhD

Jacquie Laframboise, MSc

Courtney Bean, BSc(PT)

Shiraz Kapadia, BSc(PT)

We are equally indebted to York University and Cassandra Volpe for the use of York's EMG research facilities and equipment and to Bill McIlroy from the University of Toronto for his expertise in EMG analysis. Special thanks to the owners of Player's Health and Fitness Gym for use of their facilities; to Toula Reppas, owner of the Eglinton and Bayview Physiotherapy Clinic; and to Joints in Motion for use of their facilities.

We express our appreciation to the friends and close associates who have contributed either directly or indirectly to the completion of this book:

Kelly Gallacher	Patricia Morrell
Michael Berger	Trevor Butler
John Poptsis	Carmela Caggianiello
Xena Walsh	Bernadette Taggio
Frank Covelli	Laura Binetti
Scott Milnes	Andre Elie
Sammy Wong	Melony Marsen

We thank Peter Robinson for his high professionalism throughout the hundreds of hours necessary to take thousands of photographs. Our special appreciation to Sam Wong of Sam Wong Photography for his exercise and nutrition pictures and to Ralph Dehaan for his photos.

Special thanks to all the bodybuilders and fitness models who posed for the photographs. Thanks also to Marie Kun for her help with photos and editing.

Special thanks to Stephen Holman, editor in chief of *Ironman* magazine; Tom Deters, DC, associate publisher of *Flex* (Weider Publications); and Mark Casselman, science editor of *Muscle and Fitness*.

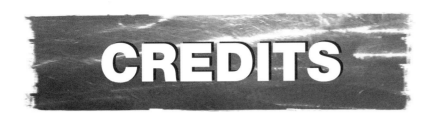
CREDITS

Figure 1.3: Reprinted, by permission, from Vander, A., J. Sherman, and D. Luciano, 1990, *Human physiology*, 5th ed. (NY: McGraw-Hill), 296.

Figures 1.4, 3.1, 3.2, 3.3., 3.4, 3.5, 3.6, 3.7, 3.8, 3.9, 3.10, and 10.1; tables 3.1, 3.3, 4.2, and 10.1; and appendixes 1, 2, and 3: Reprinted, by permission, from Bompa, T.O., 1996, *Periodization of strength*, 4th ed. (Toronto, Canada: Veritas Publishing.)

Figures 3.11, 3.12, and 3.13: Reprinted, by permission, from Bompa, T.O., 1983, *Theory and methodology of training*. (Dubuque, IA: Kendall/Hunt.)

PART I

SCIENCE OF STRENGTH TRAINING

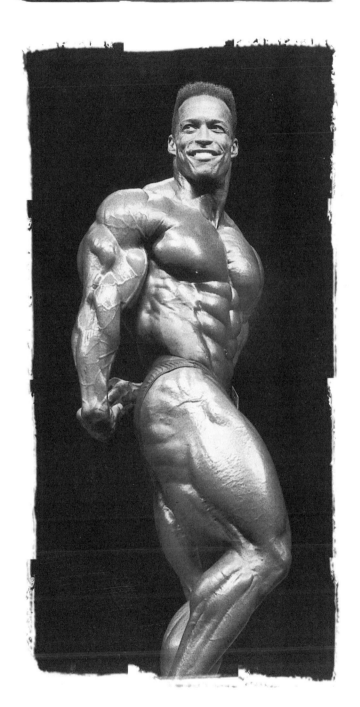

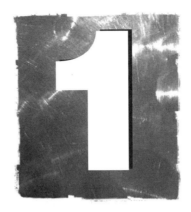

ADAPTING TO THE TRAINING STIMULUS

Everyone who engages in strength training and bodybuilding should understand certain theoretical principles and fundamental concepts of these activities. The better they understand basic principles, the better and faster they will be able not only to use the information in this book, but also to create training programs conducive to their own talents and specific situations. To comprehend the training methods discussed in this book, one must understand muscle contractions and how muscles produce work.

The Muscle and Muscle Contraction

A muscle consists of special fibers that range in length from a few inches to over three feet, and extend over the entire length of the muscle. These fibers are grouped in bundles called *fasciculi*, each separately wrapped in a sheath *(perimysium)* that holds them together.

Each muscle fiber has thread-like protein strands called *myofibrils*, which hold the contractile proteins *myosin* (thick filaments) and *actin* (thin filaments), whose actions are very important in muscle contraction (figure 1.1). The ability of a muscle to contract and exert force is determined by its design, the cross-sectional area, the fiber length, and the number of fibers within the muscle. Because genetics determines the number of fibers within the muscles, training does not affect it; but training does affect the other variables. Dedicated training increases the thickness of muscle filaments, thereby increasing both muscle size and force of contraction.

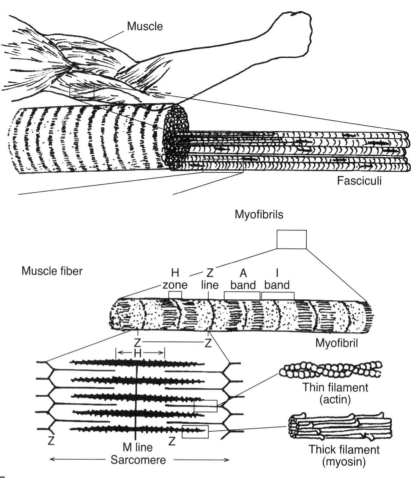

Figure 1.1 **Muscle cell.**

Mechanism of Muscle Contraction: The Sliding Filament Theory

According to the *sliding filament theory of contraction,* muscle contraction involves the two contractile proteins (actin and myosin) in a series of mechanical events. Each myosin filament is surrounded by six actin filaments. The myosin filaments contain *cross bridges,* which are tiny extensions that reach toward the actin filaments. When the impulse from a motor nerve reaches a muscle cell, it stimulates the entire fiber, creating chemical changes that allow the actin filaments to join with the myosin cross bridges. The binding of myosin to actin via cross bridges releases energy that causes the cross bridges to swivel, pulling or sliding the myosin filament over the actin filament. This sliding motion causes the muscle to shorten (contract), producing force. Once the stimulation ceases, the actin and myosin filaments separate, returning the muscle to its resting length (figure 1.2). This cross-bridge activity explains why the force that a muscle generates depends on its initial length before contraction. The optimal length before muscle contraction is resting length (or slightly greater), because all of the cross bridges can connect with the actin filaments, slowing development of maximal tension.

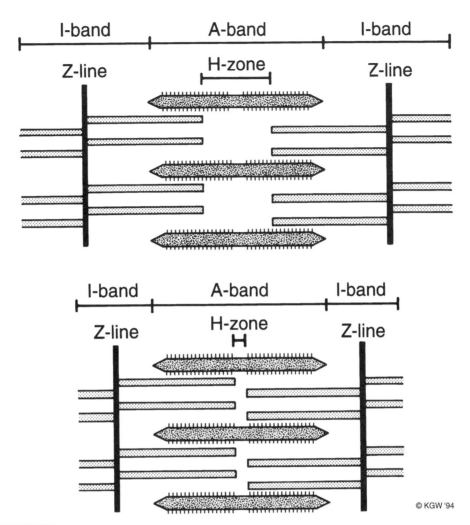

Figure 1.2 Contraction while muscle is shortened.

© K. Galasyn-Wright, Champaign, IL 1994

The highest force output occurs when contraction begins at a joint angle of approximately 110 to 120 degrees. Contractile force diminishes as the muscle length before contraction is either shorter or longer than resting length: When the length is significantly shorter than resting length (i.e., already partially contracted), the actin and myosin filaments already overlap, leaving fewer cross bridges open to "pull" on the actin filaments; when a muscle is significantly beyond resting length before contraction, the force potential is small because the actin filaments are too far away from the cross bridges to be able to join and shorten the muscle.

The Motor Unit

Each motor nerve entering a muscle can stimulate from one to several thousand muscle fibers, which contract and relax in unison to the nerve's impulses. A single motor nerve, together with the muscle fibers it activates, creates a *motor unit* (figure 1.3).

When a motor nerve is stimulated, the impulse sent to the muscle fibers within the motor unit either spreads completely or does not spread at all. This is the

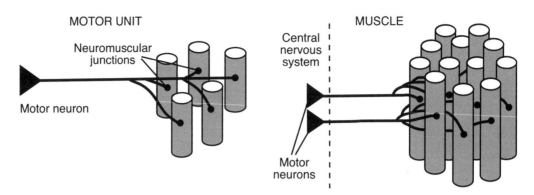

Figure 1.3 **Motor-unit source.**

Reprinted from Vander, Sherman, and Luciano 1990.

all-or-none law—that is, a weak impulse creates the same tension within the motor unit as a strong impulse.

This all-or-none law does not apply to the muscle as a whole. While all muscle fibers within a single motor unit respond to stimulation by the motor nerve, not all motor units are activated during a muscle contraction. The number of motor units involved in a contraction depends on the load imposed on the muscle, which in turn directly correlates with the force produced. If the load imposed on a muscle is extremely heavy, then all or almost all of the motor units will be recruited, resulting in a maximal force output. If the load is light, only a small number of motor units are recruited and the strength of contraction is low (Wilmore and Costill 1999). Since a muscle's motor units are recruited in sequential order, the only way to train the entire muscle is to expose it to maximum loads so that every motor unit is used for muscle contraction.

While the force exerted by a muscle depends on the number of motor units recruited during a contraction, it also depends on the number of muscle fibers within a motor unit. The number of fibers can vary between 20 and 500, the average being around 200. The more fibers in a motor unit, the higher the force output. Genetic factors determine the number of fibers. Some people can increase muscle size and strength quite easily, whereas others have to fight for the smallest gains.

Muscle Fiber Types

All motor units behave in the same way, but all muscle fibers do not. Muscle fibers differ in their biochemical (metabolic) functions: Although every muscle fiber can function under both anaerobic and aerobic conditions, some work better under anaerobic conditions; others work better under aerobic conditions.

Fibers that primarily rely on and use oxygen to produce energy are referred to as aerobic, type 1, red, or *slow twitch (ST) fibers*. Fibers that do not require oxygen are referred to as anaerobic, type 2, white, or *fast twitch (FT) fibers*. ST and FT fibers exist in relatively equal proportions within the body—proportions not thought to be greatly affected by strength training and bodybuilding. The distribution of fiber types can vary, both within the same muscle and between different muscles. The arms tend to have a higher percentage of FT fibers than the legs; biceps average about 55 percent FT, and triceps 60 percent, whereas soleus muscles (calves) average around 24 percent FT (Fox et al. 1989). The proportion of FT fibers within a muscle plays an important role in strength training and bodybuilding.

Muscles containing a higher percentage of FT fibers are capable of quicker and more powerful contractions, while those with more ST fibers resist fatigue and are useful for endurance activities.

The recruitment of muscle fibers is load-dependent. During moderate- and low-intensity activity, ST fibers are recruited as workhorses. As the load increases, a greater number of FT fibers are activated during contractions.

There are no clear differences in muscle fiber distribution between female and male athletes. Individuals with an inherited propensity toward more FT fibers are more genetically suited to strength training and bodybuilding than are people with a preponderance of ST fibers. Yet while genetics is an important factor in determining success, it is not the only one. Regardless of genetic endowment, every individual, through intensive training and proper nutrition, can improve muscle size, tone, and definition.

Muscle Contraction

The musculoskeletal frame of the body is an arrangement of bones, attached to one another by a series of ligaments, at structures called joints. The muscles crossing these joints provide the force necessary for body movements. Skeletal muscles do not contract independently of one another; movements about a joint involve several muscles, each with a different role.

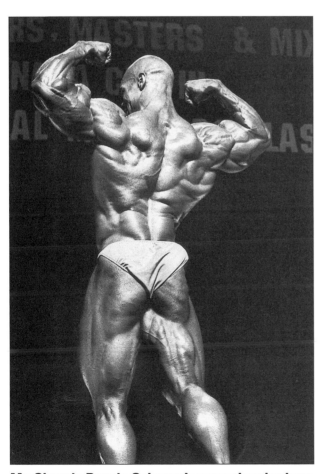

Mr. Olympia Ronnie Coleman's muscular physique.

Agonists, or *synergists*, are muscles that work together as a team, cooperating to perform a movement. *Antagonists* act in opposition to agonists during movement. The interaction between agonist and antagonist muscle groups directly influences athletic movements. In most cases, especially for skilled and experienced athletes, the antagonist muscles are relaxed, allowing motions to be performed with ease. A motion that looks jerky, or is performed rigidly, may result from improper interaction between the two groups. Only by concentrating on relaxing the antagonists can an athlete improve the flow and smoothness of a muscle contraction.

Prime movers are the muscles primarily responsible for producing a comprehensive strength movement. During a biceps curl, for example, the prime mover is the biceps muscle, while the triceps acts as an antagonist and needs to be relaxed in order to facilitate smooth flexion.

The *line of pull* for strength training and bodybuilding is an imaginary line that crosses the muscle longitudinally, connecting the two extreme heads of the muscle. A muscle contraction achieves its highest physiological and mechanical efficiency when performed along the line of pull. Here's an example: You can flex your elbow with your palm held in several different positions. With the palm turned upward, the line of pull is direct, creating the highest efficiency. With the palm facing down, efficiency of contraction decreases because the tendon of the biceps muscle wraps around the radius bone. In this case, the line of pull is indirect, which wastes a large portion of the contractile force. For maximum strength gains and optimal muscle efficiency, perform strength exercises along the line of pull.

Types of Muscle Contraction

Skeletal muscles are responsible for both contraction and relaxation. A muscle contracts when it is stimulated, and when the contraction stops the muscle relaxes. Bodybuilders and strength athletes use various types of contractions depending on the scope of their training phase and the equipment being used. There are three types of contractions—*isotonic, isometric,* and *isokinetic.*

Isotonic

Isotonic (dynamic), from the Greek *isos + tonikos* (equal tension), is the most familiar type of muscle contraction. As the term implies, during an isotonic contraction the tension should be constant throughout the entire range of motion. There are two types of isotonic contractions: concentric and eccentric.

- In *concentric,* from the Latin *com-centrum* (having a common center), the muscle shortens in length. Concentric contractions are possible only when the resistance (i.e., weight load) is less than the athlete's maximum potential. Examples of concentric contractions include the curling action of a biceps curl, or the extending motion of a leg extension.

- *Eccentric,* or *negative,* contractions reverse the process of a concentric action—that is, eccentric contractions return muscles to their starting point. During a biceps curl, the eccentric component occurs when the arm extends to the starting point after the curl. During a leg extension, eccentric work is being done when the legs bend at the knee toward the starting position. During an eccentric contraction, the muscles are yielding either to the force of gravity (as in free weights) or to the force of a machine's pull. Under such conditions, the muscle lengthens as the joint angle increases, thus releasing a controlled tension.

Isometric

In isometric (static) contractions—from the Greek *isos + metrikos* (equal in measurement)—the muscle develops tension without changing length. During an isometric contraction, the application of force against an immovable object forces the muscle to develop high tension without altering its length. For example, if you push against a wall, tension is created in your muscles although they remain the same length. The tension developed from this type of contraction is often higher than that developed during an isotonic contraction.

Isokinetic

Isokinetic, from the Greek *isos + kineticos* (equal motion), describes a contraction with constant velocity over the full range of motion. Isokinetic work needs special equipment designed to allow a constant velocity of contraction regardless of the load. During the movement, an athlete performs both concentric and eccentric

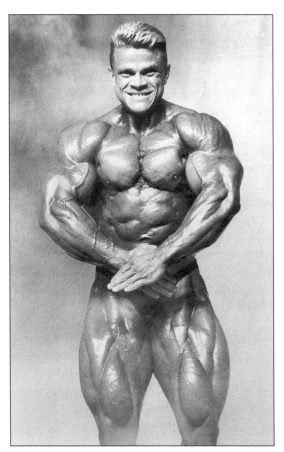

Roland Cziurlok's awesome size and strength are the result of employing maximum strength training.

contractions while the machine provides a resistance that is equal to the force generated by the athlete. The benefit of this type of training is that it allows the muscle to work maximally throughout the entire movement. It eliminates the "sticking point," or weak spot, that is present in every exercise motion.

Types of Strength and Their Significance in Training

Various types of strength training are needed to build and sculpt the most muscular, defined, symmetrical, and injury-free physique possible.

General strength is the foundation of the entire strength and bodybuilding program. It must be the sole focus of training during the early training phase of an experienced lifter, and during the first few years for entry-level strength trainers or bodybuilders. A low level of general strength can limit overall progress, leaving the body susceptible to injury—and, potentially, to development of asymmetrical shape or to diminished ability to build muscle strength and size.

Maximum strength refers to the highest force that can be performed by the neuromuscular system during a maximum contraction. It reflects the heaviest load that an athlete can lift in one attempt, and is expressed as 100 percent of maximum, or *one-repetition maximum, or 1RM*. It is crucial, for training purposes, to know one's maximum strength for each exercise, since it is the basis for calculating loads for every strength phase.

Muscle endurance is defined as the muscle's ability to sustain work for a prolonged period. It is used largely in endurance training, and also plays a crucial role in bodybuilding and strength training, where it is used extensively during the muscle definition or "cuts" phase of training.

Muscular Adaptation to Bodybuilding

Systematic training results in certain structural and physiological changes, and the size and definition of the body's muscles indicate the level of adaptation. The magnitude of these adaptations is directly proportional to the demands placed on the body by volume (quantity), frequency, and intensity (load) of training. In the following paragraphs we explore several types of muscle adaptation: hypertrophy, anatomical adaptation, nervous system adaptation, adaptation of neuromuscular coordination, metabolic adaptation, cardiovascular adaptation, and changes in body composition.

STRENGTH CUE

Training is beneficial to a strength trainer and bodybuilder only as long as it forces the body to adapt to the stress of physical work. In other words, if the body meets with a demand greater than that to which it is accustomed, it works to adapt to the stressor by becoming bigger and stronger. When the load is not high enough to challenge the body's adaptation threshold, the training effect will be nil (or at best minimal) and no adaptation will occur.

Hypertrophy

One of the most visible signs of adaptation is the increase in muscle size—*hypertrophy*. This phenomenon is due to an increase in the cross-sectional area of individual muscle fibers. A reduction in size, resulting from inactivity, is referred to as *atrophy*. Strength trainers and bodybuilders experience two kinds of hypertrophy:

Short-term hypertrophy, as the name implies, lasts for only a few hours and results from the "pump" experienced during heavy training—largely the result of fluid accumulation (edema) in the muscle. Heavy lifting results in an increased amount of water being held in the intracellular spaces of the muscle, making it look even larger. When the water returns to the blood a few hours after training, the pump disappears. This is one reason why strength is not always proportional to muscle size.

Chronic hypertrophy is the result of structural changes at the muscle level. Since it is caused by an increase in either the number or size of muscle filaments, its effects are more enduring than those of short-term hypertrophy (Bompa 1999).

People with a large number of fibers tend to be stronger and show more size than those with fewer fibers. The number, determined by genetics, traditionally has been thought to remain constant throughout one's life; however, a controversial theory now suggests that the heavy loads used in strength training may provoke "muscle splitting," or *hyperplasia*, possibly leading to an increase in the number of muscle fibers. This theory is based on animal research and the results have not yet been duplicated in research involving human subjects.

Strong evidence suggests that individual-fiber hypertrophy accounts for most of the gains in muscle size. Many researchers reported increases in the size of muscle fibers and in the number of filaments (especially the myosin filaments) (Behm 1995; McCall et al. 1996; Starkey et al. 1996). In the case of myosin, training with heavy loads increases the number of cross bridges, leading to an increase in the cross-sectional area of the fiber and to visible gains in the force of maximum contraction.

Not all of the factors responsible for hypertrophy are fully understood. It is widely believed that growth in muscle size is stimulated mainly by a disturbance in

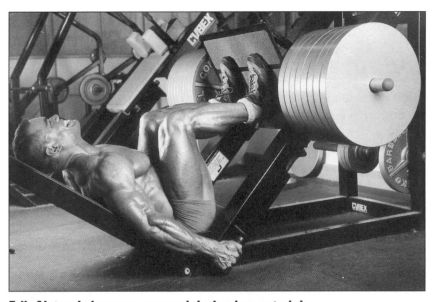

Erik Alstrup's legs are pumped during heavy training.

the equilibrium between the consumption and remanufacturing of ATP (adenosine triphosphate), called the *ATP deficiency theory* (Hartman and Tünneman 1988). During and immediately after a heavy-load training session, protein content in the working muscles is very low, if not exhausted, due to ATP depletion. As athletes recover between training sessions, their bodies replace the protein in the working muscles; but the protein content in the end exceeds the initial levels, increasing the size of the muscle fibers. A protein-rich diet will make this effect especially pronounced.

Another theory regarding hypertrophy focuses on the role of the male sex hormone testosterone (serum androgen, a substance that has masculinizing properties). Although there are no physiological differences between the muscles of women and men, male athletes usually have larger and stronger muscles. The difference is attributed to testosterone content, which is approximately ten times greater for men than for women. While testosterone seems to promote muscle growth, there is no scientific proof to indicate that it is the sole determinant of muscle size.

It is also possible that muscle hypertrophy is attributable to a conversion of ST fibers to FT fibers. Although it is mostly speculation at this point, some research indicates that the percentage of ST fibers decreases as a result of strength training (Staron et al. 1994; Wilmore and Costill 1999). Studies on this theory have been largely inconclusive, since the research is typically conducted on subjects who are not serious strength trainers or bodybuilders. The findings might be different if a research study followed these athletes from entry level to the professional level, instead of observing changes that occur in individuals of varying fitness levels during only eight weeks of training.

Anatomical Adaptation

Research in the area of anatomical adaptation suggests that training with constant and extensive high-intensity loads may decrease the material strength of the bones (Matsuda et al. 1986). This means that if the load does not vary from low to maximum, the result may be a decrease in material bone strength, which may leave the athlete prone to bone injuries. An injury-prone athlete may be one whose training exposes the bones to an intense mechanical stress without a progressive period of adaptation.

Note, however, that at an early age, or at the entry level, low-intensity training may have a positive, stimulating effect on the length and girth of one's long bones—while high-intensity, heavy-load training may permanently restrict bone growth in beginners (Matsuda et al. 1986).

Young and entry-level strength trainers and bodybuilders should follow a long-term plan in which they progressively increase the load over several years. The purpose of training is to stress the body in such a way that it results in adaptation, not aggravation. A well-monitored load increment also has a positive effect for mature athletes, as it results in increased bone density, which allows the bones to better cope with the mechanical stresses of weight training.

The adaptation of tendons is also important in strength training. Muscles do not attach to bones directly, but rather through their extensions, called tendons. The ability of a muscle to pull forcefully against a bone—and, as a result, to perform a movement—depends on the strength of the muscle's tendons. Because tendons adapt to powerful contractions more slowly than muscles, muscle growth should not exceed the rate of tendon adaptation.

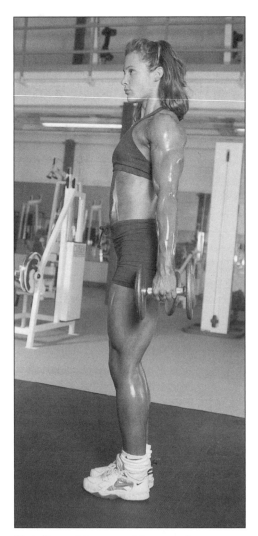

Natalie, a 19-year-old sensation.

Nervous System Adaptation

Gains in muscle strength can also be explained by changes in both the pattern of motor unit recruitment and the synchronization of the motor units to act in unison (Enoka 1996). Motor units are controlled by nerve cells, called *neurons*, which have the capacity to produce both excitatory (stimulating) and inhibitory impulses. *Excitation* initiates the contraction of a motor unit. *Inhibition* helps prevent muscles from exerting more force than the connective tissue (tendons) and bones can tolerate. These two nervous system processes perform a sort of balancing act to ensure the safety of muscle contraction. The force outcome of a contraction depends on how many motor units contract and how many remain in a state of relaxation. If the number of excitatory impulses exceeds the number of inhibitory impulses, a given motor unit is stimulated and will participate in the overall contraction and production of force. If the opposite occurs, that particular motor unit stays relaxed. The theory is that training can counteract inhibitory impulses, thus enabling a muscle to contract more powerfully. Gains in strength are largely the result of an increased ability to recruit more motor units to participate in the overall force of contraction. Such an adaptive response is facilitated only by heavy and maximum loads, and is safe only after the tendons have adapted to high-intensity training.

Adaptation of Neuromuscular Coordination

Neuromuscular coordination for strength training and bodybuilding movement patterns takes time and is a function of learning. The ability to coordinate specific sequences, which involve different muscles to perform a lift, requires the precision that can be acquired only over a long period of continuous repetition. In other words, "practice makes perfect." An efficient lift can be achieved only when the bodybuilder learns to relax the antagonistic muscles, so that unnecessary contractions do not affect the force of the prime movers. A highly coordinated group of muscles consumes less energy during contraction, providing superior performance.

Because young or entry-level strength trainers and bodybuilders lack certain necessary motor skills and muscle coordination, they cannot expect immediate hypertrophy. Within the course of four to six weeks of strength training, young athletes typically experience visible increments in strength but no concomitant increase in muscle size. The reason for strength gain without achieving muscle hypertrophy is *neural adaptation* (Wilmore and Costill 1999), which is an increase in the nervous coordination of the muscles involved. As a result of training, these entry-level athletes have learned to use their muscles effectively and economically. This motor learning effect is of major importance in the early stages of training, and athletes must realize that it is part of a necessary progression. It is

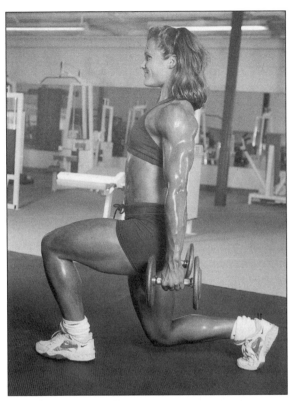

Natalie demonstrates excellent coordination and training technique.

easy to become frustrated when improvement in size is not visibly apparent, but it will come when the body is ready.

Metabolic Adaptation

The biochemical process that uses chemical energy to perform physical activity is known as metabolism. Both strength training and cardiovascular training induce physiological and metabolic adaptations within the body, eventually resulting in more effective workouts. The metabolic adaptations vary with the specifics of each type of training. No training program, no matter how well designed, can do everything for everyone. For a more comprehensive adaptation, you must use a complex training program. This is a basic premise of why a periodized, phase-specific training program works best.

Strength training increases muscles' myoglobin content, especially if done in conjunction with cardiovascular training. Myoglobin—the red pigment that gives red muscle fiber its color—stores oxygen necessary for a longer duration of physical activity. Glycogen, consisting of long chains of glucose, is the storage form of carbohydrates; during exercise it releases glucose for energy production—and since the muscles of trained individuals store more glycogen, they have increased capacity to generate energy. Moreover, long-duration training programs increase the body's ability to oxidize fat as an energy source, delaying the depletion of glycogen. Long-duration activity (i.e., that which is continuous over at least 25 minutes) uses fat as the major source of energy—a important point for anyone who intends to lose weight or enhance muscle definition and striation.

In addition to increasing the production of glycogen, adaptation to strength training increases the capacity for the muscles to store larger amounts of ATP and creatine phosphate (CP). ATP and CP reserves are used for energy during short-term and intense-strength training.

Training also helps bodybuilders adapt better to the buildup of lactate concentration in the blood—for example, when they perform intense sets over a 15- to 20-second period. Lactate is a fatiguing metabolite that results from incomplete breakdown of glucose (the form of sugar used for energy). Better adaptation to lactate results in less fatigue.

Cardiovascular Adaptation

Cardiovascular conditioning is a very important aspect of strength training and bodybuilding. The efficiency with which we perform even simple daily activities depends on the functioning of our cardiovascular systems. Conditioning this system involves the progressive adaptation of both the physiological and biochemical aspects of our bodies. Bodybuilders enhance their endurance capacity

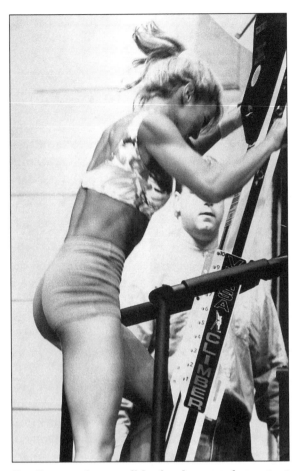

Cardiovascular conditioning is a very important aspect in strength training and bodybuilding.

when they use large muscle groups in performing activities such as running, bicycling, stair climbing, and swimming.

Cardiovascular endurance training leads to specific adaptations that increase not only competitive ability but also overall health and longevity: decreased heart rate during rest and exercise, increased heart stroke volume, lowered blood pressure, and higher lung volume.

Changes in Body Composition

One of the most visible results of an organized training program is in the area of body composition—overall body shape as well as the proportions of fat and lean muscle mass. Combining cardiovascular and strength training will lower an individual's level of body fat by using fatty acids as fuel, especially during nonstop, longer-duration activity. Another important result of combined cardiovascular and strength training is the ratio between caloric intake and caloric expenditure. When the ratio is in favor of caloric expenditure, people lose weight and their body compositions change in favor of leaner body shapes. Any fitness program that is intended to increase lean muscle mass must incorporate heavier loads, *and* it must include a cardiovascular program (longer than 25 minutes) that will cause the body to use fatty acids as fuel (Bompa 1999). This is why, in our six phases of training, we propose a maximum strength phase and a muscle definition phase, whose objectives are to increase lean muscle mass and use more fatty acids. As a result of these two specific training phases, the metabolic rate of the body will increase; and body composition and overall body form and proportions will be improved.

Principles of Strength Training and Bodybuilding

Training is a complex activity governed by principles and methodological guidelines, designed to help athletes achieve the greatest possible muscle size and definition. The principles of training explained in the next section are very important training guidelines that must be considered at the start of an organized training program.

Principle #1—Vary Your Training

Bodybuilding and strength training are highly demanding activities that require hour after hour of dedicated training. The pressure of continually increasing training volume and intensity, along with the repetitive nature of weightlifting, can easily lead to boredom that may become an obstacle to motivation and success.

The best medicine for monotonous training is variety. To add variety, you must be familiar with the training methods and with Periodization planning (see part II), and be comfortable with a multitude of different exercises for each muscle group (see part II).

Variety in training improves psychological well-being and improves training response. The following suggestions will help you to add variety to your training.

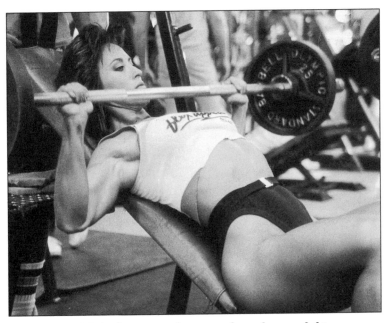

Rachel McLish isn't one to shy away from free weights.

- Choose different exercises for each specific body part instead of doing your favorite exercises each time. Change the order in which you perform certain exercises. Remember, both your mind and your body become bored; they both need variety.

- Incorporate variety into your loading system as suggested by the step-loading principle (discussed under "Principle #3").

- Vary the type of muscle contractions done in your workouts (i.e., include both concentric and eccentric work).

- Vary the speed of contraction (slow, medium, and fast).

- Vary equipment so you go from free weights to machine weights to isokinetics, and so on.

Principle #2—Observe Individual Differences

Rarely do two individuals come to training with exactly the same history and agenda. Everyone is different in his or her genetics, athletic background, eating habits, metabolism, training desire, and adaptation potential. Strength athletes and bodybuilders, regardless of their level of development, must have individualized training programs. Too often, entry-level athletes are seduced into following the training programs of advanced athletes. Advice given by these seasoned athletes is inappropriate for novices, no matter how well intentioned. Beginners, whose muscles, ligaments, and tendons are unaccustomed to the stresses of serious weight training, require a longer period of adjustment, or adaptation, in order to avoid injury.

Often the following factors influence an individual's work capacity:

- **Training background**. The work demand should be proportional to your experience, background, and age.

- **Individual capacity for work**. Not all athletes who are similar in structure and appearance have the same work tolerance. Individual work abilities

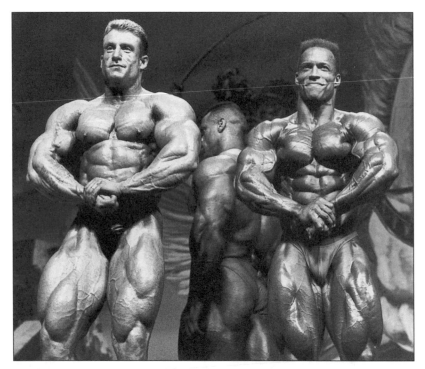

No two bodybuilders are alike. Yates and Ray—both gloriously big and symmetrical—each have their own individual look, style, and training needs.

must be assessed before determining the volume and intensity of work. This will increase the odds of becoming successful and remaining injury free.

- **Training load and rate of recovery.** When planning and evaluating the training load, consider the factors outside training that place high demands on you. For example, heavy involvement in school, work, or family, and even the distance traveled to the gym, can affect the rate of recovery between training sessions. Also account for destructive or negative lifestyle habits and emotional involvements as you create a training plan.

Principle #3—Employ Step-Type Loading

The theory of progressive load increments in strength training has been known and employed since ancient times. According to Greek mythology, the first person to apply the theory was Milo of Croton, a pupil of the famous mathematician Pythagoras (c. 580-500 B.C.), who was an Olympic wrestling champion. In his teen years, Milo decided to become the strongest man in the world, and embarked on this mission by lifting and carrying a calf every day. As the calf grew and became heavier, Milo became stronger. Finally, when the calf had developed into a full-grown bull, Milo, thanks to a long-term progression, was able to lift the bull, and was indeed the strongest man on earth. Improvements in muscle size, tone, and definition are a direct result of the amount and quality of training performed over a long period of time. From the entry level right up to the Mr. or Ms. Olympia level, the training workload must increase gradually, in accordance with each individual's physiological and psychological abilities, if gains in muscle size, tone, and definition are to continue.

The most effective technique for load patterning is the step-loading principle, because it fulfills the physiological and psychological requirements that increased training load must be followed by a period of *unloading*. The unloading phase serves as a reprieve for the body, so that it can adapt to the new, more intense stressors and regenerate itself in preparation for yet another load increase. Since everyone responds differently to stress, each athlete must plan a loading schedule that fits his or her specific needs and rate of adaptation. For instance, if the load is increased too abruptly it may exceed the body's adaptation capacity, disrupting the physiological balance of the overload-to-adaptation cycle. Once this disruption occurs, adaptation will be less than optimal, and injuries might occur.

The step-type approach involves the repetition of a microcycle, or a week of training (figure 1.4), in which the resistance is increased over several steps, followed by an unloading step to ensure recuperation.

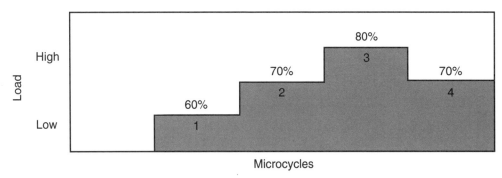

Figure 1.4 **The step-type method of increasing training load.**
Reprinted from Bompa 1996.

Note that each step represents more than one single workout, which means that the workload is not increased at every training session. One workout provides insufficient stimulus to produce marked changes in the body. Such adaptation occurs only after repeated exposure to the same training loads. In figure 1.4, each step represents one week, each vertical line indicates a change in load, and each horizontal line represents the week over which you use and adapt to that load. The percentages indicated above each step are the suggested percentages of maximum. You can see the progression for the first three weeks, as well as the decrease for the unloading phase in the fourth week.

Let's look at how your body responds to the step-loading approach. On Monday, for example, you begin a microcycle (a new step) by increasing the workload. After Monday's workout your body is in a state of fatigue—a physiological crisis, because it is unaccustomed to such stress. When the same level continues, your body will probably be comfortable with the load by Wednesday, and adapt to it in the following two days. By Friday, you should feel really good and capable of lifting even heavier loads. After the crisis of fatigue comes a phase of adaptation, which in turn is followed by a physiological rebound, or improvement.

By the next Monday, you should feel physically and mentally comfortable, which indicates that it is time to challenge the level of adaptation once more.

Each step of the microcycle will bring improvements until you reach the unloading (regeneration) phase (step 4). This phase gives your body the time it needs to replenish its energy stores, restore

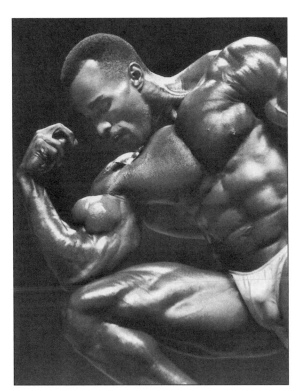

Darem Charles hits a biceps pose.

a psychological balance, and rid itself of the fatigue

that has accumulated over the preceding three weeks. The fourth step in this example becomes the new lowest step for another phase of load increments.

Figure 1.5 illustrates how the same four microcycles (steps) shown in figure 1.4 fit into the context of a longer training cycle, where the goal is to build muscle size.

Although the load increments may seem small, it is important to remember that because you are getting stronger your maximum weight values are increasing, which means that your percentages of maximum are increasing as well. For example, the first time you reached the high step of 80 percent, your 80-percent-of-maximum weight for a specific exercise may have been 120 pounds. Three weeks later, because of your adaptation and strength gains, your 80 percent may have increased to 130 pounds. Consequently, you use progressively heavier loads over the long term, despite the fact the your percentages of maximum remain the same.

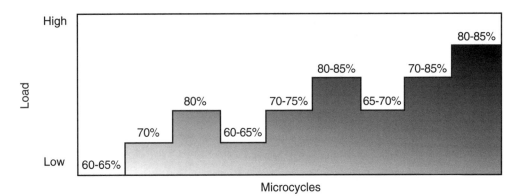

Figure 1.5 An example of how to increase the training load over a longer period.

Three Basic Laws of Strength and Bodybuilding Training

The training principles just discussed provide a loose guideline for general training. There are also three laws of strength training that must be adhered to if an athlete is to proceed, injury-free, to a more comprehensive, rigorous training program. Entry-level bodybuilders and strength athletes often begin training programs without being aware of the strain they will encounter and without understanding the progression or training methodology behind the program. These are usually the people who tend to seek advice from seasoned athletes (who may not be qualified to give it) and who, consequently, find themselves out of their league and on a collision course with injury. Adherence to the following training laws will ensure the proper anatomical adaptation of a young or untrained body, before subjecting it to the rigors of strength training.

Law #1—Before Developing Muscle Strength, Develop Joint Flexibility

Most strength-training exercises, especially those employing free weights, use the whole range of motion around major joints. In some exercises, the weight of the barbell compresses the joints to such a degree that, if the individual does not

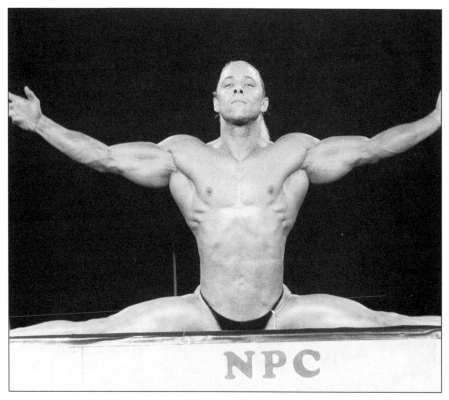

Flexibility is the cornerstone of a sound bodybuilding training program.

have good flexibility, strain and pain can result. Consider deep knee squats: during a deep squat, compression of the knee joints may cause an inflexible athlete a lot of pain, or even injury. Also, in the deep-squat position, a lack of good ankle flexibility forces the person to stay on the balls of the feet and toes, rather than on the flat of the foot where a good base of support and balance is ensured. Development of ankle flexibility (i.e., *plantar flexion*, or bringing the toes toward the calf) is essential for all strength trainers, but especially for entry-level athletes.

Law #2—Before Developing Muscle Strength, Develop the Tendons

The rate of gain in muscle strength always has the potential to exceed the rate at which tendons and ligaments can adapt to higher tensions. It is crucial that the tendons and ligaments have time to adapt, because many individuals lack a long-term vision, they prematurely use heavy loads to develop specific muscle groups without strengthening the support systems of those muscles. It's like building a house on the sand—it may look good for a little while, but at high tide the whole thing is destroyed. Build your body on a rock-solid foundation and this will not happen to you.

Tendons and ligaments are trainable and can actually increase in diameter as a result of proper anatomical adaptation training (see chapter 10), which increases their ability to withstand tension and wear. This training is accomplished via a low-load program for the first one to two years of training. Shortcuts are not the answer to achieving a well-developed, injury-free body. Patience will ultimately pay off.

Law #3—Before Developing the Limbs, Develop the Body's Core

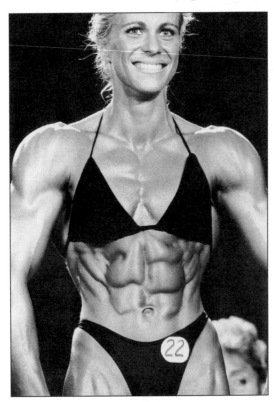

Anja Langer, the picture of symmetry, knows the importance of building a strong foundation.

It is true that big arms, shoulders, and legs are impressive, and that a lot of training must be dedicated to these areas. Yet the trunk is the link between these areas, and the limbs can only be as strong as the trunk.

The trunk has an abundance of abdominal and back muscles: bundles that run in different directions surround the core of the body with a tight and powerful support system. A poorly developed trunk represents a weak support system for the hard-working arms and legs. So in spite of temptations in this direction, an entry-level training program must not revolve around the legs, arms, and shoulders. The focus must first be on strengthening the core area of the body—the muscles of the abdomen, lower back, and spinal column.

Back muscles consist of long and short muscles that run along the vertebral column. They work together as a unit, with the rotators and diagonal muscles, to perform many movements.

Abdominal muscles run lengthwise (rectus abdominis), crosswise (transversus abdominis), and diagonally (abdominal obliques), enabling the trunk to bend forward and sideways, to rotate, and to twist. Since the abdominal muscles play important roles in many exercises, weakness in this area can severely limit the effectiveness of many strength actions.

Application of the above training principles, especially the step-type loading, will allow you to break away from the regimented bodybuilding of traditional programs and to use science and creativity to become the best you can be.

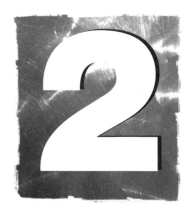

UNDERSTANDING THE PERIODIZATION SYSTEM

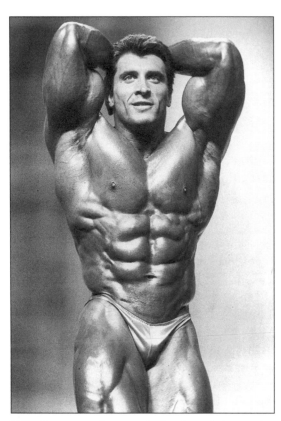

Milo Sarcev understands that in training nothing happens by accident but rather by design.

The field of strength training, especially that of bodybuilding, is saturated with methods and programs that often lack logic and are unproven. Scientific research cannot support the novel systems that pop up in magazines and on the Internet at an astounding rate. You will do well to ignore fads and follow well-tested approaches validated both by research and in competition. The following discussion about Periodization training will help you comprehend and apply the periodized training programs and nutrition plans suggested in part II.

The Periodization System

Although Periodization of Bodybuilding was copyrighted in May 1988 (as an adaptation for bodybuilding of an earlier-developed Periodization of Strength), many individuals—athletes and authors alike—still do not fully understand this very successful training system. Some authors describe Periodization

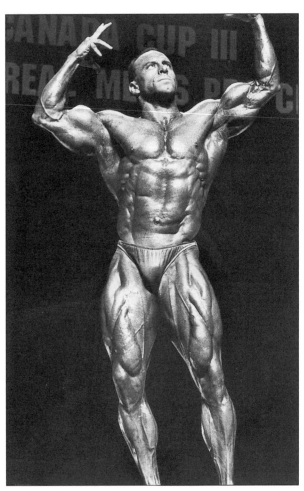

John McGough reaches for the stars.

as the "science behind reps and sets" or the principle of "progression of the training load per week," while others characterize it as a "philosophy." Others have simply decided, without research, understanding, or testing, that Periodization doesn't work! In fairness to the Periodization system of training, I have to say, "Try it first and then draw your own conclusions."

One of the major goals of this book is to help athletes learn to plan their own training program, allowing them to gain independence from others and eventually to help others properly use the Periodization system. Periodization, which is the most effective way to organize a training program, refers to two major elements:

1. How to structure a longer period of time, such as a year of training, into smaller and more manageable phases.

2. How to structure the program into specific training phases, such as

   • **anatomical adaptation,** or the beginning and progressive training performed after a break or extended absence from the sport;

   • **hypertrophy,** or a training phase where the objective is to increase muscle size;

• **maximum strength,** where the objective is to increase muscle tone and density;

• **muscle definition,** a training phase using specific training methods, where the objective is to burn fat and in the process further improve muscle striation and vascularization; and

• **transition,** where the objective is recovery and regeneration before beginning another phase.

The above sequence of training phases is essential because it outlines an entire training cycle. First, it facilitates the development of muscle size via the hypertrophy phase. It then improves muscle tone and muscle separation during a maximum-strength phase. Once muscle size and tone reach the level you want, training focuses on the development of muscle definition, where muscle striation is enhanced.

Periodization is not a rigid system in which only the basic model is the legitimate one. On the contrary—since there are several variations of the basic model, you can choose the one that best suits your own training goals. At the end of the book there are suggested phase-specific training and nutritional programs that will facilitate your ability to fit a true Periodization program to your specific needs.

In addition to presenting highly organized and phase-specific training programs, Periodization provides a variety of year-round training methods—plus the use of phase-specific training loads that employ different variations of both muscle stimulation and contractions for optimum muscle growth and strength.

Very few strength trainers and bodybuilders follow a well-adjusted and carefully designed plan. Through Periodization we intend to promote a new type of athlete—one who is in control of his or her body and whose training leads to complete body development. The new athlete will have impressive muscular development and will cultivate muscle density, tone, definition, symmetry, and strength superior to that of traditional bodybuilders who use antiquated training philosophies. Regardless of whether you are training just to look gorgeous or to compete professionally, the ideal for every athlete is to acquire the desired amount of muscle mass without sacrificing physical appearance.

Periodization is a training concept that allows you to accomplish your goals through the strategic implementation of specific phases: anatomical adaptation (AA), hypertrophy (H), mixed training (M), maximum strength (MxS), muscle definition (MD), and transition (T). Figure 2.1 illustrates the basic model of Periodization. Many variations of this plan are possible, however, to meet the different needs of each bodybuilder and strength trainer.

The basic model of Periodization presented in figure 2.1 illustrates the proper sequence of training phases and may be adapted to address the specific needs of individual athletes. This particular plan uses September as the starting point, although you can use any month of the year when developing your own plan. The small blocks beneath each month represent the weeks, or microcycles. You must plan in advance how many weeks are appropriate for each phase. The bottom row of the chart divides the year into training phases. Organize these phases in a way that assures you of meeting your goals at the appropriate time. For example, a competitive athlete might design an annual plan to peak for major shows. Recreational bodybuilders and strength trainers more concerned with aesthetics might wish to plan for vacations and other activities.

Dates	Sept	Oct	Nov	Dec	Jan	Feb	Mar	Apr	May	June	July	Aug
Weeks												
Phase	AA	H1	T	H2	T	M	T	MxS	T	MD1	T	MD2	T

Figure 2.1   The basic model of the annual plan for Periodization of Bodybuilding and Strength Training. AA = anatomical adaptation; H = hypertrophy; M = mixed training; MxS = maximum strength; MD = muscle definition; T = transition.

Periodization of Training for Increased Size

Periodization is not a rigid concept. Figure 2.1 is a basic structure that will not apply to every bodybuilder and strength trainer. We recognize that each athlete has different personal and professional commitments, so we offer different variations of training plans. Please keep in mind that the suggested variations do not exhaust all of the possible options. You should construct an individualized Periodization plan according to your unique set of needs and obligations. The

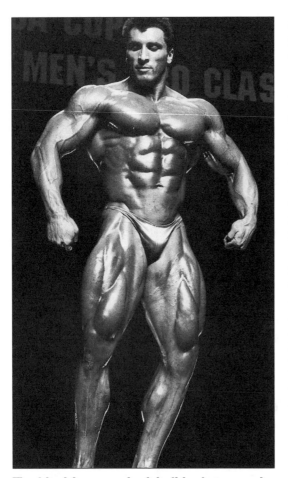

The ideal for every bodybuilder is to acquire the desired amount of muscle mass without sacrificing physical appearance.

options presented below are intended to help implement the concept of Periodization according to individual needs.

Double Periodization: Design and Duration

Double Periodization is an option for individuals who cannot commit themselves to the year-round training program recommended in figure 2.1. It is also an option for individuals with better training backgrounds, or for those seeking more variety in training.

In the double-Periodization model (figure 2.2), the months of the year are numbered rather than named, to allow you to commence training at any time throughout the year. The phases in this model follow the same sequence as those in the basic model (figure 2.1), except that the annual plan is divided into two halves and the sequence is repeated. Also, for each training phase in figure 2.2, there is a number on the upper right-hand side that refers to the number of weeks for each phase.

1	2	3	4	5	6	7	8	9	10	11	12
4		6		6		6	2	4		6		6		6	4
AA	H	T	MxS	MD		T	AA	H	T	MxS	MD	T

Figure 2.2 A double-Periodization model. Numbers in top row refer to months. Numbers in upper right of boxes indicate number of weeks to devote to the phase.

Double Periodization for Athletes With Family Obligations

Figure 2.3 presents another variation of the basic model that revolves around the busiest times of the year for a family person. During Christmas and summer vacation periods, training is often disorganized and interrupted because of family commitments. In order to avoid the frustration that accompanies periods of

Sept	Oct	Nov	Dec	Jan	Feb	Mar	Apr	May	June	July	Aug
4	6	6	2	4	6		6	6		6	4
AA	H	MxS	T	AA	H1	T	H2	MxS	T	MD	T

Figure 2.3 A double-Periodization model revolving around the holidays of the year. Numbers in top row refer to months. Numbers in upper right of boxes indicate number of weeks to devote to the phase.

fragmented training, it is better to actually structure an annual plan around the main holidays of the year.

As figure 2.3 indicates, mini-transition phases are planned during holiday times. The second part of the plan prescribes two hypertrophy phases in which the purpose of training is to increase muscle size.

Certainly, other variations of the basic structure are possible, for instance:

- H2 could be replaced by a mixed program of H and MxS in proportions decided by the athlete.
- H2 could be replaced by MxS, if the development of this strength quality is the goal.
- H2 could be divided into three weeks of MxS followed by three weeks of H.

Periodization Program for Entry-Level Bodybuilders

We strongly recommend that entry-level bodybuilders and strength trainers create their own programs or follow a model such as figure 2.4 presents. This figure presents months by number—month 1 represents the first month of training with a new program. Resist the temptation to copy the programs of experienced bodybuilders. Entry-level athletes have fragile bodies that are not ready for the challenge designed for experienced individuals. Beginners must be extra careful to progressively increase the training load by performing a lower number of training sessions and hours per week, planning longer AA phases, and confronting the body with less overall stress in training.

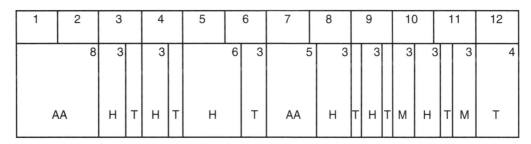

1	2	3	4	5	6	7	8	9	10	11	12
	8	3	3		6	3	5	3	3	3 3	3	4
AA		H	T	H	T	H	T	AA	H	T H T M	H T M	T

Figure 2.4 A recommended Periodization program for entry-level bodybuilders or strength trainers. Numbers in top row refer to months. Numbers in upper right of boxes indicate number of weeks to devote to the phase.

In this entry-level program, AA is eight weeks long, giving the muscle tissues, ligaments, and tendons adequate time to prepare for the phases to come.

In order to make adaptation to hypertrophy a careful and gradual process, the first two H phases are only three weeks long, separated by a one-week regeneration T phase.

After four months, the anatomy of an entry-level athlete should have progressively adapted to training, permitting longer H phases. The first half of the program ends with a three-week T phase, giving the body a long period of regeneration before a new and slightly more difficult program begins.

Periodization Program for Recreational Bodybuilders

Those who have completed one to two years of bodybuilding or strength training could follow an annual plan such as figure 2.5 presents. T phases occur during the Christmas and summer holidays to allow recreational bodybuilders time to enjoy other activities. Note that, except for the first AA and H phases, a T phase of one to two weeks is planned throughout to avoid high levels of fatigue and overtraining.

1	2	3	4	5	6	7	8	9	10	11	12
	8	3	3		6	3	5	3	3	3	3	3	4
AA		H	T	H	T	H		T	AA	H	T	H	T	M	H	T	M	T

Figure 2.5 A recommended Periodization program for recreational bodybuilders or strength trainers. Numbers in top row refer to months. Numbers in upper right of boxes indicate number of weeks to devote to the phase.

Non-Bulk Program for Female Athletes

Figure 2.6 describes a program for athletes who want more variety in training. This high-variety program has many alternations of training phases. It was created for bodybuilders and strength trainers (especially female athletes) who

Sept	Oct	Nov	Dec	Jan	Feb	Mar	Apr	May	June	July	Aug
3	3	3	3	3	3	4	3	3	3	3	3	3	4	4
AA	H	MxS	T	M	MD	T	AA	H	M	T	MD	MxS	T	MD	M	T	MD	T

Figure 2.6 A recommended Periodization program for female bodybuilders or strength trainers or those who do not want to train for bulk. Numbers in upper right of boxes indicate number of weeks to devote to the phase.

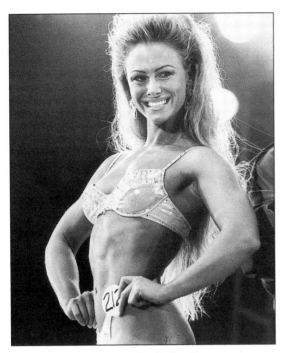

A toned and symmetrical physique.

want to sculpt a toned, muscular, and symmetrical body without packing on bulky muscles.

Triple-Periodization Plan: Design and Duration

We suggest the triple-Periodization plan for recreational bodybuilders or strength trainers or for busy professionals who cannot easily commit themselves to a year-long plan such as the basic model or even to a double-Periodization plan.

Shorter modules, such as the ones that figures 2.6 and 2.7 present, help these athletes to achieve the basic goals of well-developed bodies and good fitness, while taking into account their social needs during the main holidays of the year.

Hypertrophy (Mass) Program

An athlete whose primary training objective is building muscle size could use the program outlined in figure 2.8. It follows a double-Periodization plan, whereby most of the training program is dedicated to developing muscle hypertrophy. Longer H phases, alternated with M training towards the end of each segment, will stimulate the highest possible development of muscle size.

Sept	Oct	Nov	Dec	Jan	Feb	Mar	Apr	May	June	July	Aug
7	3	3 2	3		6	3	3 2	3 3		3 3	5
AA	H T	M T	AA		H	T M	MD T	AA	H T	MxS MD	T

Figure 2.7 Triple Periodization: a recommended program for recreational or busy professional bodybuilders or strength trainers. Numbers in upper right of boxes indicate number of weeks to devote to the phase.

1	2	3	4	5	6	7	8	9	10	11	12
3	6	6	3	3	3 2	3	6	3	3	4	4
AA	H	T H	T	M	H M	T AA	H	T	M	H	M T

Figure 2.8 A hypertrophy (mass) training program. Numbers in top row refer to months. Numbers in upper right of boxes indicate number of weeks to devote to the phase.

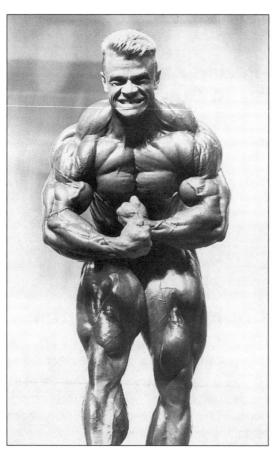

Roland Cziurlok knows how to gain muscle mass.

Our periodized approach to mass training differs from traditional programs in that the M phases, which mix hypertrophy with maximum strength training, have the important merit of developing short-term and, more significantly, chronic hypertrophy.

Periodization Plan Stressing Maximum Strength

Many bodybuilders would like to develop large muscles and, more importantly, muscle tone, high muscle density, and certainly stronger muscles. Increased chronic hypertrophy results from following a training program such as that in figure 2.9.

As figure 2.9 illustrates, the program to maximize strength follows a double-Periodization plan. The fact that MxS dominates this program means that the training recruits more fast twitch muscle fibers—resulting in chronic hypertrophy and muscles that are well defined and visibly striated.

Periodization Plan Stressing Muscle Definition

Some athletes have already reached their desired level of muscle hypertrophy; they now want to improve muscle definition in order to achieve total body development. People who have already tested our program (especially women) have reported incredible changes in their bodies. The majority found that they drastically trimmed their waist, while at the same time significantly increasing muscle definition in the upper body, buttocks, and legs. Some have even reported increments in strength. In one of our female groups, 68 percent lost substantial weight and changed their overall body shape so much that they had to change their wardrobe. They achieved this weight loss by natural means and not as a result of some diet gimmick—just natural, honest, and dedicated training. This is the healthy way.

1	2	3	4	5	6	7	8	9	10	11	12
3	6	6		3	3	3 2	3	3	3 3	3	5
AA	H	MxS	T	MxS	M	MxS T	AA	H	MxS T	MxS	M T MxS	T

Figure 2.9 A Periodization plan stressing maximum strength. Numbers in top row refer to months. Numbers in upper right of boxes indicate number of weeks to devote to the phase.

1	2	3	4	5	6	7	8	9	10	11	12
3		6		3			4			6		2		3		6		3			4		3		4	
AA	H	MxS	T	MD	T	MD	T	AA	H	MxS	T	MD	MD	T

Figure 2.10   **A periodization plan stressing muscle definition. Numbers in top row refer to months. Numbers in upper right of boxes indicate number of weeks to devote to the phase.**

This plan, shown in figure 2.10, is a double-Periodization program that focuses on burning subcutaneous fat, thus allowing for better-striated and more visible muscles.

The purpose of periodized bodybuilding training is to sequence specific types of strength training in order to obtain maximum gains. These phases can be combined to create a certain type of adaptation, allowing bodybuilders to model their bodies to reach maximum hypertrophy, muscle tone, or muscle definition. After the first year of using periodized training plans, bodybuilders become better accustomed to creating models of training that fit their own needs.

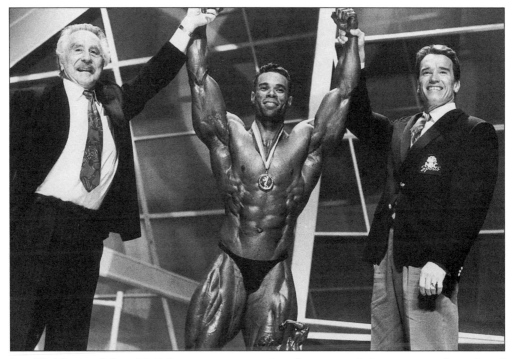

Joe Weider and Arnold Schwarzenegger raise the arms of the awesomely striated physique of Kevin Levrone.

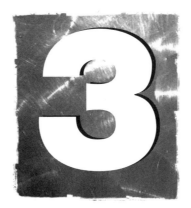

DESIGNING THE PERFECT PROGRAM

In order to obtain both continuous improvement and the necessary balance between work and regeneration, athletes must pay constant attention to the amounts of work (volume) and the loads (intensity) they use in training. They must ceaselessly monitor the loads, number of exercises, sets, rest intervals, and the types of split routines they employ. Athletes who wish to design their own training program need to understand all of these training elements and combine them effectively for their own body.

Volume and Intensity

Training *volume* is the quantity of work performed and incorporates the following integral parts:

- The duration of training (in hours)
- The cumulative amount of weight lifted per training session or phase
- The number of exercises per training session
- The number of sets and repetitions per exercise or training session

Bodybuilders should maintain training logs in order to correctly monitor the total volume of work performed, and to help plan the total volume of training for future weeks and months.

Training volume varies among individuals according to their training background, work tolerance, and biological makeup. Mature athletes with a solid background in strength training will always be able to tolerate higher volumes of training. Regardless of a person's experience, however, any dramatic or abrupt

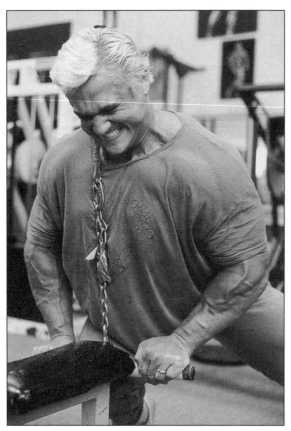

Now there's intensity: Tom Platz gives it his grunting, vein-bulging, teeth-gnashing best.

increase in training volume can be detrimental. Such increases can result in high levels of fatigue, inefficient muscular work, and greater risk of injury. This is why a well-designed, progressive plan, along with an appropriate method of monitoring load increments, is crucial to your well-being and training success.

Training volume also changes with the type of strength training performed. For instance, high-volume training is planned during the muscle definition phase in order to burn more fat and, consequently, develop better muscle striations. Medium-volume training, on the other hand, is typical for maximum strength or power training. Muscle size and definition improve only as a result of careful and constant physiological adaptation, which depends on the proper manipulation of the quantity or volume of training.

One adaptation that occurs as a result of progressively higher volumes of training is a more efficient and faster recovery time between sets and between training sessions. Faster recovery permits more work per training session and per week, encouraging even further increases in training volume.

In strength training, *intensity* is expressed as a percentage of 1RM. Intensity is a function of the power of the nervous stimuli employed in training. The strength of a stimulus depends on the load, the speed at which a movement is performed, the variation of rest intervals between repetitions and sets, and the psychological strain that accompanies an exercise. Thus, the intensity is determined by the muscular effort involved and the energy spent by the central nervous system (CNS) during strength training. Table 3.1 gives the intensities and loads employed in strength training.

Supermaximum is a load that exceeds one's maximum strength. In most cases, loads between 100 and 125 percent of 1RM are used by applying eccentric force, or by resisting the force of gravity. When using supermaximum loads you should have two spotters, one at each end of the barbell, to assist you and protect you from accident or injury; if you use the eccentric method in a bench press without

Table 3.1	Intensity Values (Loads) Used in Strength and Bodybuilding Training		
Intensity value	**Load**	**Percent of 1RM**	**Type of contraction**
1	Supermaximum	>105	Eccentric/isometric
2	Maximum	90-100	Concentric
3	Heavy	80-90	Concentric
4	Medium/submaximum	50-80	Concentric
5	Low	30-50	Concentric

Reprinted from Bompa 1996.

spotters, the barbell could fall on your chest because the weight is actually heavier than you can lift.

During the maximum-strength phase, only bodybuilders with a strong background or base in strength training can use supermaximum loads. Most other athletes should restrict themselves to a load of up to 100 percent, or 1RM.

The load, however, should also relate to the type of strength being developed, as scheduled in the Periodization plan.

Number of Exercises

One of the keys to an effective training program is to have an adequate repertoire of exercises from which to choose. Athletes should build their repertoire around several key principles.

Exercises That Stimulate the Greatest Amount of Electrical Activity

The greater the electrical activity, the more muscle fibers are recruited, resulting in greater increments in muscle strength and size (see chapter 11). In order to maximize this effect, it is critical to know which loading pattern to use, how that pattern should vary in a given training phase, the lifting technique to use, and how the load increments can vary in order to induce supercompensation.

Level of Development

One of the main objectives of an entry-level bodybuilding program is the development of a strong anatomical and physiological foundation. Without such a base, consistent improvement will be unlikely. Entry-level strength trainers and bodybuilders need a number of exercises (about 12 to 15) that collectively address the major muscle groups of the body. The duration of this type of training may be from one to three years, depending on the individual's background (and level of patience!).

Training programs for advanced bodybuilders follow a completely different approach. The main training objective for these athletes is to increase muscle size, density, tone, and definition to the highest possible levels.

Individual Needs

As training progresses over the years, some bodybuilders develop imbalances among different parts of the body. When this occurs, they should adapt their programs by giving priority to exercises that stress the underdeveloped parts of the body.

Training Phase

As outlined by the Periodization concept, the number of exercises varies according to the phase of training (see part III, chapters 10 to 15).

The order of exercises in bodybuilding must be phase-specific, taking into account the scope of training for each particular phase. Just as the rest interval, volume of training, exercises, and so on, vary according to the different kinds of strength being developed, so must the order of performing exercises.

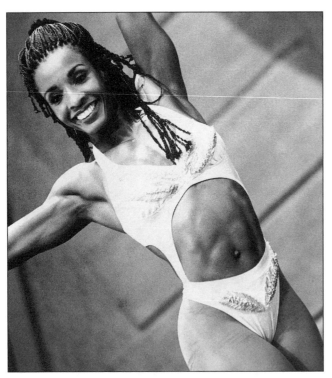

The superfit body of Madonna Grimes.

For example, in the maximum strength training phase, exercises are cycled in vertical sequence as they appear on the daily program sheet. The athlete performs one set of each exercise, starting from the top and moving down, and repeating the cycle as often as prescribed. The advantage of this method is that it allows for better recovery of each muscle group. By the time exercise #1 is repeated, enough time has elapsed to promote almost full recovery. When you are lifting 90 to 105 percent 1RM, this much rest is necessary if training is to remain at a high intensity throughout the session.

If, however, the phase of training is hypertrophy, then all of the sets for exercise #1 are performed before moving on to the next exercise—this is the horizontal sequence. This sequence exhausts the muscle group much faster, leading to greater increases in muscle size. Local muscle exhaustion is the main training focus of the hypertrophy phase.

Technique of Lifting and Range of Motion

Correct form and good technique increase the effectiveness of targeting a given muscle group. Good technique also ensures that muscle contraction occurs along the line of pull. Any contraction that is performed along the line of pull increases the mechanical effectiveness of that particular exercise. For instance: a squat performed with the feet apart and the toes pointed diagonally (often done in powerlifting) is not mechanically effective, since the quadriceps muscles are not contracting along the line of pull. Placing the feet at shoulder width, with toes pointed forward and slightly to the side, is more effective since the contraction of the muscles is along the line of pull. Similarly, arm curls intending to target the biceps muscle are performed along the line of pull only when the palm is facing up (supination), as in preacher curls.

For an exercise to be effective and have good fluidity, it must be performed throughout the entire range of motion (ROM). Using the full range of motion ensures maximum motor-unit activation. In addition, bodybuilders must constantly stretch to maintain a good range of motion and excellent flexibility at the end of the warm-up, during the rest interval between sets, and as part of the cooldown. Good stretching practice keeps the muscle elongated and speeds the rate of recovery between workouts. Stretching also helps the overlapped myosin and actin to return to their normal anatomical state where biochemical exchanges are optimized.

Loading Patterns

The serious training program should follow a number of variations of distinct loading patterns that pertain to the pyramid loading formation. These variations

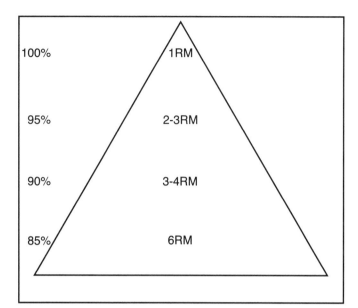

Figure 3.1 **An example of the pyramid loading pattern. The number of repetitions (inside the pyramid) refers to their number per training session.**

Reprinted from Bompa 1996.

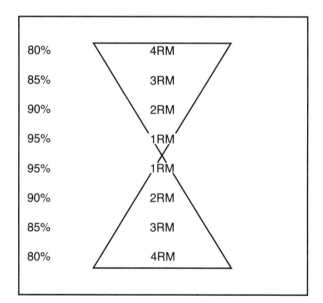

Figure 3.2 **An example of the double pyramid loading pattern.**

Reprinted from Bompa 1996.

include the pyramid loading pattern as well as the double, skewed, and flat pyramid loading patterns.

The Pyramid

The pyramid (figure 3.1) is one of the most popular loading patterns in bodybuilding. Notice that as the load progressively increases to maximum, the number of sets decreases proportionately. The physiological advantage of using the pyramid is that it ensures the activation or recruitment of most, if not all, of the motor units.

The Double Pyramid

The double pyramid (figure 3.2) is two pyramids, one mirroring the other. In this loading pattern, beginning at the bottom, the load increases progressively up to 95 percent 1RM and then decreases again for the last sets. Note that as the load increases the number of repetitions, shown inside the pyramid, decreases and vice versa.

The Skewed Pyramid

The skewed pyramid (figure 3.3) is an improved variant of the double pyramid. In this pattern, the load constantly increases throughout the session, except during the last set when it is lowered. The purpose of this last set is to provide variation and motivation, since the athlete must perform the set as quickly as possible.

The Flat Pyramid

The flat pyramid loading pattern (Bompa 1999) can provide maximum training benefits. A comparison between the traditional pyramids and the flat pyramid shown in figure 3.4 will explain why this is the most effective loading pattern. In the traditional pyramids the load varies too much, often ranging between 60 percent to over 100 percent of 1RM. Load variations of such magnitude cross over three intensity (load) borders—medium, heavy, and maximum.

In order to produce hypertrophy, the load must range between 60 to 80 percent 1RM, whereas for maximum strength the load must be 80 to 100+ percent 1RM. The flat pyramid gives the physiological advantage of providing the best neuromuscular adaptation for a given type of strength training, because it keeps the

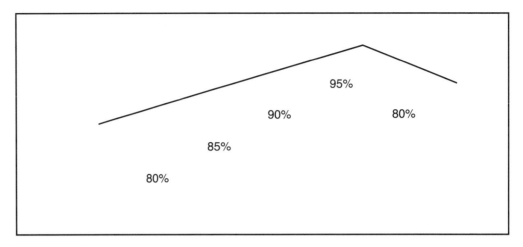

Figure 3.3 A suggested loading pattern for the skewed pyramid.
Reprinted from Bompa 1996.

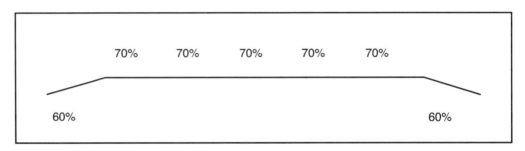

Figure 3.4 An example of the flat pyramid loading pattern.
Reprinted from Bompa 1996.

load within one intensity level. This prevents the body from becoming confused by several different intensities.

The flat pyramid begins with a warm-up set (60 percent 1RM), and then the load stabilizes for the entire exercise at 70 percent 1RM. Another set at 60 percent 1RM may be performed at the end of each exercise for variety.

Variations of the flat pyramid are possible depending on the phase and scope of training, as long as the load stays within the boundaries of the required intensity for a given phase:

70% - 80% - 80% - 80% - 80% - 70%
80% - 90% - 90% - 90% - 90% - 80%
85% - 95% - 95% - 95% - 95% - 85%

Repetitions per Set

Strength trainers and bodybuilders who follow traditional thinking about the number of repetitions performed per set—that is, those who go to the gym every day and always perform 8 to 12 sets—will be shocked by the numbers recommended in table 3.2. Very few people have thought of performing 150-rep sets. We will show you that this is possible, because each training phase is different and requires a separate approach to loading rest intervals, number of reps, and exercise order.

Table 3.2	Number of Repetitions Appropriate for Each Training Phase	
Training phase	**Training purpose**	**Number of repetitions**
Maximum strength	Increase muscle strength/tone	1-7
Hypertrophy	Increase muscle size	6-12
Muscular endurance	Increase definition	30-150

Lifting Speed

The speed of lifting is an important component of strength and bodybuilding training. For the best results, some types of work must be executed quickly, while others must be performed at a medium pace. The speed with which you intend to lift, however, is not necessarily reflected in the appearance of the lift. For example, when you lift a heavy load that is 90 percent of 1RM, the performed motion might look slow; however, the force against the resistance must be applied as quickly as possible. Only under this condition will you be able to synchronize and recruit all of the motor units necessary to defeat the resistance. The FT muscle fibers are recruited for action only when the application of force is fast and vigorous.

You can usually maintain optimum speed throughout the first half of a set. Once fatigue sets in, speed often declines and a great deal of mental concentration is required to complete the intended number of repetitions.

Number of Sets

A set represents the number of exercise repetitions followed by a rest interval. The number of sets prescribed per exercise and workout depends on several factors, including how many exercises you perform in a training session, the phase of training, how many muscle groups you want to train, and how experienced you are.

Exercises in a Training Session

As the number of exercises increases, the number of sets per exercise declines—for as energy and work potential decrease, the ability to perform numerous exercises and repetitions for a very high number of sets declines. As work potential improves, however, the number of sets per workout that you can tolerate will improve.

Training Phase

As explained in chapter 2, an athlete goes through several training phases during a year of training. Each phase has a specific objective related to creating the best possible body shape. In the adaptation phase, where the scope of training is just overall adaptation, the number of sets per exercise is not high (2-3). In the hypertrophy phase, however, where the objective is to increase muscle size, it is necessary to perform the highest number of sets you can tolerate.

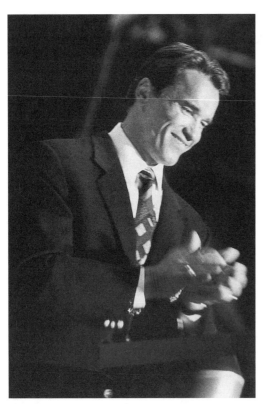

From super-bodybuilder to mega-movie star, Arnold Schwarzenegger still finds time to keep in shape and motivate others.

Muscle Groups Trained per Session

If training only one or two muscle groups in a given session, you can perform more sets per muscle group than if you are training three or four muscle groups. But when selecting the muscle groups per training session, you must consider how many training sessions are planned per week and how much time you can dedicate per workout. The more time available per week, the lower the number of muscle groups on which each session must focus. If there is a shortage of time, use multijoint (compound) exercises.

Bodybuilder's Experience

The classification of the bodybuilder (i.e., entry-level, recreational, advanced) also plays a part in determining the number of sets that will be included in the training session. As you become more experienced and achieve a high state of adaptation to weight training, you can perform more sets per body part per workout. For example, while an advanced bodybuilder might prepare for a contest by performing 20 or 30 sets for two or three muscle groups, a recreational athlete might train the same muscle groups with only 15 or 20 sets.

Rest Interval

Energy is a crucial commodity in bodybuilding. The type of energy system used during a given workout depends on the phase of training (e.g., hypertrophy vs. muscle definition, etc.), the load employed, and the duration of the activity. High-intensity training can completely deplete your energy stores. To complete the workout, you must take a *rest interval (RI)* between each set in order to replenish the depleted fuel stores before you perform the next set.

Bodybuilders must realize that the RI and restoration of energy between sets and training sessions are as important as the training itself. The amount of time allowed between sets determines, to a high degree, the extent to which the energy source will be replenished before the next set. Careful planning of the RI is crucial if you are to avoid needless physiological and psychological stress during training. See also the discussions of recovery in chapter 4 and of nutrition in chapter 5.

Steps for Designing a Training Program

In order to design an effective training program, the bodybuilder should follow these steps, which are described in the following section:

1. Select the type of strength sought.
2. Select the exercises.

3. Test maximum strength.

4. Develop the actual training program

5. Test to recalculate 1RM.

First, strength training should be phase-specific and designed to meet the needs of the individual. Decide on the appropriate percentage of 1RM to be used and the number of reps and sets based on the type of strength sought. Details on training methods and progression are provided in part II.

Next, select the exercises. Identify the prime movers and then select the exercises that can best stimulate these muscles to meet your individual needs. These needs might depend on your background or foundation, your individual strengths and weaknesses, or the disproportionate development among your muscle groups and body parts. For example, if you have the capacity to develop massive legs

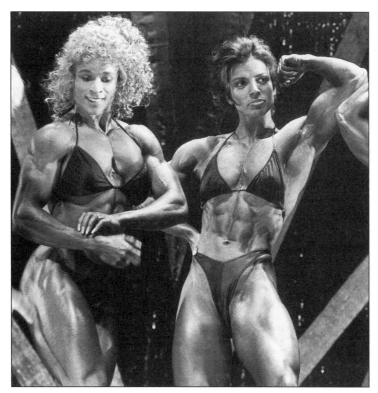

Crevalle and Bruneau strut their stuff.

quickly but your upper body takes longer to grow, then select exercises to compensate the weaker part to encourage growth and restore symmetry.

Selection of exercises is also phase-specific. For example, during the anatomical adaptation phase, most muscle groups are worked in order to develop a better overall foundation; whereas in the muscle definition phase, training becomes more specific and exercises are selected to target the prime movers.

Third, test maximum strength. This value is referred to as the *one-repetition maximum (1RM)*, and is the highest load that you can lift in one attempt. Knowing your 1RM for each exercise is crucial to the concept of Periodization, as each workout is planned using percentages of 1RM.

If for some reason you are unable to test 1RM for each exercise, try to test 1RM for at least the dominant exercise within the training program. Often the load and number of repetitions are chosen randomly, or by following the programs of others, instead of using your own objective data, which is 1RM for each exercise. Such data are valid for only a short period of time, since there is continual improvement in maximum strength, recovery ability, lifting techniques, and other factors from phase to phase.

Among some members of the bodybuilding world, there is an unfounded belief that testing for 1RM is dangerous. Some trainers maintain that injury will result if an individual puts forth a maximal effort; but an adequately trained athlete can lift 100 percent once in a four-week period without danger. Keep in mind, however, that a very thorough and progressive warm-up must precede any test for 1RM. If an athlete is still reluctant to test for 100 percent, another option is to test for a 3RM or 5RM (i.e., maximum weight that can be lifted 3 or 5 times before exhaustion) and then extrapolate to what the 1RM would be (see appendix 3 for a chart that gives the estimated 1RM for submaximal values).

The fourth step is to develop the actual training program. By this point, you know which exercises are to be performed, the 1RM for each exercise, and the type of strength to be developed. With this information, you can select the number of exercises, the percentage of 1RM, the number of reps, and the number of sets.

This program cannot be the same, however, for each training phase. The training demand must be progressively increased so you are forced to adapt to increasing work loads—such adaptation is required in order to increase muscle size, tone, and strength. You can increase the training demand by any of the following means: increase the load, decrease the rest interval, increase the number of repetitions, or increase the number of sets.

Table 3.3 illustrates a hypothetical program to demonstrate how to set up your own program. Before looking at the chart, be sure that you understand the notation used to express the load, number of reps, and number of sets.

$$80/10 \times 4 = \text{load}/\# \text{ of reps} \times \text{sets}$$

The 80 in the numerator represents the load as a percentage of 1RM.

The denominator of 10 represents the number of repetitions per set.

The multiplier of 4 represents the number of sets.

Table 3.3 **A Hypothetical Training Program to Illustrate Format Design**

Exercise #	Exercise	Load/# reps × sets	RI (minutes)
1	Leg press	80/6 × 4	3
2	Flat bench press	75/8 × 4	3
3	Leg curl	60/10 × 4	2
4	Half squat	80/8 × 4	3
5	Abdominal curl	15 × 4	2
6	Dead-lift	60/8 × 3	2

Reprinted from Bompa 1996.

While many books and articles on this subject actually take the liberty of prescribing the load in pounds or kilograms to be used, please notice that we do not. There is little basis on which someone could legitimately suggest the weight that an athlete should use, without knowing anything about the athlete! The load must be suggested as a percentage of 1RM. This allows strength trainers and bodybuilders to objectively calculate the load for each exercise according to their individual potential, within the parameters of a given training phase.

The first column of table 3.3 lists the exercises by number, or the order in which they are performed during the training session. The second column lists the exercises. The third column shows the load, number of reps, and number of sets. The last column gives the RI required after each set.

Finally, test to recalculate 1RM. Another test for 1RM is needed before the beginning of each new phase, to ensure that progress is acknowledged and new loads are based on the new gains made in strength.

Training Cycles

A good bodybuilding program improves muscle size, tone, density, and definition. A training program is successful only when it has these characteristics:

- It is a part of a longer plan.
- It is based on the scientific knowledge available in the field.
- It uses Periodization as a guideline for planning training throughout the year.

The program must have short-term goals and long-term goals that are phase specific. Each training phase has it own objectives, so it is necessary to design the daily and weekly programs to meet these objectives, while coinciding with the overall plan.

The compilation of a plan with both short- and long-term goals must take into account an individual's background, physical potential, and rate of adaptation to the physiological challenges imposed by training. Of all possible plans that can be used, we will make reference in this chapter only to the training session plan and the microcycle. In chapters 10 to 15, we introduce you to several types of plans; and since planning theory is very complex, we discuss annual planning only as it pertains to bodybuilding.

The Training Session Plan

The training session, or daily program, includes a warm-up, the main workout, and a cool-down. Each of these three parts of the training session has its own goals. The first part prepares you for the training planned that day; the work is done in the second, or main, part of the workout; and the third part cools you down and speeds up your recovery before the next training session.

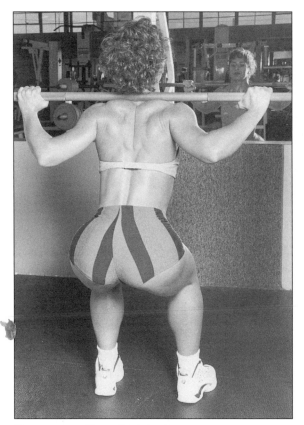

Fitness star Zena Walsh always warms up.

Warm-Up

The purpose of the warm-up is to prepare you for the program to follow. During the warm-up your body temperature rises, enhancing oxygen transport and preventing, or at least reducing, ligament sprains and muscle and tendon strains. It also stimulates CNS activity, which coordinates all the systems of the body, speeds up motor reactions through faster transmission of nerve impulses, and improves coordination.

For the purpose of strength and bodybuilding training, the warm-up consists of two parts. *General warm-up* (10-12 minutes) consists of light jogging, cycling, or stair climbing, followed by stretching exercises. This ritual prepares the muscles and tendons for the workout by increasing blood flow and body temperature. During this time, you can mentally prepare for the main part of the training session by visualizing the exercises to be performed, and motivating yourself for the eventual strain of training.

The second part, the *specific warm-up* (3-5 minutes), is a short transition period that consists of performing a few repetitions of each planned exercise using significantly lighter loads. This prepares your body for the specific work to be done during the main part of the workout.

Main Workout

This part of the training session is dedicated to performing the actual bodybuilding exercises. For the best results, make up the daily program well in advance of the workout and write it down on paper or, better yet, in a log book. To know the program in advance is of psychological benefit, because it enables you to better motivate yourself and focus more clearly on the task at hand.

The *duration* of a training session depends on the type of strength being developed, and the specific training phase of the model of Periodization that you have developed. For example, the longest workouts are needed for the hypertrophy phase, because there are many sets to perform. As a result, a hypertrophy workout may be as long as one to two hours, especially if there are a large number of exercises. Multijoint exercises are beneficial in a hypertrophy workout because they save you time.

The recommended duration of a workout, both in specific sports as well as in bodybuilding, has shifted dramatically over the years. From the 1960s to the early 1970s the duration of suggested workouts was often two and a half to three hours. The results from numerous scientific investigations have had a dramatic influence on the recommended duration of a workout, and have demonstrated that one may improve more over the course of three one-hour workouts than during a single three-hour workout. In the case of strength training and bodybuilding, longer workouts result in a hormonal shift. Specifically, testosterone levels decrease, promoting breakdown (catabolism) of protein, which has a negative effect on muscle building. The type of strength or bodybuilding training dictates, to a very high degree, the duration of a workout. It is also important to realize that the rest intervals employed greatly influence the duration of a training session. The following durations are suggested for each type of strength-training session:

- 1 to 1.25 hours for anatomical adaptation and general conditioning
- 1 to 2 hours for hypertrophy training
- 1 to 1.5 hours for maximum-strength training
- 1.5 hours for muscle definition training

Cool-Down

Just as the warm-up is a transition period to take the body from its normal biological state to a state of high stimulation, the cool-down is a transition period that produces the opposite effect. The job of the cool-down is to progressively bring the body back to its normal state of functioning.

A cool-down of 10 to 25 minutes consists of activities that facilitate *faster recovery and regeneration*. After a tough workout, the muscles are exhausted, tense, and rigid. To overcome this, you must allow for muscle recovery (see chapter 4). Hitting the showers immediately after the last exercise, though tempting, is not the best activity.

Removal of lactic acid from the blood and muscles is necessary if the effects of fatigue are to be eliminated quickly. The best way to achieve this is by performing 20 to 25 minutes of light, continuous aerobic activity, such as jogging, cycling, or rowing, which will cause the body to continue perspiring. This will remove about half of the lactic acid from the system and help you recover more quickly between training sessions. Remember, the faster you recover, the greater the amount of work you can perform in the following training session.

The Microcycle

The *microcycle* refers to the weekly training program and is probably the most important tool in planning. Throughout the annual plan, the nature and dynamics of the microcycles change according to the phase of training, the training objectives, and the physiological and psychological demands of training.

Variations of Load Increments per Microcycle

To plan a program you must understand how the microcycle fits into a longer training phase—namely, the *macrocycle,* or four weeks of training—and how to plan the load of training per microcycle. Well-organized bodybuilders should also seriously consider load variations. Furthermore, low-intensity days represent a crucial concept in training—one which not only aids in reaching recovery and supercompensation but also helps prevent overtraining, which is so common among many bodybuilders who follow the traditional "no pain, no gain" philosophy.

Load Increments per Macrocycle

Load increments within the macrocycle must follow a step-type progression. Figure 3.5 illustrates the standard approach. With regard to intensity, microcycles follow the principle of step-type loading.

The load progressively increases over three microcycles (weeks), and then declines for a regeneration cycle to facilitate recuperation and replenishment of

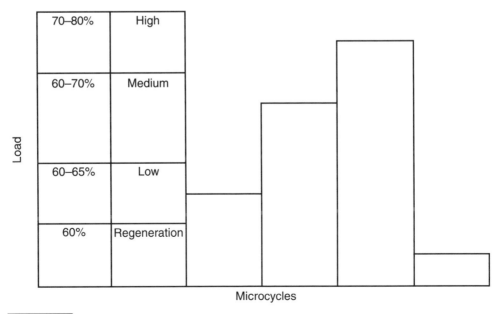

Figure 3.5 **The dynamics of increasing the training load over four microcycles (a macrocycle).**

Reprinted from Bompa 1996.

energy before another macrocycle begins. Based on the model shown in figure 3.5, figure 3.6 gives a practical example suggesting load increments and using the notation explained in this chapter.

Figure 3.6 illustrates that the work, or the total stress in training, increases in steps, with the highest point being in step 3. To increase the work from step to step, there are two options: increase the load (the highest one being in step 3) or increase the number of sets (from five sets in step 1 to seven sets in step 3).

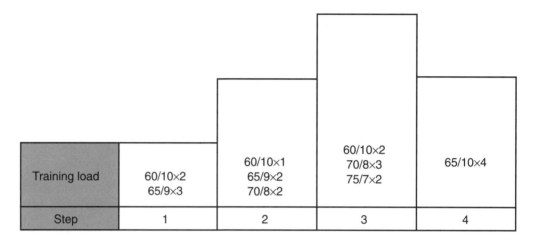

Training load	60/10×2 65/9×3	60/10×1 65/9×2 70/8×2	60/10×2 70/8×3 75/7×2	65/10×4
Step	1	2	3	4

Figure 3.6 **A practical example of load increments in training (a macrocycle).**
Reprinted from Bompa 1996.

In this example, both options are used at the same time—an appropriate approach for athletes with a solid background in training. Other options will suit the needs of different classifications. Entry-level athletes, for example, have difficulty tolerating higher loads and an increased number of sets, so it is more important for them to increase the number of exercises. This approach will develop their entire muscular system and help the ligaments and tendons adapt to strength training.

Step 4 is a regeneration cycle in which the load and number of sets are lowered. This lessens the fatigue that has developed during the first three steps and allows the body to replenish its energy stores. This step also allows the athlete to psychologically relax.

Load Increments per Microcycle

The work, or the total stress per microcycle, is increased mainly by increasing the number of training days per week.

Before discussing options of training per microcycle, we must mention that the total work per week follows the principle of step-type loading. Figures 3.7 to 3.9 illustrate the first three microcycles of the macrocycles shown in figures 3.5 and 3.6.

The Role of Low-Intensity Days

Due to unscientific theories—such as "no pain, no gain" and "overloading"—that have dominated the sports of bodybuilding and strength training, most athletes believe in training hard day-in and day-out regardless of the season. It is not surprising that most of them constantly feel exhausted and frustrated because

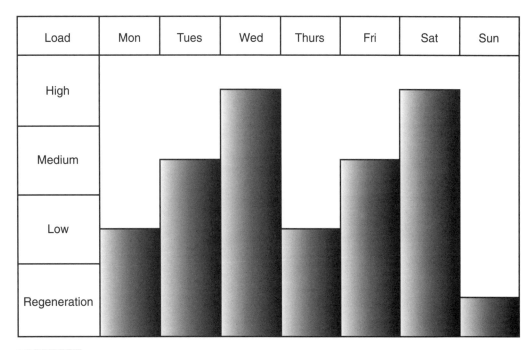

Figure 3.7 **A low-intensity microcycle.**

Reprinted from Bompa 1996.

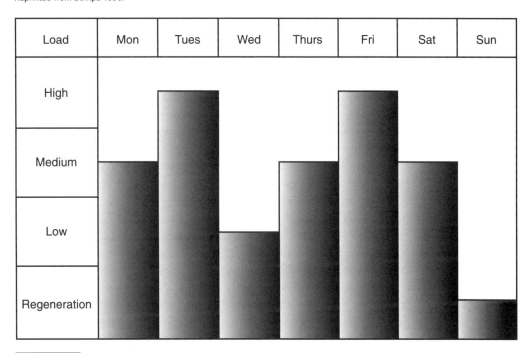

Figure 3.8 **A medium-intensity microcycle.**

Reprinted from Bompa 1996.

they do not achieve expected gains, and many quit because they stop enjoying their sport.

To avoid such undesirable outcomes, athletes need to follow the step-type loading pattern and alternate intensities inside each microcycle. Figures 3.7 to 3.9 illustrate three such intensity variations. Other variations are possible, depending on individual circumstances.

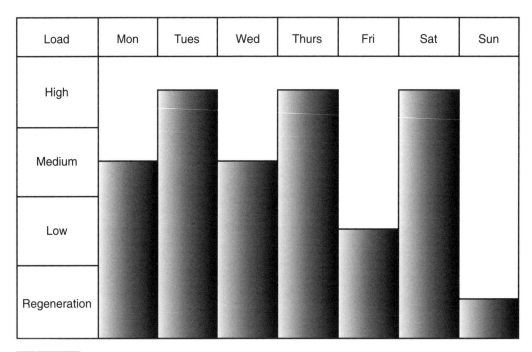

Load	Mon	Tues	Wed	Thurs	Fri	Sat	Sun
High							
Medium							
Low							
Regeneration							

Figure 3.9 **A high-intensity microcycle.**

Reprinted from Bompa 1996.

In any microcycle variations, there are low-intensity days, and athletes might legitimately question their role. We will explain. The body uses the fuels ATP/CP and glycogen to provide energy. For high-intensity workouts that consist of low-rep sets, and rest intervals of at least two to three minutes, which are typical of maximum-strength training, the ATP/CP system provides the energy. Under these conditions, energy stores can be replenished in about 24 hours, which means that the next day's workout could also be of high intensity.

Every high-intensity workout session, however, creates physiological strain and mental or psychological stress, caused by the intense concentration that is necessary to tackle the challenging loads. Consequently, after such a workout the athletes must be concerned with two things: whether their energy pools will be replenished before the next workout and whether they will be mentally ready for the next session. These factors make it necessary to plan in advance for low-intensity days following one to two days of hard training. Figure 3.10 gives another option for planning a microcycle, where two challenging days are planned back to back. Please note that this type of microcycle is only for highly trained strength trainers and bodybuilders who have a high adaptive response and are capable of tolerating intense physiological and psychological strain.

If, however, the session consists of high-rep sets, as proposed for the muscle definition ("cuts") phase, or if the workout is especially long (2-3 hours), the glycogen system supplies a large proportion of the fuel. After these long and exhausting workouts, the complete restoration of glycogen often takes 48 hours. The same duration of time is necessary for protein synthesis, implying that only after 48 hours is the same muscle group ready for another workout. Figure 3.9 suggests an appropriate microcycle structure for this type of training.

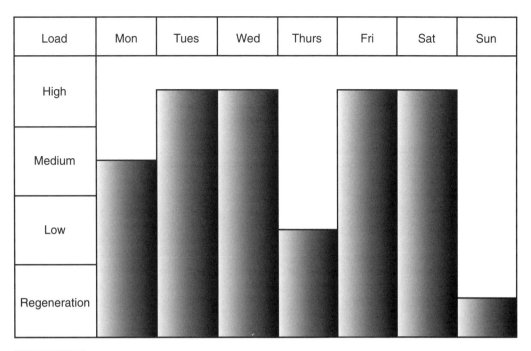

Load	Mon	Tues	Wed	Thurs	Fri	Sat	Sun
High							
Medium							
Low							
Regeneration							

Figure 3.10   **A suggested microcycle for the third, high-intensity step of a macrocycle for elite strength trainers and bodybuilders.**

Reprinted from Bompa 1996.

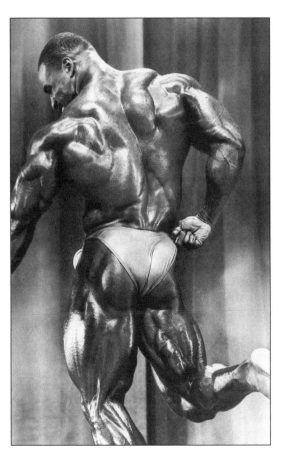

Supercompensation

Supercompensation is the state of physiological and psychological arousal that ideally occurs before a day of high-intensity training. Supercompensation can only be achieved, however, if work and regeneration are timed perfectly.

Mistakes in timing are what turn supercharged workouts into daily-grind sessions. Figure 3.11 illustrates the supercompensation cycle of a training session.

This is how it works. Under normal conditions of rest and proper diet, an individual is in a balanced state *(homeostasis)*. As figure 3.11 illustrates, a certain level of fatigue is reached, both during and at the end of a training session. This fatigue is caused by the depletion of fuel stores, lactic-acid accumulation in the working muscles, and psychological stress. The abrupt drop of the homeostasis curve illustrates the reduction of functional capacity to perform high-quality work,

During the maximum-strength workouts that are necessary to create a body this massive, the energy system taxed (ATP/CP) can be replenished in approximately 24 hours.

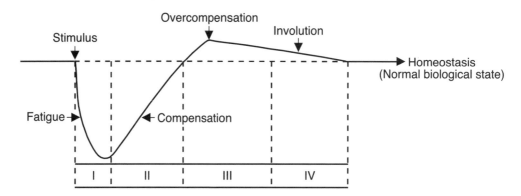

Figure 3.11 The supercompensation cycle of a training session modified from Yakovlev (1967).
Reprinted from Bompa 1983.

the depletion of glycogen stores, and the fact that the muscles are in a state of catabolism, or a posttraining state of protein degradation. Levels of insulin, which increases the rate of glucose transport to the working muscles, decline in the blood, thereby reducing cellular uptake of glucose.

After each session, and between two sessions, there is a phase of compensation during which the biochemical sources of energy are replenished. The return of the curve toward the normal biological state, or homeostasis, is slow and progressive, indicating that the replenishment of lost energy stores requires several hours. If the rest interval between two high-intensity training sessions is planned correctly, the energy sources (especially glycogen) are fully replaced and the body also acquires some fuel reserves. This energy rebound puts athletes into a state of supercompensation and gives them the energy needed to train even harder. Furthermore, the state of compensation represents the beginning of the anabolic state of the muscles, when protein is resynthesized and blood insulin levels return to normal. This compensation phase is essential for adaptation to training and, consequently, for improving muscle size, tone, and definition.

If the time between two workouts is too long, the supercompensation will fade away *(involution)*, resulting in little, if any, improvement in work capacity. The optimal recovery period needed for supercompensation varies according to the type and intensity of training. See table 3.4.

The way in which loads are planned directly affects how the body responds to training. For example, if the athlete follows the philosophy of lifting as heavy a load as possible day-in and day-out, and the intensity of training per microcycle does not vary, then the supercompensation curve changes drastically. Under these conditions the body never has time to replenish its energy stores, and comes closer to exhaustion with every workout. Figure 3.12 illustrates what happens to the

Table 3.4	Time Needed for Supercompensation to Occur Following Different Types of Training	
Type of training	**Energy system**	**Time needed for supercompensation (hours)**
Aerobic/cardiovascular	Glycogen/fats	6-8
Maximum strength	ATP/CP	24
Hypertrophy/muscle definition	Glycogen	36
Protein synthesis	?	48

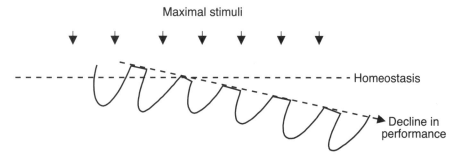

Maximal stimuli

Homeostasis

Decline in performance

Figure 3.12 **The effect of continuous overload training on one's body and working capacity.**
Reprinted from Bompa 1983.

body and to training potential when continuous exhaustive training is employed over a prolonged period of time.

As we can see from figure 3.12, it is still possible to reach supercompensation during the first two to three days of constant overloading, because fatigue has not yet affected the body's overall potential. As constant overload training continues, however, fatigue increases, taking the body further away from its balanced state (homeostasis). After about three or four days, every workout begins in a state of residual fatigue. At this stage supercompensation is never reached, and the bodybuilder's training capacity and growth potential are inhibited. Eventually the athlete reaches a very high level of exhaustion and a very low level of motivation. From this point, overtraining and breakdown are only steps away.

In comparison, when one alternates heavy training days with light training days, as suggested in figures 3.7 to 3.9, and follows the step-loading principle, the supercompensation curve forms a wave-like pattern (figure 3.13) that hovers around and above the body's homeostasis level. Energy stores are being continuously replenished, and the body is not striving to operate in a state of exhaustion or fatigue. When the body is rested and full of fuel, it can be pushed to heights never dreamed of before. By training this way, you can expect supercompensation to occur every two to four days.

Improvements in your working potential and feelings of overall well-being occur mostly on the days when you experience supercompensation. This is also the time when growth and muscle size increase. Since every bodybuilder and strength trainer wants these positive outcomes, you should carefully plan your training program so that heavy and intense training is followed by an easy day that encourages supercompensation.

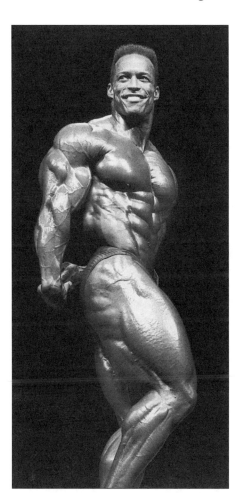

A body that is rested and full of fuel can be pushed to the limits.

Training Frequency per Microcycle

The frequency of training sessions depends on the athlete's classification, training phase, and training background. Recreational bodybuilders must progressively introduce training.

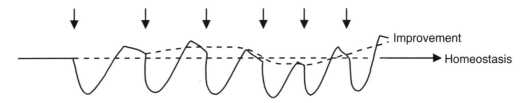

Figure 3.13 Alternating heavy workouts with low- and medium-intensity workouts produces a wave-like curve of improvement.
Reprinted from Bompa 1983.

At first they can plan two relatively short strength-training sessions per microcycle. Once this training regime is handled easily, the frequency can gradually be increased to three to four sessions per microcycle. Higher-level athletes who are taking part in shows can plan 6 to 10 training sessions per microcycle.

As part II illustrates, the number of training sessions also depends on the phase of training: three to five for anatomical adaptation, four to six or even higher for professional bodybuilders and strength trainers, and six to ten during the maximum-strength and hypertrophy phases.

The athlete's training background and resulting work tolerance are important factors in determining the frequency of training sessions per microcycle. Obviously well-trained athletes with two to three years of experience can train with ease at least four times per microcycle, which translates into visible improvements in size and muscle tone. These athletes can tolerate more work than novices.

The Split Routine

Although split routines are a virtual necessity for seriously committed bodybuilders, they are not necessarily appropriate for recreational athletes whose goals are to look fit, strong, and toned. These recreational bodybuilders will probably get the best results from training three times a week with a total-body routine. Lower training frequency would decrease training efficiency and reduce the necessary adaptive responses.

Most serious bodybuilders train very frequently, from four to six times a week. But it is difficult to challenge the same muscles in consecutive training sessions. Split routines are very important to these athletes, because they allow them to train the various muscle groups every second day or so in order to achieve better recovery between workouts. Table 3.5 is a classic example of a six-day split routine.

Many athletes believe that a program such as the classic split routine shown in table 3.5, which trains each muscle group twice per week, is sufficient to stimulate an optimal adaptive response to training. Others believe that training a muscle group to exhaustion only once a week is sufficient stimulus to make the desired gains in muscle size, tone, and definition. We seriously question both these modes of thinking: in our opinion, twice a week is not enough. For continual improvements, workouts must *constantly challenge* your present state of adaptation. In order to provoke a new adaptive response, you should progressively increase your training load using the step-type loading method. Depending on

Table 3.5	Classic Six-Day Split
Day	**Body part**
1	Legs, calves, and shoulders
2	Chest and biceps
3	Back and triceps
4	Legs, calves, and shoulders
5	Chest and biceps
6	Back and triceps
7	Rest

Table 3.6	Suggested Sets per Workout
Muscle	**Number of sets per workout**
Chest	8
Back	10
Quadriceps	6
Hamstrings	4-6
Calves	6-8
Biceps	6
Triceps	6
Shoulders	10-12
Abdominals	6

Table 3.7	High-Adaptive Response Six-Day Split
Day	**Body part**
1	Chest, back, and arms
2	Legs, calves, shoulders, and abdominals
3	Chest, back, and arms
4	Legs, calves, shoulders, and abdominals
5	Chest, back, and arms
6	Legs, calves, shoulders, and abdominals
7	Rest

the load used, this approach will stimulate an increase in muscle size or an increase in tone and strength. Competitive bodybuilders should work some muscle groups three times a week during certain training phases. (Please note that this is feasible only if you decrease the number of sets and exercises per muscle group to the lowest level realistically possible, to ensure that your energy is spent most effectively). Table 3.6 suggests the number of sets for each muscle or muscle group per workout.

The high-adaptive response six-day split outlined in table 3.7 trains each body part three times per week and allows each muscle group 48 hours of recovery before it is trained again.

The same approach can be used on a double-split routine. Table 3.8 shows one of many possible combinations.

Although most bodybuilders believe that the split routine allows sufficient recovery between training sessions, this belief does not accord with the reality of the energy systems' requirements. While a split routine helps eliminate local muscle fatigue (the fatigue acquired by a group of muscles worked to exhaustion), it does little to facilitate overall replenishment of the body's energy stores. If athletes perform exhaustive workouts every day, their glycogen stores become depleted regardless of whether they used

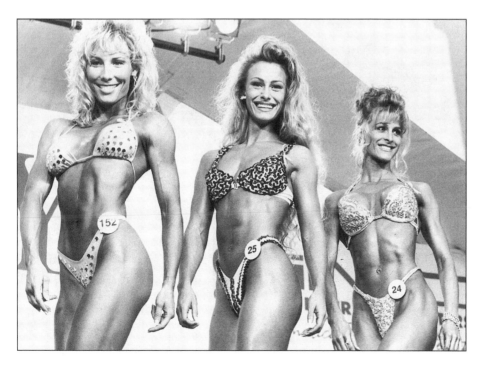

The sexy and strong fitness look can be achieved with total body routines as opposed to the split routines favored by many hard-core bodybuilders.

Table 3.8	High-Adaptive Response Six-Day Double Split				
Day		**Body part**	**Day**		**Body part**
1	A.M.	Legs and calves	**4**	A.M.	Shoulders and triceps
	P.M.	Chest and biceps		P.M.	Back and abdominals
2	A.M.	Shoulders and triceps	**5**	A.M.	Legs and calves
	P.M.	Back and abdominals		P.M.	Chest and biceps
3	A.M.	Legs and calves	**6**	A.M.	Shoulders and triceps
	P.M.	Chest and biceps		P.M.	Back and abdominals
			7		Rest

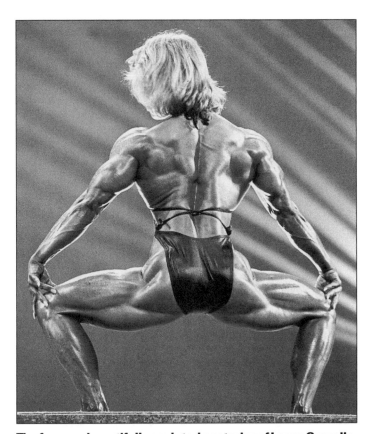

The famous, beautifully sculpted posterior of Laura Crevalle.

a split routine. Remember: exhaustive workouts use glycogen as the main fuel source, taking it from the working muscles as well as from the liver. The body needs 48 hours to fully restore glycogen levels and synthesis of protein, and cannot operate optimally if a person trains to exhaustion every 24 hours.

A well-structured, periodized training program is essential to success. Of all the concepts discussed above, consider the importance of alternating intensities during the microcycle. Traditional bodybuilding programs, where the highly regarded "no pain, no gain" theory is the norm, consistently result in overtraining. This book offers new concepts and ideas that will help you prevent overtraining, such as low-intensity days and supercompensation. Use them to enjoy a different type of bodybuilding training.

4

ACCELERATING MUSCLE RECOVERY

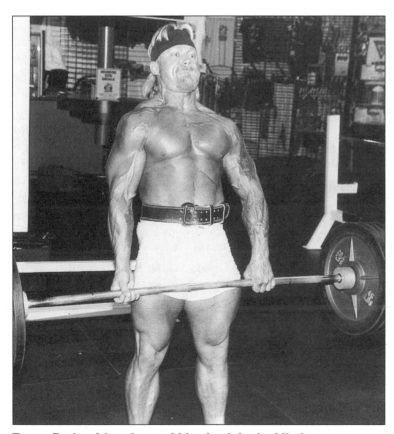

Trevor Butler drives beyond his physiological limits.

Recovery is one of the most important elements of successful training. Athletes who understand the concept avoid critical fatigue and overtraining. Strength athletes are constantly exposed to various types of training loads, reps, and sets, some of which can exceed their threshold of tolerance. As a result, the ability to adapt to the desired training load decreases and detracts from overall performance.

When athletes drive themselves beyond their physiological limits, they risk going into a state of fatigue—and the greater the level of fatigue, the greater the training after-effects such as low rate of recovery, decreased coordination, and diminished power output. Personal factors—such as stressful conditions in social, school, or work situations—also can increase levels of fatigue that athletes experience during training.

Muscle Fatigue

Muscle fatigue is a decrease in the peak tension and power output, resulting in reduced work capacity. Such fatigue depends on many factors, including a person's state of fitness, the fiber-type composition, and the sport that the person is performing. For example, fatigue in an endurance athlete is different from fatigue in a powerlifter.

Discussion of muscle fatigue can be broken into central and peripheral components. *Central fatigue* is related to events of neural input to the higher brain centers and to central command centers; to recruitment of the alpha motor nerve pool; and to the alpha motor nerves themselves. *Peripheral fatigue* involves the neuromuscular junction, the process of excitation-contraction (E-C) coupling (which involves the activation of the surface membrane), the propagation of that activation down the T-tubules (which brings the activation into the depths of the cell), the release of calcium, and the activation of contractile elements involved in the generation of force and power.

The degree to which the central and peripheral mechanisms contribute to fatigue is not fully known, although the peripheral mechanisms involved with fatigue, the cellular aspects in the muscle cell, may be the primary causes of muscle fatigue in the experienced weight trainer.

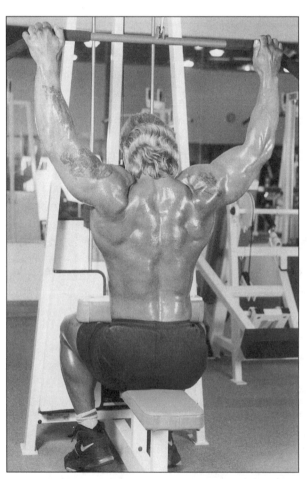

Muscular fatigue is associated with exercise-induced muscle damage.

Muscle fatigue is commonly associated with exercise-induced muscle damage. As we have seen, this is a very complex physiological and psychological phenomenon. Although much research has been devoted to muscle fatigue, neither the exact sites nor the exact causes are well known. A number of hypotheses exist, however, and it's likely that the real cause of fatigue involves many mechanisms.

A recent study has shown that human muscle fibers have a substantial reserve capacity for ATP consumption, and that fiber-type differences in the reserve capacity for ATP consumption exist (Han et al. 2001). Certainly this reserve capacity for ATP consumption becomes important under conditions where ATP production may be insufficient to meet the demands for cross-bridge cycling. Such an energetic imbalance has been suggested as an underlying mechanism of muscle fatigue. The lower reserve capacity for ATP consumption, together with the higher ATP consumption rates, may explain, at least in part, the greater fatigue susceptibility of fibers. Under conditions of greater workloads, as energy utilization increases in proportion to work, reserve capacity for ATP consumption decreases and susceptibility to fatigue increases (Ameredes et al. 2000).

While we have several working theories on the possible causes of fatigue and of overtraining syndrome and injuries, at this point we don't know which of these theories are important. It is probable that a number of different factors are involved in most instances of fatigue. For example, it is sometimes difficult to determine whether performance is decreasing because of muscle fatigue or as a result of muscle damage. We find it helpful to distinguish between muscle fatigue, from which a person can recover in about one or two hours, and muscle damage, from which it may take seven to ten days to recover. In high-intensity weight training, muscle damage will affect performance in subsequent training days, whereas muscle fatigue will generally disappear by the next training session.

Avoiding Fatigue, Overtraining, and Injury

In order to improve muscle size and strength, training loads must be as high as necessary to provide a stimulus for adaptation. But in order for the adaptation to occur, training programs must incorporate periods of rest with work while alternating different levels of intensity. These factors will result in a good balance between work and rest. It is important to avoid large increments in training loads. Using heavy loads far beyond your capacity or miscalculating necessary rest will result in decreased ability to adapt to the new load. Failing adaptation triggers biochemical and neural reactions that take you from a state of fatigue to chronic fatigue and ultimately to the undesirable state of overtraining.

Whatever the true physiological basis of fatigue, it is certain that it results from physical work that reduces the capacity of the neuromuscular and metabolic systems to continue physical activity.

The focus of the following section is neuromuscular and metabolic aspects of fatigue. We will also discuss fatigue on the basis of its central and peripheral components.

Central and Neuromuscular Fatigue

While the general assumption is that fatigue originates in the muscles, clearly the central and peripheral nervous systems play an important role in fatigue, since temperature as well as psychological factors (e.g., incentive and stress) can cause fatigue. Increasing evidence suggests that the CNS may be involved in limiting performance to a greater extent than once assumed.

A recent study, for example, demonstrated that hyperthermia reduces voluntary force development during prolonged maximal voluntary contractions, and this reduction is highly associated with decreased central activation (Nybo and Nielsen 2001). Since total muscle force appears not to differ in hyperthermic and normothermic individuals, hyperthermia-induced central fatigue seems to fully account for attenuated voluntary force development.

The CNS and peripheral nervous system have two basic processes for modulating muscle function—excitation and inhibition. Throughout training, the two processes constantly alternate. For stimulation, the CNS sends a nerve impulse to the working muscle, causing it to contract and perform work. The speed, power, and frequency of the nerve impulse directly depend on the state of the CNS.

The nerve impulses are most effective (as evidenced by good performance) when controlled excitation prevails. When the opposite occurs, as a result of fatigue, the nerve cell is in a state of inhibition and the muscle contraction is slower and weaker. The force of contraction relates directly to the electrical activation sent by the CNS and the number of motor units recruited; and as fatigue increases, the recruitment of motor units decreases.

Nerve cells cannot maintain working capacity for a very long time. Under the strain of training or demands of competition, the working capacity decreases. If high intensity is maintained in spite of fatigue, nerve cells assume a state of inhibition to protect themselves from external stimuli. Fatigue, therefore, should be seen as the body's way of protecting itself against damage to the contractile mechanism of the muscle.

Skeletal muscles produce force by activating their motor units and regulating their firing frequency, and these factors must progressively increase in order to enhance force output. The body can neutralize fatigue to some degree by signaling motor units to change their firing frequency, thereby permitting muscles to maintain force more effectively under a certain state of fatigue. If the duration of sustained maximum contraction increases, the frequency of motor-unit firing decreases, and inhibition becomes more prominent (Sherwood 1993; Nybo and Nielsen 2001).

Marsden et al. (1971) demonstrated that in a 30-second maximum voluntary contraction firing frequency decreased by 80 percent from beginning to end. Grimby et al. (1992) made similar observations: as the duration of contraction increased, activation of large motor units decreased, lowering the firing rate below the threshold level. Any continuation of contraction beyond that level was possible only through short bursts (phasical firing) that are not appropriate for constant performance.

The above findings should send a strong message of caution to those who promote the theory (especially in football and bodybuilding) that muscle size and strength can only be achieved by performing each set to exhaustion. The fact that as a contraction progresses the firing frequency decreases discredits this highly acclaimed method.

When analyzing the functional capacity of the CNS during fatigue, one must consider the bodybuilders' perceived fatigue and their past physical capacity achieved in training. When athletes' physical capacities are above the level of fatigue they experienced in testing or competition, it enhances their motivation and, as a result, their capacity to overcome fatigue.

Local Muscular and CNS Fatigue

Most research findings point to the following causes and sites of fatigue. The motor nerve is the first. The nervous system transmits nerve impulses to muscle fibers via the motor nerves. A nerve impulse has certain characteristics of force, speed, and frequency. The higher the force impulse, the stronger the muscle contraction, which gives greater ability to lift heavier loads. Since fatigue greatly affects the force of nerve impulses, rising levels of fatigue lead to declining force of contraction. This is why longer rest intervals (RIs) of up to seven minutes are necessary for CNS recovery during the maximum strength phase.

The second site is the neuromuscular junction. This is the nerve attachment on the muscle fiber that relays the nerve impulses to the working muscle. This type of fatigue is largely due to increased release of chemical transmitters from the nerve endings (Tesch et al. 1986). After a set, a two- to three-minute RI usually returns the electrical properties of the nerve to normal levels. After work of powerful contractions (such as maximum strength training), however, an RI of longer than five minutes is needed for sufficient recovery to occur.

Finally, the contractile mechanisms, actin and myosin, are also sites of fatigue. This fatigue is related to the following factors:

- Lactic acid (LA) accumulation decreases the peak tension, or the power of the muscle to contract maximally.
- LA accumulation leads to a high acidic concentration in the muscle, which in turn affects the muscle's ability to react to the nerve impulses.
- Depletion of the muscle glycogen stores, which occurs during prolonged exercise (i.e., over 30 minutes), causes the fatigue of the contracting muscle.

Other energy sources available to the muscle, including glycogen from the liver, cannot fully cover the energy demands of the working muscle.

Metabolic Sources of Fatigue

Force decline during fatigue in skeletal muscle is attributed mainly to progressive alterations of the intracellular milieu. Metabolite changes and the decline in free myoplasmic calcium influence the activation and contractile processes. Thus muscle fatigue may be associated with the mechanism of calcium flux in skeletal muscle, although the relationship between them still remains a mystery. The complex cycle of muscle contraction is triggered by the nerve impulse that depolarizes the surface membrane of the muscle cell, and is then conducted into the muscle fiber. This is followed by a series of events in which calcium is bound together with protein filaments (actin and myosin), resulting in contractile tension.

The functional site of fatigue is suggested to be the link between excitation and contraction, which results in either reducing the intensity of these two processes or in decreasing the sensitivity to activation. Changes in the flux of calcium ions affect the operation of excitation-contraction (Sherwood 1993).

In isolated skeletal muscle fibers, a marked reduction in sarcoplasmic reticulum (SR) Ca^{2+} release occurs during the latter stages of fatigue induced by repeated tetanic stimulation (Westerblad et al. 1998). Although this has been the subject of many previous studies, the mechanism underlying failure of the SR Ca^{2+} release mechanism remains uncertain. It has been suggested that fatigue-induced changes in the cytosolic environment might directly influence the sensitivity of the SR Ca^{2+} channel. In particular, cytosolic levels of H^+, lactate, Ca^{2+}, adenine nucleotides, and Mg^{2+} are known to change during fatigue, and all of these factors influence the gating properties of the SR Ca^{2+} channel (Coronado et al. 1994). However, recent work has failed to establish a clear link between release failure and any of these intracellular factors. Below we will discuss some of these factors, giving the traditional explanations first and then the recent work that is throwing some doubt on the status quo theories.

Fatigue Due to Lactic Acid Accumulation

Accumulation of lactic acid in a muscle decreases contractile activity in response to stimulation (Fox et al. 1989). As bodybuilders predominantly use anaerobic systems, they produce and accumulate high levels of lactic acid, which is the major end product of anaerobic metabolism (i.e., of glycolysis). The onset of fatigue varies with the type of muscle fiber. Heavy loads cause FT fibers to produce high levels of lactates, causing these fibers to be affected first.

The biochemical exchanges during muscle contraction result in the liberation of hydrogen ions, which in turn produce acidosis (lactate fatigue), which seems to determine the point of exhaustion (Sherwood 1993).

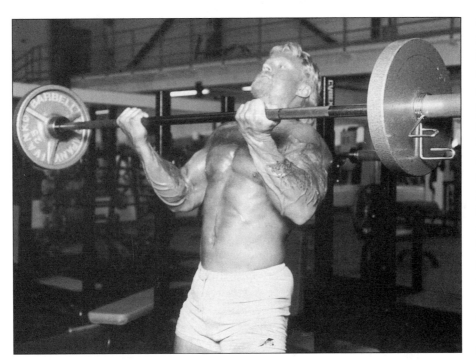

Fatigue due to lactic acid accumulation.

Increased acidosis also inhibits the binding capacity of calcium through inactivation of troponin, a protein compound. Since troponin is an important contributor to the contraction of the muscle cell, its inactivation may expand the connection between fatigue and exercise. The discomfort produced by acidosis can also be a limiting factor in psychological fatigue.

Recent studies, however, have questioned this fatigue hypothesis. One study looked at the effects of lactate on normal excitation-contraction coupling in skeletal muscle and found that the presence of lactate does not inhibit excitation-contraction coupling in mechanically skinned fibers (Posterino et al. 2001).

Nielsen and colleagues (2001) observed quite the opposite. This study looked at the combined effect of a reduction in muscle pH and loss of muscle potassium (K^+)—that lead to higher concentrations of extracellular K^+ (reduced pH and increased K^+ have both been suggested to contribute to muscle fatigue)—on function of isolated rat soleus muscles. The study showed that acidification had no effect on the membrane potential or on Ca^{2+} activity within the muscles. The authors concluded that acidification counteracts the depressing effects of elevated K^+ on muscle excitability and force. Since intense exercise increases levels of K^+, this indicates that, in contrast to the often suggested role for acidosis as a cause of muscle fatigue, acidosis may actually protect against fatigue.

Although some of the research data mentioned here are conflicting, the bottom line is that fatigue is a reality that must be accepted during training. If you correctly design your training program, you will increase your threshold to tolerate fatigue. Well-trained athletes are always capable of working more, with higher efficiency, and with visible results. Equally important is to avoid fatigue by applying some of the techniques suggested in this book, among which a periodized program is essential.

Fatigue Due to the Depletion of ATP/CP and Glycogen Stores

The energy system experiences fatigue when creatine phosphate (CP), muscle glycogen, or the carbohydrate stores are depleted from the working muscle (Sahlin 1986). The result is obvious: the muscle performs less work, possibly because its cells are consuming adenosine triphosphate (ATP) faster than they are producing it. Endurance capacity during prolonged moderate-to-heavy body-building activity varies directly with the amount of glycogen in the muscle before exercise, indicating that fatigue occurs as a result of muscle glycogen depletion (Fox et al. 1989). For high-intensity sets, the immediate source of energy for muscular contraction is ATP and CP. Complete depletion of these stores in the muscle will certainly limit the ability of the muscle to contract (Sherwood 1993). Muscle ATP loss with exercise has implications both to the causes of fatigue and muscle damage (Harris et al. 1997).

When an athlete performs high numbers of reps with prolonged submaximum levels of work, the fuels used to produce energy are glucose and fatty acids. The availability of oxygen is critical throughout this type of training because, in limited quantities, carbohydrates are oxidized instead of free fatty acids. Maximum oxidation of free fatty acids is determined by the inflow of the fatty acids to the working muscle and by the aerobic training status of the athlete. The diet to which an athlete has adapted (see discussion of the Metabolic Diet in chapter 5) is also an important factor determining substrate oxidation. Lack of oxygen, poor oxygen carrying capacity in the blood, and inadequate blood flow all contribute significantly to muscle fatigue (Grimby 1992).

Muscle Soreness

Two basic mechanisms explain how exercise initiates muscle damage. One is associated with the disturbance of metabolic function, while the other stems from mechanical disruption of muscle cells. Whenever you experience muscle soreness, you should immediately change your training program—for pursuing it at the same level will bring you one step closer to overtraining.

Metabolic damage to muscle occurs during prolonged submaximum work to exhaustion. Direct loading of the muscle, especially during the eccentric contraction phase, can cause muscle damage, and that metabolic change may aggravate the damage. Disruption of the muscle-cell membrane is one of the most noticeable damages.

Eccentric muscle contraction can produce more heat than concentric contraction at the same workload, and the increased temperatures can damage structural and functional components within the muscle cell (Armstrong 1986; Ebbing and Clarkson 1989).

Both mechanisms of muscle damage occur in stressed muscle fibers. If they have been stressed slightly, they quickly return to normal length without injury. If the stress is severe, the muscle becomes traumatized. Discomfort sets in 24 to 48 hours after the exercise. The sensation of dull aching pain, combined with tenderness and stiffness, tends to diminish within five to seven days after the initial workout.

For years, lactic acid buildup was considered the main cause of muscle soreness. It is now believed, however, that soreness results from an influx of calcium ions into muscle cells (Armstrong 1986; Ebbing and Clarkson 1989; Evans 1987; Fahey 1991).

Calcium is very important in a muscle contraction. It stimulates the fiber to contract, and is rapidly pumped back into the calcium storage area after completion of the contraction. Accumulation of calcium ions within the muscle fiber causes release of *proteases*—protein-degrading enzymes that break down muscle fibers. The soreness is primarily due to the formation of degraded protein components, or dead tissue. The body initiates a "clean-up" phase to eliminate muscle cells of dead tissue; and the muscle starts producing stress protein, which is a protective mechanism to stop further damage. This explains why muscle soreness is not felt every day.

Traumatized muscle accumulates substances—such as histamine, serotonin, potassium, and others—that are responsible for the inflammation of the injured muscle fibers (Prentice 1990). Once the concentrations of these substances have reached certain levels, they activate the nerve endings. Perhaps muscle soreness is felt about 24 hours after exercise because of the time required for the damaged cells to accumulate these substances (Armstrong 1986; Ebbing and Clarkson 1989).

Discomfort and soreness are felt intensely in the region of the muscle-tendon junction because, since tendon tissue is less flexible than muscle tissue, there is a high chance of injury from intense contraction. During high-intensity training greater damage occurs in fast twitch (FT) than in slow twitch (ST) fibers, because FT fibers play a greater role in more intense contraction.

Athletes' most important preventive technique is to use the principle of progressive increase of load. Furthermore, applying the concept of Periodization will avoid discomfort, muscle soreness, and any other negative training outcomes.

An extensive overall warm-up will result in better preparation of the body for work. Superficial warm-ups, on the other hand, can easily result in strain and pain. Good stretching sessions at the end of the warm-up, between sets, and at the end of the workout, aid in preventing muscle soreness.

After extensive muscle contraction that is typical in strength training, muscles can take up to two hours to reach their resting length without being intentionally stretched. Five to ten minutes of stretching allows muscles to reach their resting length much faster. This is optimal for biochemical exchanges at the muscle fiber level. At the same time, stretching also seems to ease muscle spasm.

It has been proposed that ingesting 100 milligrams of vitamin C per day may prevent or reduce muscle soreness. Similar benefits seem to result from taking vitamin E. Taking anti-inflammatory medication, such as aspirin or ibuprofen, may help combat inflammation of muscle tissue (Sherwood 1993). Diet is also an important element in aiding recovery from muscle soreness. Strength trainers and bodybuilders exposed to heavy loads require more protein, carbohydrates, and supplementation of their diets.

Recovery From Strength Training

Whether recovering from fatigue, overtraining, or just an exhausting training session, athletes should be aware of the various techniques that can speed or ease their recovery. Using these techniques is just as important as training effectively. As athletes continually strive to implement new loads into their training programs, they often do not adjust their recovery methods to match the new loads. And this imbalance can lead to serious setbacks. Approximately 50 percent of an athlete's final performance depends on the ability to recover effectively and quickly.

It is vital for athletes to be aware of *all* the factors that aid the recovery process, because it is the *combination* of all the factors that leads to the most successful recovery. The main factors for consideration are listed below.

- Age affects the rate of recovery. Older athletes generally require longer periods of recuperation than their younger counterparts.
- Better-trained, more experienced athletes generally require less time to recuperate, as they have quicker physiological adaptation to a given training stimulus.
- Female athletes tend to have a slower rate of recovery than males, apparently because of differences in their endocrine systems.
- Environmental factors such as jet lag, short-term changes in altitude, and cold climates tend to slow the recovery process.
- Replenishment of nutrients at the cellular level affects recovery. Muscle cells require constantly adequate levels of proteins, fats, carbohydrates, and ATP/CP for efficient general cellular metabolism as well as for production of energy (Fox et al. 1989).
- Negative emotions such as fear, indecisiveness, and lack of willpower tend to impair the recovery process.
- The recovery process is slow and depends directly on the magnitude of the load employed in training.

Recovery time depends on the energy system that is being used. Table 4.1 provides recommended recovery times after exhaustive strength training. The timing of recovery techniques strongly influences their effectiveness—whenever possible, they should be performed *during and after* each training session (Bompa 1999).

Table 4.1 Suggested Recovery Times After Exhaustive Training

Recovery process	Recovery time
Restoration of ATP/CP	3-5 minutes
Restoration of muscle glycogen	
After prolonged exercise	10-48 hours
After intermittent exercise (such as strength training)	24 hours
Removal of lactic acid from muscle and blood	1-2 hours
Restoration of vitamins and enzymes	24 hours
Recovery from high-intensity strength training (both metabolic and CNS to reach overcompensation)	2-3 days
Repayment of the alactacid oxygen debt	5 minutes
Repayment of the lactacid debt	30-60 minutes

Recovery From Short-Term Overtraining

To overcome the effects of short-term overtraining, sessions must be interrupted for three to five days. After this rest period, training can be resumed by alternating a training session with a rest day. If overtraining is more severe and the initial rest period is extended, then for every week of rest it will require roughly two weeks of training to attain the athlete's previous physical condition (Bompa 1999; Terjung and Hood 1986).

Repair of damaged muscle tissue falls under the category of short-term overtraining, requiring at least five to seven days to complete the process, while regeneration of muscle tissue takes up to 20 days (Bompa 1999; Ebbing and Clarkson).

During the acute phase of recovery from muscle damage, the best treatments are ice, elevation, compression, and active or complete rest (depending on the extent of the damage). After three days, the coach should begin to introduce other modalities such as massage. Alternation of hot and cold temperatures can also help loosen the stiffness associated with exercise-induced muscle damage (Arnheim 1989; Visconti 2001).

According to Fahey (1991) and DiPasquale (2001), diet may play an important role in muscle-tissue recovery. In addition to the obvious need for protein, particularly animal protein, carbohydrates are also required. Recovery from muscle injury is delayed when the muscle carbohydrate stores are not adequate.

The use of some vitamin supplements is generally popular when it comes to dealing with muscle damage. Fahey (1991) and DiPasquale (2001) both feel that vitamins E and C can be of great benefit to the athlete in terms of assisting in the recovery process. At the end of this chapter we comment on the use of nutritional supplements for both preventing and dealing with fatigue, overtraining, and injuries; and we discuss the particulars of JointSupport, a complex formulation meant to assist in the prevention and healing of injuries.

An important note: *anytime* you are injured, it is important that you seek the advice and assistance of qualified personnel such as physicians and physiotherapists. Misdiagnosing or mistreating an injury can lead to serious long-term consequences, and you should no more self-treat an athletic injury than you should self-treat a serious infection.

Rest Intervals Between Sets

An inadequate RI between sets causes an increased reliance on the lactic acid (LA) system for energy. The degree to which ATP and CP, a high-energy compound stored in muscles, are replenished between sets depends on the duration of the RI. The shorter the RI, the less ATP/CP will be restored and, consequently, the less energy will be available for the next set. If the RI is too short, the energy needed for the following sets is provided by glycolysis—the anaerobic metabolic pathway that produces lactic acid as its end product. The obvious problem with this energy system is that it always increases LA accumulation within the working muscles, leading to pain and fatigue and thereby impairing one's ability to train.

It is during the RI, not during the work, that the heart pumps the highest volume of blood to the working muscles. A short RI diminishes the amount of blood reaching the working muscles; and without this supply of fuel and oxygen, the athlete will not have the energy to complete the planned training session. A longer RI is required to combat excessive LA accumulation.

Several factors influence the appropriate duration of the RI between sets:

- Type of strength the athlete is developing
- Magnitude of the load employed
- Speed of contraction
- Number of muscle groups worked during the session
- Level of conditioning
- Amount of rest taken between training days
- Total weight of the athlete (heavy athletes with larger muscles usually regenerate at a slower rate than lighter athletes)

See table 4.2 for guidelines on RIs between sets.

Table 4.2 **A Guideline for RIs Between Sets for Various Loads**

Load percent	Speed of performance	RI (minutes)	Applicability
>105 (eccentric)	Slow	4-5/7	Improve maximum strength and muscle tone
80-100	Slow to medium	3-5/7	Improve maximum strength and muscle tone
60-80	Slow to medium	2	Improve muscle hypertrophy
50-80	Fast	4-5	Improve power
30-50	Slow to medium	1-2	Improve muscle definition

Reprinted from Bompa 1996.

REST INTERVAL CUES

- A 30-second RI restores approximately 50 percent of the depleted ATP/CP.
- An RI of 3 to 5 minutes or longer allows almost entire restoration of ATP/CP.
- After working to exhaustion, a 4-minute RI is not sufficient to eliminate lactic acid from the working muscles or to replenish the energy stores of glycogen.

Rest Interval Between Strength-Training Sessions

The athlete's fitness level and recovery ability influence the RI between strength-training sessions. Well-conditioned athletes recover more quickly than those with lower fitness levels. We strongly recommend that strength trainers and bodybuilders train their aerobic systems through cardiovascular training, in addition to their muscular systems.

Another benefit of aerobic training is that it helps bodybuilders and strength trainers to stay relatively lean throughout the entire annual plan, not just during contest preparation.

The energy source used during training is probably the most important factor to consider when planning the RI between sessions. For example, during the maximum-strength phase, when you are taxing primarily the ATP/CP system, daily training is possible because ATP/CP restoration is complete within 24 hours. If, on the other hand, you are training for muscle endurance (for muscle definition), you should schedule workouts every second day—it takes 48 hours for the full restoration of glycogen. Even with a carbohydrate-rich diet, glycogen levels will not return to normal levels in less than two days.

Activity During Rest

Most athletes do nothing during the RI to facilitate recovery between sets. There are, however, some things that can be done to enhance both the rate and completeness of recovery.

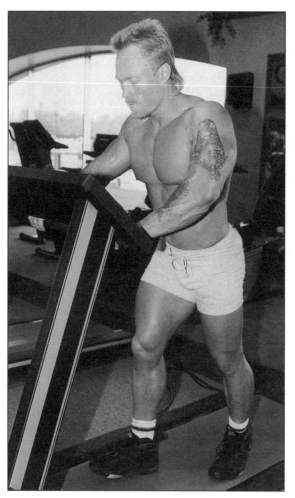

Aerobic training helps a bodybuilder's recovery process.

• **Relaxation exercises:** Simple techniques such as shaking the legs, arms, and shoulders, and a light massage, are effective ways to facilitate recovery between sets. Exercises using heavy loads cause an increase in the quantity of muscle protein, which causes muscle rigidity (Baroga 1978). These basic recovery techniques aid in its removal by improving blood circulation within the muscle.

• **Diverting activities:** Diversions involve such activities as performing light contractions with the nonfatigued muscles during the RI (Asmussen and Mazin 1978). Such physical activities can facilitate a faster recovery of the prime movers. The message of local muscle fatigue is sent to the CNS via sensory nerves. The brain then sends inhibitory signals to the fatigued muscle that reduce its work output during the RI. As the muscle becomes more relaxed, its energy stores are more easily restored.

Nutritional Supplements for Recovery

Energy supplements can prevent or alleviate various aspects of fatigue (see discussions in chapter 6 under the headings "Preworkout Stack" and "Workout Stack").

A large number of nutritional supplements can positively affect the immune system and can both help prevent and help treat injuries due to overtraining. An example of a comprehensive, multifaceted, synergistic supplement that can be useful for all of these conditions is JointSupport (see **www.MetabolicDiet.com**). JointSupport contains the following ingredients:

Betaine HCl

BioCell Collagen II (containing several ingredients including chondroitin sulfate and hyaluronic acid)

Boron

Boswellia serrata extract

Bromelain

Calcium

Cayenne

Ginger

Glucosamine sulfate

Glutathione

Harpogosides

Kavalactones

L-arginine

L-methionine

Magnesium

Manganese

Methyl-sulfonyl-methane (MSM)

N-acetyl-cysteine

Niacin

Omega-3 fish oil - EPA DHA

Papain

Quercetin dihydrate

Rutin

Shark cartilage

Silicon

Stinging nettle extract

Turmeric

Vitamin C

Vitamin D

Vitamin E

White willow

Yucca extract

Zinc

While most soreness results from muscle tissue trauma, stress is also induced on tissues connected to the muscles: bones, tendons and ligaments. These tissues are also subject to aging. Connective tissue trauma is a major source of physical discomfort in athletes. This is not surprising, considering that connective tissue is widely distributed in the body—it forms our bones, surrounds our organs, holds our teeth in place, cushions and lubricates our joints, and connects the muscles to our skeleton.

Most connective tissue injuries involve damage to structural components of the tissue. In sports activities, injuries are classified into two types: acute and overuse injuries. Acute trauma occurs from lacerations and from partial or complete rupture of the tissue. Overuse injuries, the most common, result from chronic overloading or repetitive motion.

Inflammation is the most prominent symptom of both types of injuries. While inflammation is a natural part of the healing process, chronic inflammation may lead to increased tissue degradation and impair the repair process. Indeed, chronic inflammation is a major factor in several connective tissue diseases, especially within articular joints. Pharmaceuticals are often used to manage or alleviate symptoms of connective tissue inflammation—yet many of these substances may alter the healing process, and they offer only temporary relief. Many of the medications used cause side effects (such as gastrointestinal upset) and may even accelerate joint degradation in the long run.

Many herbal remedies have been used over the centuries that have not only alleviated symptoms of tissue stress but also have shown to help rebuild tissue and restore function in joints. Many of these natural substances aid in recuperation, help heal sore muscles and joints, increase recovery from injuries such as strains and sprains, and help strengthen musculoskeletal support tissues.

JointSupport is formulated to support cartilage and joint function. It helps maintain healthy joints and relief for minor aches and pains after exercise. By providing ingredients that are essential for the body's natural synthesis and maintenance of joints, ligaments, muscles and tendons, it aids in protection against the effects of excessive exercise.

5

MAXIMIZING NUTRITION FOR MUSCLE GROWTH

Over the past five decades nutrition has been increasingly recognized as an important part of any sport, including bodybuilding and the power sports. In the past, many felt that athletes did not need to eat any differently from anyone else—after all, our diets (at least if they were carefully planned) provided everything athletes needed to develop their bodies and compete. Overwhelming scientific and medical information has demonstrated, however, that special approaches to nutrition are vital to athletic success. Unfortunately, there are still people today who feel that athletes don't need any more nutrients than the average person. But they are wrong and that's what this chapter is all about.

This chapter discusses the special nutritional needs of bodybuilders, and how you can use diet and nutritional supplements to maximize your muscle mass and strength gains and minimize your body fat. It is obvious that those who exercise regularly need more calories than those who are sedentary. But it is not so obvious that they need more protein and other macronutrients, micronutrients, and

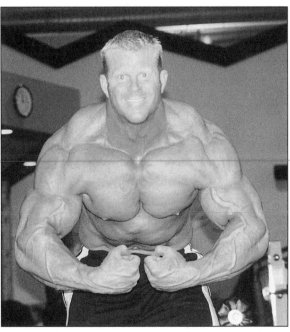

Scott Milnes' caloric intake at times exceeds 7,000 calories per day.

nutritional supplements. First, consider just what it takes to maximize gains in muscle and strength and to minimize body fat.

Factors Involved in the Training Solution

Diet and nutrition are important parts of the training solution that also includes genetics, lifestyle, and training. All the parts of this chain depend on having the other links of the chain in place.

Genetics

In order to excel in any sport or to develop extensive muscularity, you must be born with the potential to do so—and this potential involves not only physical but also mental capabilities. The enthusiasm, fortitude, and drive needed for success are as important as the physical attributes. While elite athletes have a genetic head start, what they actually accomplish depends on the other factors. The environment shapes the flow of genotype to phenotype. All four environmental factors— lifestyle, training, diet, and nutritional supplements—must be in sync before you can reach the upper limits of your natural genetic potential.

Good genes was one key to Laura Binetti's success.

Lifestyle

Lifestyle changes to maximize anabolic and minimize catabolic hormones and to maximize the anabolic effects of exercise include getting adequate sleep, minimizing stress, and avoiding use of recreational drugs, alcohol, and tobacco.

In order to manipulate the body's endogenous hormones to insure that anabolic edge, a person's lifestyle must be brought under control. Reducing emotional and psychological stress leads to increased testosterone and decreased cortisol levels (cortisol breaks down muscle tissue). Stated most simply: stress makes it more difficult to excel and shape your body and easier to break it down.

You also need sleep. While some people can get away with as little as six hours or less a day, most people need at least seven and sometimes up to ten hours a day. This can be done straight through at night, or with a six- to eight-hour stretch at night plus a one- to two-hour nap in the afternoon. Sleep deprivation adversely affects hormone function (Opstad and Asskvaag 1983).

Recreational drug use is out of the question. Marijuana and cocaine can decrease serum testosterone (Diamond et al. 1986). Alcohol lowers critical hormone levels, such as the sex hormones and growth hormone (Babichev et al. 1989; Chung 1989; Noth and Walter 1984; Soszynski and Frohman 1992).

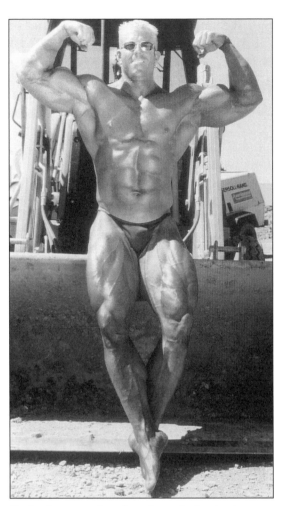

Reducing emotional and psychological stress leads to increased testosterone and decreased cortisol levels.

Training

Training should result in an adaptive response that in turn will lead to results. Other chapters of this book describe the best ways to train. Remember that it is also important to allow adequate recovery, to recognize when you are overtraining and make appropriate changes to your training, and to train in such a way as to minimize injuries.

Diet

The third component of the training solution is to determine the best diet that will give you the results you want in the shortest time and that will fit into the various Periodization phases. In this chapter we discuss some dietary guidelines that are of special interest to anyone who is physically active. In particular, we introduce the Metabolic Diet, a new paradigm in dieting for people interested in increasing strength and lean muscle mass.

Nutritional Supplements

Nutritional supplements are the fourth part of the training solution. Once your lifestyle, training, and diet are in order, the next step is to identify and use the right nutritional supplements for the job at hand, depending on your goals and your phase of training. Nutritional supplements can help you train more effectively, gain muscle mass and strength, and lose body fat.

Diet Basics for the Athlete

A good diet must be in place before you even consider nutritional supplements. It is important to remember that nutritional supplements are just that—they do not replace the diet, but only supplement it. Many studies have shown that the nutritional needs of athletes are above those of the general public. The first source for needed macro- and micronutrients should be a proper diet—one that satisfies the needs for energy, water, protein, and most of the vitamins and minerals, such as thiamine, riboflavin, niacin, iron, zinc, and chromium. Varying the diet can also be productive. Several studies have shown that an appropriate diet started several days before a competition can assist in loading the glycogen stores of muscle and improve performance (Durnin 1982). At times, special dietary practices, such as carbohydrate loading, offer a competitive advantage (Malomsoki 1983).

While hormones play an important role in the muscle hypertrophic response to resistance training (Borer 1994), the hormonal response will not result in a maximal anabolic response without an optimal dietary intake of protein and other nutrients. Thus, the anabolic effects of training are dependent not only on the resulting immediate and delayed hormonal changes but also on the presence of a systemic and cellular environment during both training and recovery that provides the nutrients needed to translate the training effect into increased protein synthesis. Ingesting certain nutrients around the training period and in the recovery period can accentuate the hormonal response of training, thus increasing protein synthesis and further maximizing the anabolic response to training.

Dietary protein appears to stimulate muscle growth directly by increasing muscle RNA content and inhibiting proteolysis, as well as by increasing insulin and free T3 (triiodothyronine—a thyroid hormone whose major metabolic function is to control metabolic rate and growth) levels. A diet high in protein appears to enhance the anabolic effects of intense training. When intensity of effort is maximal and stimulates an adaptive response, protein requirements rise in order to provide increased muscle mass.

Taking in Enough Calories

The first rule in gaining muscle mass is to make sure you are consuming enough calories. You cannot gain significant amounts of lean body mass by starving yourself. Your body will break down other tissues, including your muscle, to make up for the lack of dietary calories.

Amino acids are not efficiently incorporated into protein without enough energy sources from other foods, in part because incorporation of amino acids into peptides requires prodigious amounts of energy derived from ATP. Any excess of dietary energy over basic needs thus improves the efficiency of dietary nitrogen utilization.

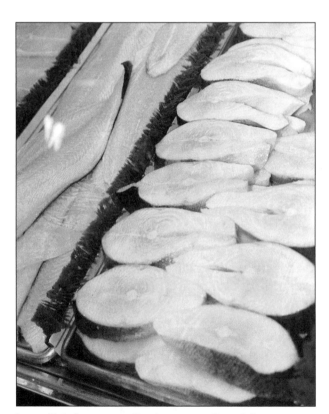

Lean fish is an excellent source of protein.

Your caloric input should match your calorie output and your goals. If you are trying to lose body fat and still are gaining or maintaining muscle size, you can drop your calories somewhat; but if you drop them too much, you will lose some lean body mass. The trick to losing body fat and maintaining or even increasing muscle mass is to gradually drop the calories as you increase your protein intake and increase your supplement intake.

Protein

Does exercise increase protein needs? Athletes have been claiming this for years while eating protein-rich foods and adding protein supplements to their daily routine. Recent research has confirmed this view (Lemon 2000): studies involving both strength and endurance in athletes have found that exercise actually does increase protein needs (Lemon 1998). Higher intake of protein and amino acids also has beneficial effects on the anabolic hormones, especially insulin-like growth factor 1 (IGF-1) (Sanchez-Gomez et al. 1999).

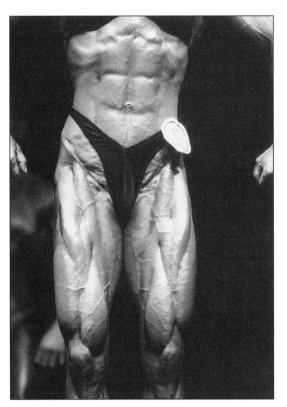

Bodybuilders' protein intake at times reaches levels of two to three grams per pound of body weight.

Besides IGF-1, bioavailable testosterone is increased by diets high in fat and protein, decreased in vegan diets (as is IGF-I), and decreased in diets high in carbohydrates. Not only is dietary protein important to optimize serum testosterone levels—the *kind* of protein is also important. A recent study substituted soy protein for meat protein, for example, and found that SHBG (serum hormone binding globulin) was higher (less bioactive testosterone) and serum testosterone was lower on the tofu diet (Habito et al. 2000).

While RDA levels for protein in standard diets may be acceptable for couch potatoes, they aren't sufficient for athletes. The intense muscle stimulation of weightlifting seems especially likely to increase both protein catabolism and its use as an energy source. By providing another energy source for use during exercise, a high-protein diet protects the protein to be used for building muscle mass. The body will burn this protein instead of the protein inside the muscle cells.

It is our belief that once a certain threshold of work intensity is crossed, dietary protein becomes essential in order to maximize the anabolic effects of exercise. Exercise performed under that threshold, however, may have little anabolic effect and may not require increased protein. While serious athletes can benefit from increased protein, other athletes who don't undergo similar, rigorous training may not benefit.

For competitive or recreational athletes who want to maximize lean body mass but don't wish to gain weight or have excessive muscle hypertrophy, we recommend consuming at least one gram of high-quality protein per pound of body weight every day. This applies to athletes who wish to stay in a certain competitive weight class or those involved in endurance events.

For athletes involved in strength events such as Olympic field and sprint events, however, or for football or hockey players, weightlifters, powerlifters, or bodybuilders, we recommend 1.2 to 1.6 grams of high-quality protein per pound of body weight per day. That means that if you weigh 200 pounds and want to put on a maximum amount of muscle mass, then you'll have to take in as much as 320 grams of protein daily.

If you are trying to lose weight or body fat by restricting calories, it is important to keep your dietary protein levels high: the body oxidizes more protein on a calorie-deficient diet than on a diet with adequate calories. For people who want to lose weight but maintain or even increase lean body mass in specific skeletal muscles, we recommend daily intake of at least 1.5 grams of high-quality protein per pound of body weight. The reduction in calories needed to lose weight should be at the expense of the fats and carbohydrates, not protein.

Carbohydrates

You must control carbohydrate intake if you want to achieve maximum lean body mass and strength with a minimum of body fat. We will discuss various aspects of carbohydrates in the section on the Metabolic Diet.

Fats

One key to success is to understand the difference between "good fats" and "bad fats"—maximizing the former, minimizing the latter, and eating the different kinds of fat in the proper proportions. While some of the information in this chapter may be somewhat technical, the recommendations and applications will be easy to understand and apply.

In spite of widespread negative publicity about ills of dietary fat, the fact is that dietary fat is essential for good health. Fat is necessary for the proper absorption, transportation, and function of the fat-soluble vitamins A, D, E, and K. The body uses lipids (a general term for all types of fats) to produce hormones and other substances that can aid good health and protect against degenerative diseases. Fats are also an excellent energy source.

Components of lipids known as *essential fatty acids* (EFAs) are necessary building blocks for all cell membranes in the body (see figure 5.1). They also make up many of the more intricate structures inside the cells. The retina (which turns light into nerve impulses in the eye) and nerve synapses (which join the body's individual nerve cells) rely on EFAs for structure. These are the types of fat that are essential to life. However, there are other fats that can actually destroy good health and lead to serious problems down the road.

Good Fats

The two essential fatty acids—linoleic acid (LA) and linolenic acid (LNA) (also called omega fats)—are critical to health and must be supplied in a person's diet since the human body can't manufacture them.

Many people get insufficient amounts of EFAs in their diets, which can cause health problems because these EFAs are necessary for growth, for the integrity of

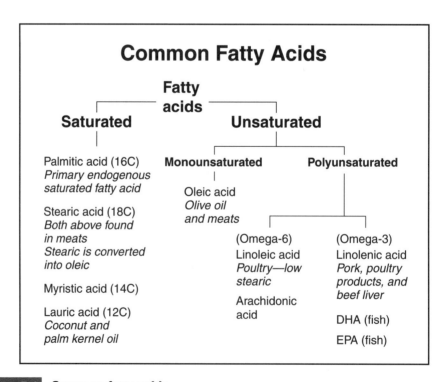

Figure 5.1 Common fatty acids.

cell membranes, and for the synthesis of many important compounds. Getting enough LNA (an omega-3 fatty acid) seems to be more of a problem, while deficiency of linoleic acid (an omega-6 fatty acid) is less common: the diets of most people are much higher in LA than LNA. The excess LA seems to affect the biological action of LNA, creating an even greater relative deficiency of LNA. This is a serious problem, since LNA and the other omega-3 FAs are responsible for most of the health benefits of EFAs.

Supplemental EFAs can be beneficial even if a deficiency doesn't exist; if used properly, they can increase overall health, help you avoid heart disease, and lose body fat. Overall, the increased processing of foods in our society has significantly lowered the amount of EFAs in the average diet. Foods rich in EFAs are highly perishable and not deemed practical or profitable for most commercial preparations. The Metabolic Diet, as explained below, provides extra EFAs.

For people on the Metabolic Diet, which calls for high levels of fat and protein, the omega-3s can provide an excellent hedge against worries about cholesterol. Omega-3 fatty acids positively affect blood pressure, clotting, immune response, insulin resistance, and triglyceride levels (Simopoulos 1999). Even in cases where dietary cholesterol is increased, omega-3s may aid in actually lowering serum cholesterol (Garg et al. 1989). There is some evidence to suggest that in higher-fat diets aerobic exercise also reduces serum cholesterol and thus may improve the effects of omega-3-rich fish oil on cholesterol (Schurch et al. 1979).

LNA, eicosapentaenoic acid (EPA), and docosahexaenoic acid (DHA) can also enhance lipolysis (body fat breakdown) (Awad and Zepp 1979; Parrish et al. 1991) and decrease lipogenesis (body fat formation) (Belzung et al. 1993; Parrish et al. 1990). The combined breakdown of stored body fat and decrease in additional body fat can have very positive results for the dieter. You actually end up making less fat and breaking down more of what's already on the body when using these oils. We wholeheartedly support adding portions of fish and fish oil to your daily diet, as fish oil is high in these beneficial fatty acids. Moreover, while many foods contain more than one type of fatty acid, plant oils usually contain much more unsaturated fatty acids than do animal fats. Flaxseed oil, nuts, seeds, and unprocessed vegetable oil are also rich in essential fatty acids.

Bad Fats

Commercial vegetable oils are not a good source for essential fatty acids. The problem for processors is that natural poly- and monounsaturated fatty acids are reactive to light and heat—they can quickly become rancid. Most of the vegetable oils on the shelf of your local supermarket—including corn, canola, and soybean oils—have been hydrogenated or very heavily refined, and are so overly processed that they can be harmful to your health. Processing not only removes any useful properties the oil had, such as EFAs or antioxidants; depending on the processing method, they can even cause immune problems and predispose people to certain cancers.

Even natural polyunsaturated fats, because they are unstable and oxidize readily, appear to have two serious drawbacks. First, they seem to promote certain cancers at a dietary concentration of 5 percent or more (Philip et al. 1992). Second, while they can lower total cholesterol, they can also lower levels of high-density lipoprotein (HDL, the so-called "good cholesterol") (Lichtenstein et al. 1993), and thus increase the chances of coronary artery disease.

To make matters worse, polyunsaturated fats are usually *hydrogenated* in order to make them more solid and stable at room temperature, to give a longer shelf life, and to make them easier to use in certain foods and baked goods. Hydrogenation involves heating the oil in a vacuum and then forcing hydrogen through it under pressure. Unfortunately, hydrogenation—along with other refining methods such as use of chemical solvents, bleaches, and heat—tends to destroy any healthful qualities present in the natural oils and to create by-products that can be harmful to your health. Trans fatty acids, crosslinked fatty acid chains, and fragments of fatty acid chains produced secondary to hydrogenation can have significant adverse effects on blood cholesterol, increasing the risk of heart disease. By competing with EFAs, moreover, these fats lead to EFA deficiencies and subsequently to a host of other health problems including diabetes, cancer, and weight gain.

In summary, bad fats are those that have been altered by processing; because they compete with essential fatty acids, they negatively affect cellular metabolism and structure. There is also some speculation that trans fatty acids may adversely affect insulin sensitivity, decrease fat oxidation, and increase fat synthesis.

Foods containing significant amounts of trans fatty acids usually list hydrogenated or partially hydrogenated products in their ingredients. These foods include baked goods, crackers, candies, almost all fried fast foods, potato chips, and other foods made with shortening, margarine, or refined oils. Keep away from them as much as possible.

Fats to Avoid

- All margarines except those with low trans fatty acid content
- Hydrogenated and partially hydrogenated oil products and foods (check the labels)
- Shortening
- Old fats and oils of any type

Amount and Type of Fats

In a diet where fat plays the key role as it does in the Metabolic Diet, it's important to get a handle on just what kind of fats you should look for and in what proportion you should eat them. The following guidelines will be helpful:

- Eat fewer processed baked goods and fried foods, especially fast foods.
- Bake, boil, microwave, poach, or steam foods instead of frying them.
- Buy oils that are predominantly monounsaturated (olive or canola oils).
- Consume only fresh oils.

Twenty-five percent of your fat intake should come from olive oil and EFA-rich foods such as nuts, seeds, fish, flaxseed oil, salmon oil, and unprocessed vegetable oils. The other 75 percent of your fat intake should come from high-quality meats, chicken, eggs, cheese, pork, butter, shell- and other fish, and associated foods. Also, use omega-3 enriched eggs and dairy products if they are available in your area. Table 5.1 provides an easy way to judge the various fats in some common foods and oils.

You should supplement your diet with oils containing gamma linolenic acid (GLA) (such as evening primrose or borage seed oils), unspoiled fish oil (if your intake of fish is lacking), and to a lesser extent flaxseed oil. Make liberal use of extra virgin olive oil for preparing foods, salads, protein drinks and any other items that you find palatable. Following is more information on some recommended fats.

Flaxseed Oil   One of the best-known sources of LNA (and a good source of LA) is flaxseed oil (also known as flax oil or linseed oil). Hemp oil, another rich source of LNA (and LA and to a lesser extent GLA) is slowly becoming more available.

Table 5.1 Fatty Acid Composition of Commonly Consumed Foods (as Percentage of Total Fatty Acids)

Food	Saturated	Monounsaturated	Polyunsaturated
Butter, cream, milk	65	30	5
Beef	46	48	6
Bacon and pork	38	50	12
Lard	42	45	13
Chicken	33	39	28
Fish	29	31	40
Coconut oil	92	6	2
Palm kernel oil	86	12	2
Cocoa butter	63	34	3
Olive oil	15	76	9
Peanut oil	20	48	32
Cottonseed oil	27	20	53
Soybean oil	16	24	60
Corn oil	13	26	61
Sunflower seed oil	11	22	67
Safflower seed oil	10	13	77

Flaxseed oil consists of 45 to 65 percent LNA, 15 percent LA, and a lesser amount of monounsaturated and saturated fatty acids.

If you use flaxseed oil, make sure it's fresh. Refrigerate after opening, and use it soon after opening—flaxseed oil, like other perishable foods, becomes rancid very quickly. Look for it in the refrigerated section of any good health food store or nutritional center. If you keep it refrigerated, flaxseed oil will generally last up to six weeks after it is opened.

We usually recommend a minimum of five grams of flaxseed oil per day to ensure that you get the necessary EFAs. In addition to the liquid form, flaxseed oil capsules are available and generally come in doses of one gram per capsule. Fresh unrefined flaxseed oil can also be added to a protein drink or salad (one to three tablespoons) as a tasty way to supplement LNA.

Evening Primrose Oil and Borage Seed Oil Both oils are rich in linoleic acid, vitamin E, and GLA. Since GLA is a precursor for DGLA (dihomogamma linolenic acid—an essential fatty acid), which has been shown to be depleted by steroids, alcohol, and other drugs, it has been suggested that GLA provides protection for the liver. DGLA is easily produced from GLA; use of GLA supplements may lead to increased production of the good prostaglandins that help fight musculoskeletal inflammation, decrease cholesterol and fluid retention, and have beneficial effects on several hormones in the body.

We usually recommend at least 500 mg of GLA daily. That usually translates to six or more capsules of evening primrose oil or three or more capsules of borage seed oil daily (evening primrose oil usually contains just less than half the amount of GLA as borage seed oil).

Fish and Fish Oils   Fish oils belong to the alpha-linolenic omega-3 series of fatty acids and are rich in eicosapentaenoic acid. While the body is able to convert alpha-linolenic acid to the longer-chained EPA and DHA, it does so slowly. It makes good sense to use fish oils since they are rich sources of EPA and DHA. While increasing fat-burning capabilities and lessening the amount of fat on the body, fish oils also help limit the breakdown of muscle tissue and add muscle tone for increased body shaping.

The best way to obtain fish oil is to regularly eat fresh fatty fish. For example, a mere 100 grams (3.5 ounces) of Atlantic salmon has about 1,400 milligrams of omega-3 fatty acids (EPA and DHA). A half pound of Atlantic salmon provides an amount of omega-3s equal to or more than what you would obtain with 10 capsules of fish oil.

Although freshwater, ocean, and shellfish all contain some omega-3 fatty acids, there is evidence that ocean fish is a better source than freshwater fish (except for lake trout); fish from colder northern waters such as the North Atlantic have more omega-3s than those caught near the equator, and shellfish have less than other fish. Of the commonly available fish, the ones that are highest in omega-3s are salmon, tuna, herring, sardines, mackerel, and bluefish. We recommend that one or all of these fish be eaten at least three to four times a week.

If you have problems with eating fish on a regular basis, then we recommend a fish oil supplement such as salmon oil capsules. Generally, we recommend 2,000 milligrams of EPA a day. Since fish oil usually contains about 20 percent EPA and a lesser amount of DHA, 10 capsules a day of 1,000 milligrams of fish oil should give you the recommended amount. If you want, or if you have a personal or family history of coronary artery disease, you may consume more fish oil—long-term fish oil supplementation appears to have no adverse metabolic effects (Eritsland et al. 1995).

Whatever the amount that you use, be careful to buy fresh fish oil capsules in an opaque container. If the capsules are fishy tasting, chances are they're partially rancid and shouldn't be used. Keep the fish oil capsules in the refrigerator and away from light and use them up as soon as possible, or at least within a few months of purchase.

Monounsaturated Fats   Monounsaturated fatty acids (oleic acid is the main one that concerns us) are produced by the body and are found in fats of both plant and animal origin. Animal sources of oleic acid usually occur along with saturated fatty acids and include beef, pork, lamb, chicken, turkey, dairy products, eggs, and some fish (like eel and trout). Although the common belief is that the fats found in the above foods are all saturated, this is not the case. Oleic acid makes up from 20 to 50 percent of the fats in these foods.

Plant sources include olive, canola (rapeseed), hazelnut, and peanut oils, as well as almonds, avocados, pistachios, and macadamia nuts. Many of the foods that contain or are cooked in the above oils have significant levels of oleic acid, including fried foods, salad dressings, baked goods, and certain soups.

Monounsaturated fatty acids, especially oleic acid, seem to have some advantages over other fatty acids. Monounsaturated fatty acids won't increase your risk of heart disease and may even decrease it by their effects on total cholesterol, HDL, and low-density lipoprotein (LDL, the so-called "bad cholesterol") (Wahrburg et al. 1992). The body also metabolically handles oleic acid more easily than the other monounsaturated fatty acids.

Olive oil is one of the better fats to consume on the Metabolic Diet. But only certain olive oils are candidates. As with any other oil, any heat, chemical solvents, or other refining process ruins the health effect of olive oil. The best olive oils are cold-pressed extra virgin oils, since they are extracted by the use of gentle pressure rather than with the use of heat and solvents.

Saturated Fats   Many of the foods recommended in the Metabolic Diet, such as red meat, eggs, cheese, and butter, contain saturated fats. These fats tend to raise total serum cholesterol and LDL levels in some individuals, especially those with previous blood cholesterol problems. The increase in total cholesterol is mainly from an increase in LDL, although there is also a small increase in HDL (McNamara 1992).

However, not all saturated fatty acids adversely affect total cholesterol. For example, stearic acid (the main saturated fatty acid found in beef) and medium-chain saturated fatty acids have little or no effect on total cholesterol. Replacement of carbohydrates with stearic acid (as is done to some extent in the high-fat, low-carbohydrate phase of the Metabolic Diet) appears to have little effect on lipid and lipoprotein concentrations in plasma (Denke and Grundy 1991; Katan et al. 1994). In these studies, oleic and linoleic acids had beneficial effects on blood lipids by raising HDL and lowering LDL.

Natural saturated fats do not have the toxic harmful effects of trans fatty acids. They are mainly an effective and compact source of energy. Most of us have no real problem with these saturated fats—our bodies know how to deal with them.

Saturated fats are an integral part of the Metabolic Diet. If used properly, natural saturated fats will help you to lose weight and body fat. Any adverse effects they might have on people susceptible to cholesterol problems are usually diminished by the fact that, in highly-trained athletes, these fats don't have a chance to do any harm because the body uses the saturated fats as a primary energy source. Moreover, other recommended fats in the Metabolic Diet can decrease or eliminate any adverse changes due to raised levels of total cholesterol, HDL, and LDL.

The Metabolic Diet

In the past, most bodybuilders and power athletes followed nearly year-round diets that were high in protein and complex carbohydrates and low in fat. The only thing that varied, except when they fell off the diet, was the calories—higher when they were trying to gain muscle mass and lower when they were cutting up. The staple diet, especially among bodybuilders, consisted of a lot of high-protein foods, such as egg whites, broiled or baked skinless chicken, tuna packed with water, and of course lots of oatmeal and rice.

All that has changed in the past decade. Since Mauro DiPasquale introduced the Metabolic Diet in the early 1990s, many power athletes, and especially bodybuilders, have gotten off the high-carbohydrate and low-fat bandwagon and have maintained the high-protein edge by cycling lower-carbohydrate, higher-fat diets. These bodybuilders have found that they can get more massive on this diet than on the traditional bodybuilding diet. Although we cover the basics of the diet in this chapter, see DiPasquale's book *The Metabolic Diet* for more details.

The Metabolic Diet is easy to follow. It has three main benefits:

1. It stimulates your metabolism to burn fat instead of carbohydrates as its primary fuel.
2. It maintains the fat burning as you lower your caloric intake, so that your body obtains its energy mainly from fat instead of glycogen or muscle protein.
3. It spares and maintains protein, allowing you to build muscle mass.

The first step in the Metabolic Diet is to induce your metabolism to burn fat as its primary fuel. This is done by limiting dietary carbohydrates and consuming ample amounts of fat. During this adaptation stage you don't really need to change your normal caloric intake—simply substitute protein and fat for your former carbohydrate calories.

The second step, once you are fat adapted, is to vary your calories to suit your goal. To increase muscle mass, increase your daily caloric intake by consuming more fat and protein. To lose body fat while maintaining muscle mass, slowly decrease both your caloric and fat intake. Because your body receives fewer calories and less dietary fat, it will increasingly use its fat stores, not muscle, to make up any energy deficits. In some circumstances, because of lower dietary fat levels, your diet may contain only moderate or even low levels of fat, mainly in the form of the essential and monounsaturated fatty acids.

Cycling between low-carbohydrate, high-fat to high-carbohydrate, lower-fat regimens manipulates the anabolic and fat-burning processes in the body so that they maintain or increase muscle mass while decreasing body fat. You are training the body to burn mainly body fat in preference to carbohydrates and protein. By shifting from a low-carbohydrate diet on weekdays to a higher-carbohydrate diet on weekends, you manipulate the muscle-building and fat-burning processes and hormones.

Purpose of the Metabolic Diet

In this chapter, we discuss how the Metabolic Diet can help maximize strength and lean body mass; in later chapters, we cover details of using the diet in the various training phases. But first, we will explain how and why it works and clear up a few common misconceptions about the diet.

First we must emphasize that, unlike with other diets that espouse a constant low-carbohydrate intake, insulin is not the enemy. In fact, insulin is a problem only when it is chronically high or extremely variable, as happens with carbohydrate-based diets. In fact, in the Metabolic Diet we make use of the anabolic effects of insulin while at the same time avoiding its bad effects on body fat and insulin sensitivity.

Insulin works its anabolic magic hand-in-hand with testosterone and growth hormone (GH). GH is very important because it increases protein synthesis and decreases muscle breakdown. During the weekdays when you are on the higher-fat, higher-protein, lower-carbohydrate portion of the diet, insulin levels stay fairly steady and don't fluctuate wildly, and growth-hormone secretion increases. Along with stimulating a great environment for body shaping, GH also induces cells to use fat instead of sugar for energy, thus increasing the burning off of body fat and limiting its production.

Insulin usually decreases the secretion of GH, but it appears that the body sees the great increase in carbohydrates and insulin during the weekend portion of the Metabolic Diet as a stressful situation, much like exercise, and GH can actually increase with insulin. In this way, we potentially can get the positive effects of increased growth hormone both during the week and on at least part of the weekends. Testosterone, also critical to increasing muscle mass and strength, responds well to the Metabolic Diet.

Overall it has been our experience that there is an acute anabolic effect on muscle when a short-term lower-carbohydrate diet is alternated with carbohydrate loading. Cellular hydration is maximized by the water and carbohydrate loading, and insulin sensitivity is increased, leading to an intense anabolic stimulus. Constant fluctuations make for an anabolic effect unparalleled by any other diet. This anabolic effect allows you to tone and shape your body as you lose weight.

Controlling Catabolism (Muscle Breakdown)

Along with increasing the anabolic process in the body, it is also important to insure that the muscles you have developed are not broken down. To do this you want to maximize the anabolic hormones, such as testosterone and GH, and minimize the production and effects of catabolic hormones, the most critical of which is cortisol (cortisol also promotes fat storage). Much of this is done naturally through the Metabolic Diet. Since body fat stimulates cortisol production (Fossati and Fontaine 1993), less cortisol is secreted as body fat is lost.

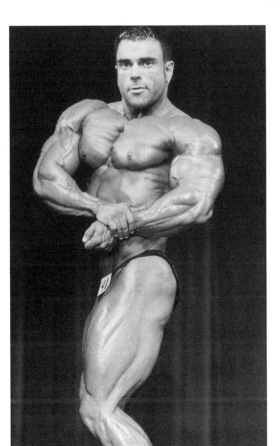

Controlling muscle breakdown while dieting is a key factor in a bodybuilder's success.

Along with the hormonal control, you'll also find that the Metabolic Diet helps with psychological control. The wide mood swings and irritability you can get on a carbohydrate-based diet can also increase cortisol levels—and psychological stress can be a prime result of cortisol production.

The Complete Picture

In order to give the Metabolic Diet your maximum effort, you need to optimize your training and your use of nutritional supplements. The diet will melt away the body fat and give you the basics for creating a fit, attractive body. Exercise will give you a leg up on increasing muscle mass and decreasing body fat, while providing good cardiovascular health and protection from heart disease. Supplements will give you an extra edge to help get the maximum anabolic and fat-loss effects out of your diet and training.

These three tools used together—the Metabolic Diet, a solid exercise program, and a savvy approach to nutritional supplements—provide a "can't miss" scenario for success. And to think it all occurs without the starvation and insanity that accompany the carbohydrate-based diets!

Getting Started

Before going on the Metabolic Diet, you should get a complete physical from your doctor. You should also have a blood workup—including a complete blood count, cholesterol levels (total, LDL, and HDL), TSH (a test for thyroid function), fasting blood sugar, serum uric acid, serum potassium, liver function array, and blood urea nitrogen (BUN). Your doctor may want to go beyond this, but he or she will let you know if you should have more done.

Remember that because you are burning fat for energy, much of the cholesterol and saturated fats that could cause a problem are used up in the process. Along with increasing the utilization of fat as an energy source and providing for weight loss, the Metabolic Diet can even reduce serum cholesterol (Schurch et al. 1979).

We also urge you to weigh yourself and get a body fat analysis before you begin the diet. Weight loss is important but so are inches. There are times when, for a variety of reasons, you might not be losing much weight but you are nevertheless subtracting unsightly body fat. Such knowledge will help keep your enthusiasm high if you know that, even though you are not losing weight, you are making progress in other areas and your body is toning up.

You might also want to keep track of your body measurements. Especially important are your waist, hips, upper thighs, chest, and upper arms. These measurements will give you an idea of how your body is responding to the diet and where you're losing weight the fastest. It will also give you an idea of where your problem areas are and where you may need to concentrate exercise to get the body you want. Measurements also help motivate you when you're retaining fluid or not losing weight—for if you see those waist and hip measurements going down despite the lack of weight loss, you will know that you are making progress.

Finally, you should review the medications you take. If you are on diuretics, you may want to use them only as needed due to the higher-fat, lower-carbohydrate diet's ability to help you shed water.

Eating Plan

We suggest that those who want to maximize strength and muscle mass and minimize body fat take a strict, uncomplicated approach to the diet. This strict, low-carbohydrate phase can last anywhere from two to several weeks and allows you to determine if you're an efficient fat user and as such can do quite nicely without too many carbohydrates.

If you are an efficient fat burner, then you're all set to carry on with the low-carbohydrate five-day, two-day phase-shift regimen. By carefully monitoring how your body reacts to the carbohydrate level you're on and then making any necessary adjustments in carbohydrate intake, you will eventually arrive at that magic dietary carbohydrate level that's just right for you.

The initial part of the Metabolic Diet, in which you determine just how your body functions under carbohydrate deprivation, is meant to be a testing ground for your ability to use fat as a primary fuel. People who are efficient fat oxidizers will do very well in this phase of the diet. Those who aren't may find that they won't cope as well on this strict part of the diet and will do much better as the carbohydrate levels are raised in subsequent weeks.

The Metabolic Diet is designed to be a phase-shift diet. That is, on weekdays you consume a lower-carbohydrate diet, while weekends are for higher carbohydrate levels. But that's not the way it works in the first two weeks.

The best way to approach the first two weeks is to stay low-carbohydrate for the first 12 days and then increase carbohydrates on Saturday and/or Sunday. Doing it this way will give your body the incentive to make the shift from burning carbohydrates to burning fat as its primary fuel. It will also tell you very quickly if you're totally unsuited for bottom-level "low carbing."

Metabolic Diet basic steps

1. Replace the carbohydrates you're eating now with protein and fat; don't change the calorie level at first.
2. At first, stick to the low-carbohydrate phase for a full 12 days before beginning the high-carbohydrate phase.
3. End carbohydrate loading the minute you start smoothing out.
4. Once you're fat adapted, change the calorie level depending on the training phase you're in.

The initial, adaptation phase of the Metabolic Diet is really quite simple. It calls for a dedicated higher-fat/high-protein/low-carbohydrate diet from Monday of the first week through Friday of the second week (a total of 12 days) before "carbing up" (see table 5.2).

Table 5.2	**Grams of Carbohydrates Allowed and Percentage of Calories From Fat, Protein, and Carbohydrates**			
	Carbohydrate intake	Percent fat	Percent protein	Percent carbohydrate
Weekday maximum	30 grams	40-60	40-50	4-10
Weekend (12-48 hour carbohydrate load)	No real limit	20-40	15-30	35-60

During those first 12 days, unless you are exceptionally uncomfortable (fatigue, weakness etc.), you will be limited to 30 grams of carbohydrates per day. Fat should be set at roughly 50 to 60 percent and protein set at 30 to 40 percent of your caloric intake. Follow these criteria during the initial 12-day phase of the diet and for the ensuing five weekdays of following weeks, assuming you're biochemically suited to this low level of carbohydrates.

Guidelines for the strict or assessment phase

Fat: 50 to 60 percent of caloric intake

Protein: 30 to 40 percent of caloric intake

Carbohydrates: 30 grams

Then, beginning on the second Saturday and on subsequent Saturdays, you perform the big turnaround. You go through a higher-carbohydrate phase of the diet for a period lasting anywhere from 12 to 48 hours over the weekend and on following weekends. Set your fat intake at 25 to 40 percent, your protein intake at 5 to 30 percent, and carbohydrate intake at 35 to 55 percent of the calories you consume. As you will understand from following paragraphs, you should adjust these levels to match and maximize individual body chemistry and needs.

The whole process is very similar to what athletes call "carbohydrate loading." You hit the carbohydrates relatively heavily, and this allows you to be very sociable in the dietary sense—you can eat those foods you've been missing during the week.

Guidelines for the carbohydrate-loading period

Fat:	25 to 40 percent of caloric intake
Protein:	15 to 30 percent of caloric intake
Carbohydrates:	35 to 55 percent of caloric intake

Here's what's happening: In the adaptation phase (the first two weeks), you limit carbohydrates. Then the second weekend hits and all of a sudden you're stuffing yourself with carbohydrates. *Insulin levels will rise dramatically.* In fact, it's been shown that the higher-fat/low-carbohydrate phase of the diet makes the insulin response to the high carbohydrates even greater than it normally would be (Bhathena et al. 1989; Sidery et al. 1990).

Needless to say, your body goes through a big transition every week with this diet, whether or not you stick to the strict carbohydrate levels or increase your dietary carbohydrates to a level where you function best. That's why it's important to know when to stop on the weekend. If you find that you have an unlimited appetite on the weekend, that's OK: you'll kick the insulin into gear that much faster. But you must be careful, because some people begin laying down body fat faster than others. That's why you must be aware of the point at which you begin to feel puffy and bloated. This point will vary greatly from person to person. Some people feel hardly any response in appetite from the increased insulin. Others, however, experience wide insulin swings and find themselves hungry and eating all the time. That is why we list 12 to 48 hours as the carbohydrate load on weekends. This could be cut back to even less than 12 hours for people whose appetites become insatiable or for people who tend to begin laying down body fat relatively early in the carbohydrate loading phase. The important thing is knowing when you've had enough. When you start feeling puffy and bloated and can even sense the fat coming on, it's time to go back to your weekday high-fat/low-carbohydrate routine.

Granted, it may take you a while to learn to know your body and realize when it's telling you it is time to change phases. This point varies widely among individuals and, while it may be easy for one person to interpret body cues, it may be harder for another. If you have trouble with this, make the change earlier in the weekend and see how you look and feel the next week. As always, patience is the order of the day. Experience will eventually teach you to interpret your body very well and know when you're putting on fat.

Also, keep in mind that the percentages listed above for fat, protein, and carbohydrate consumption are optimal numbers. If you've never done any real diet planning before, you may have a bit of trouble reaching them at first. If so, don't worry. By aiming for the 30-gram carbohydrate limitation and 40-percent minimum fat level in the diet during the early weeks, you'll make the metabolic shift necessary for initial success.

Increasing Dietary Carbohydrates

It usually takes people about three to four weeks on the phase-shift part of the Metabolic Diet to determine if they can survive and thrive on this low level of dietary carbohydrates or if they need more carbohydrates throughout or just at

Problem-Solving Guide

Steps to take in determining your carbohydrate set point.

If you are feeling fine:

1. You are starting on a 2-week assessment phase of the strict Metabolic Diet to see how well you do with 30 g carbohydrate on weekdays, 130 to 150 g of carbohydrate on weekends.
2. You have been following the guidelines in item #1 for 2 weeks now and you are doing well. What do you do now?
3. Continue with a further 2-week assessment phase of the strict Metabolic Diet to see how well you do.
4. It's now been 4 weeks on the strict Metabolic Diet assessment phase, and you feel great. What do you do now?
5. Now your strict Metabolic Diet begins in earnest: so stay on the schedule of 5 weekdays at 30 g carbohydrates and 2 weekend days at 130 to 150 g carbohydrates.

If you're feeling tired:

You need some help with the carbohydrate part of your diet.

1. You have only low to moderate tiredness at this time, so you should do another 2-week assessment phase to see how well you do.
2. You have moderate to severe tiredness so you need to introduce variations into your diet to overcome this tiredness.
3. You are at the "variations in diet" junction and need to review the options to combat this tiredness.
4. You have mid- to late-week tiredness, so what do you need to do? Try a mid-week carbohydrate spike of an additional 120 g of carbohydrates just on Wednesday and see how well you do.
5. You did the mid-week carbohydrate spike but now you lack energy during training. What should you do? Take 30 to 100 g of carbohydrates half an hour after training to combat this lack of energy on training days.
6. You still lack energy during training, so what can you do? Increase your carbohydrate intake on training days by 30 g again, and do this every week until you feel normal during your workouts.
7. You lack energy all week, so what can you do? Increase your daily intake of carbohydrates by 30 g.
8. You increased your daily carbohydrate intake by 30 g for a 1-week period and you still feel tired all week. So what can you do next? Add another 30 g of carbohydrates to your daily intake for a 1-week assessment and again every week until you feel normal.

one time or another. However, for the sake of assessing whether or not the strict Metabolic Diet suits you, we decided to do it two weeks at a time. If you feel OK after the first two weeks, then carry on with the 5+ days at 30 grams and 1 to 2 days in the higher carbohydrate phase.

If you are mildly to moderately tired and otherwise negatively affected, go through another two-week assessment phase to see if things even out. If you are severely affected then, go to one of the variation diets where you selectively take in more carbohydrates depending on when you're feeling punk.

If you feel good from Saturday to Wednesday and start to get tired and generally unwell by the time Thursday rolls around, then a Wednesday carb-spike day should do the trick—so on Wednesday you should increase your carbohydrates to at least 100 grams and probably more. You might try incorporating from 0.5 to 1.0 gram of carbohydrates per pound of body weight and see how you respond.

If you're OK most of the time but just don't have enough energy for your workouts, then try consuming around 50 to 100 grams of carbohydrates after your training. Vary the amount of carbohydrates you use after exercise—anywhere from 10 to 150 grams—to see what works for you. The type of carbohydrate you use also makes a difference in this case. We have found that the use of a combination of high-glycemic and low-glycemic carbohydrates works best.

If you are tired and feel bad for most of the low-carbohydrate weekdays, double the carbohydrate intake to 60 grams per day on the weekdays to see if this helps. If that doesn't help, increase the carbohydrate intake by 30 grams per day once a week for as many weeks as it takes for you to feel normal and function optimally.

Most people who have to increase their daily carbohydrates usually level off between 100 and 200 grams per day. We have found that about 0.5 to 1.0 gram of dietary carbohydrates per pound body weight per day is the norm in those who are relatively poor fat oxidizers. In a small number of cases it may be necessary to work up to as much as 3 grams of carbohydrates per pound of body weight, depending on the individual and the activity that he or she is involved in.

When you have to increase the level of carbohydrates in your diet, it will take a while before you discover your carbohydrate set point. It takes people about two months on average to find their ideal dietary carbohydrate level. Once you discover your *metabolic set point,* you can fix your diet at that level for several months while you work on changing your body composition.

Choosing Foods

For weekdays, there are plenty of options for high-fat/high-protein/low-carbohydrate foods (see table 5.3). Virtually any meat is OK. Most people focus on steak, hamburger, pork, and other red meats; but venison, fish, lamb, shrimp, lobster, chicken, turkey, and other white meats are also OK. So are canned sardines, tuna, shrimp, herring, and anchovies.

Almost any kind of cheese is acceptable. Use the full-fat varieties. Keep in mind that cheese spreads, cottage, and ricotta cheese are fairly high in carbohydrates. Brie, Camembert, Muenster, mozzarella, cheddar, Gruyere, and Monterey Jack are very low in carbohydrates and good for the diet.

Whole eggs are great. Deviled eggs can be a good snack food to keep in the refrigerator. Butter and poly- and monounsaturated oils are fine (subject to certain restrictions). Nuts and seeds like walnuts and sunflower seeds are also good, but keep track of the carbohydrates. So are condiments such as salt, vinegar, oil, and mayonnaise, although we urge you to use oil (especially olive oil) and vinegar dressing most of the time. Most other commercial salad dressings contain about 7 percent carbohydrates.

Sugar is a problem for people with a sweet tooth. You can end up craving it, especially during the assessment phase of the diet. Look to appease any cravings along this line with low-carbohydrate drinks and desserts with artificial sweeteners. However, avoid sorbitol and fructose (which is a sugar)—remember that "sugar-free" doesn't necessarily mean carbohydrate-free. Check the labels. Diet soft drinks are fine.

You can also put sugar-free Jell-O (no carbohydrates, uses artificial sweetener) to good use. Topping it with carbohydrate-free whipped cream may be just what you're looking for to gain control. It has no carbohydrates, and many Metabolic

Table 5.3	Some High-Fat/Low-Carbohydrate Weekday Foods for the Metabolic Diet				
Steak	Bacon	Cheese*	Shrimp	Salt	Herring
Salmon	Jell-O***	Walnuts	Tuna	Sunflower seeds	Butter
Chicken	Hamburger	Mayonnaise	Eggs	Venison	Pastrami
Anchovies	Lamb	Hamburger	Pot roast	Lobster	Diet soda
Oils**	Turkey	Sausage			

* Full fat/low-carbohydrate

** Poly- and monounsaturated fats such as found in nuts, olive oil, flax seed oil

*** Sugar-free

dieters have found it quite capable of appeasing their cravings for sweets. Just check the labels on whipped topping containers to make sure carbohydrates haven't been added.

Another factor to consider is that, even if you have cravings, you are only putting off satisfying them until the weekend. You can eat basically anything then. We are just partitioning, or separating, foods here. We're not saying you can't have lasagna—you just have to wait for the weekend! That's a lot better than other diets that basically strand you on Low-Fat or, in some cases, Low-Carb Island for the rest of your life.

At first you'll probably overdo the carbohydrates on the weekends. However, once they have been on the diet awhile, most people don't have that strong desire for a heavy-duty intake of carbohydrates anymore. They eat them but they don't pig out, and, as they start adjusting their diets and dialing them in for maximum progress, they begin to see real improvement and to acquire some real knowledge about the way their bodies work and how adjustments can be made to achieve their goals.

KEYS TO EARLY DIET SUCCESS

- Don't worry about calories.
- Take a fiber supplement.
- Watch for hidden carbohydrates.
- Don't mix diets.
- The first week is the toughest—stick it out.

The First Week

In the first week of the diet, you will be going through the metabolic shift from being a carbohydrate- and muscle-burning machine to being a fat burner. It can be difficult, and you may need more than one week to really adjust. While some people suffer few symptoms, others are highly affected. Bowel irregularities are common. You will experience some fatigue and get foul- or fruity-smelling breath caused by increased production of ketones (compounds that result from the initial steps of fat oxidation).

Emotionally, you may feel irritable and mentally foggy in the first week. You can also experience pre-flu-like symptoms where you feel like "something's coming on" or you're "fighting something off." Your energy level can drop and you can feel frequently hungry. Don't be alarmed. Basically, your body is just going through a readjustment phase. It will soon pass.

If you are like most people, you will continue with the "start-up" phase of the diet and not worry about calories or anything else until you have all your energy back and have no other symptoms. This usually takes two to four weeks, and you'll know when it's time: you'll be feeling very, very good.

On the other hand, if the tiredness is severe and continues, there is no point in persevering. That's what the Metabolic Diet is all about—finding the optimal level of dietary carbohydrates that works *for you.* So if you are feeling tired and worn out, then it's a good idea to introduce some extra carbohydrates. The best approach is to go through the Problem-Solving Guide on page 83 and figure out the best way to introduce those extra carbohydrates.

Once you have settled on what works best for your metabolism, you can begin to zero in on that weight loss and body shaping you've been dreaming of.

KEYS TO SUCCESS ON THE METABOLIC DIET

- Don't seek to lose weight at the beginning.
- Understand that caloric needs will vary among individuals.
- Try to lose 1.5 to 2.0 pounds weekly.
- Keep track of inches as well as pounds.
- Use calipers to measure body fat.
- Weigh and measure no more than once weekly.
- Don't pick an ideal weight.
- Goals are 18 percent body fat for women and 10 percent body fat for men.
- Rely on the mirror more than the scales.
- Don't change your lifestyle or habits once you reach your target weight.
- Experiment with caloric intake to find a proper maintenance level.
- Experiment with foods.

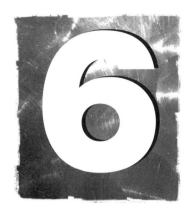

USING NUTRITIONAL SUPPLEMENTS

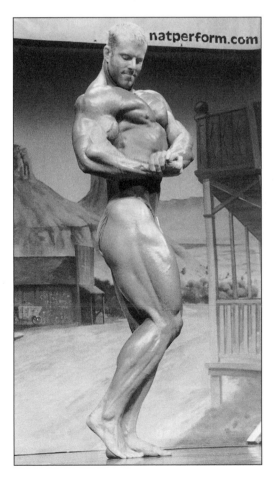

While nutritional supplements can play a vital role in maximizing the effects of exercise, they do not work in a vacuum. They must be coupled with a reasonable lifestyle, proper training routines, and a good diet.

Once those three are in order, nutritional supplements can provide an added edge. By using appropriate nutritional supplements in the right way and at the right time, you can take athletic performance and body composition to new heights.

Supplements can increase an athlete's anabolic drive and workload capacity and decrease recovery time. In order to accomplish these things, you have to take the right supplements at the right time and in the right amounts. Unfortunately, most people don't use them properly and thus don't get any significant benefits. Largely due to mistrust and ignorance, they do not use supplements with the same seriousness as they use prescription drugs.

Twenty-five-year-old Scott Milnes believes that nutritional supplements play a vital role in maximizing the effects of training.

Many supplements that have some anabolic potential do so by one or more of these ways:

- They increase one's ability to train (for example by increasing endurance or by enhancing muscular contraction).
- They increase production of endogenous testosterone or growth hormone, or they decrease secretion of cortisol.
- They increase protein synthesis.

Under specific conditions many nutritional supplements can have some positive effects on lean body mass, strength, and endurance. Targeting these supplements is the key to gaining significant amounts of lean body mass and improving athletic performance. The trick to using supplements is to know enough about them in order to use them effectively.

Popular Nutritional Supplements

Following are some commonly used nutritional supplements. This list is not exhaustive and does not include many commonly used herbal and homeopathic compounds.

- Acetyl-L-carnitine
- Alanine
- Alpha lipoic Acid
- Alpha-ketoglutarate (AKG)
- Andro and norandro prohormones
- Antioxidants (amino-acid based); the more popular ones are listed by name
- Antioxidants (vitamin and mineral); the most popular ones are listed by name
- Arginine
- Beta-hydroxy-beta-methylbutyrate (HMB)
- Biotin
- Branched-chain amino acids (BCAA); leucine is also listed
- Caffeine
- Calcium
- Carnitine
- Casein protein
- Chitosan
- Choline (CDP choline)
- Chondroitin sulphate
- Chromium
- Coenzyme Q-10
- Conjugated linoleic acid (CLA)
- Creatine monohydrate
- Di- and tripeptides
- Dimethylacetylethinol (DMAE)
- Echinacea
- Ephedrine (ephedra)
- Essential fatty acids (including EPA and DHA)
- Evening primrose oil
- Fish oil (EPA and DHA)
- Folic acid
- Gelatin
- GHB (gamma-hydroxybutyrate)
- Ginkgo biloba
- Ginseng
- GLA (gamma-linoleic acid)
- Glucosamine
- Glutamine
- Glutathione
- Glycerol
- Gotu kola
- Grape seed extract
- Green tea extract
- Guarana
- Guggelsterone
- HCA (hydroxycitrate)
- Inosine
- Inositol
- Iron
- Ketoisocaproic acid (KIC)
- Ketones
- Kola nut
- Lactate
- Lecithin
- Leucine
- Magnesium
- Manganese
- MCTs (medium-chain triglycerides)
- Meal replacements
- Melatonin
- Methionine
- N-acetyl-cysteine (NAC)

- Naringinin (grapefruit)
- Niacinamide (niacin, or vitamin B3)
- Norandrostenediol
- Norandrostenedione
- Octacosanol
- Olestra (fat substitute—not absorbed)
- Omega-3 fatty acids
- Omega-6 fatty acids
- Ornithine
- Ornithine-alpha-ketoglut-arate (OKG)
- Oryzanols (gamma oryzynal)
- Pantocrine
- Pantothenic acid
- Para-aminobenzoic acid (PABA)
- Phenylalanine
- Phophates (sodium, calcium, potassium)
- Phosphatidylcholine

- Phosphatidylserine
- Potassium
- Proanthocyanidin (grape seed extract)
- Pro-biotics
- Proline and hydroxyproline
- Pyridoxine (vitamin B6)
- Pyruvate
- Quercetin
- Riboflavin (vitamin B2)
- Ribose
- RNA
- Saw palmetto
- Selenium
- Serine
- Silymarin (milk thistle)
- Soy protein isolate
- St. John's wort
- Synephrine
- Taurine
- Thiamine (vitamin B1)
- TMG (trimethylglycine)

- Tribestan
- Tribulus terrestris
- Tryptophan
- Turmeric
- Type II collagen
- Tyrosine
- Valerian root
- Vanadium
- Vanadyl sulfate
- Vitamin B12
- Vitamin B6
- Vitamin C
- Vitamin E
- Vitamine D
- Weight gain powders
- Whey protein
- Whey protein concentrate
- Whey protein isolate
- White willow bark
- Xylitol
- Yohimbine (yohimbe)
- Zinc

Many of these nutritional supplements, as either single ingredients or in formulations, can be found in offerings from various nutritional supplement companies.

Brief Overview of Some Nutritional Supplements

In this chapter, we include a brief overview of some of the more popular nutritional supplements. We have done this so that you will be better informed about their individual properties and about how you can combine supplements to increase their overall effects on performance and body composition.

Vitamins and Minerals

Most members of our society commonly use vitamins and minerals, either as part of fortified foods or as supplements. When you mention nutritional supplements, most people think of the ubiquitous daily vitamin pill. Vitamins and minerals are indeed important—but there are many other important nutritional supplements.

The vitamin and mineral "stack" is the most pervasive example of combining a number of supplements together for ease of use and, in some cases, for additive or synergistic effects.

Zinc

Zinc deficiency in humans is widespread, and athletes may be particularly prone to lower plasma zinc levels (Cordova 1995; Prasad 1996). Because zinc is a constituent of more than a hundred fundamentally important enzymes, zinc deficiency can negatively affect nearly every body function (Kieffer 1986).

Especially where a deficiency may be present, supplemental zinc has resulted in increased secretion of growth hormone, IGF-I (Dorup et al. 1991), and testosterone (Ghavami-Maibodi et al. 1983); and it has been observed to raise plasma testosterone and sperm count (Hartoma et al. 1977; Hunt et al. 1992). Zinc deficiency can adversely affect the reproductive hormones (Oteiza et al. 1995).

In an unpublished study (Brilla and Conte 1999), supplemental use of zinc and magnesium resulted in increased strength and higher levels of testosterone. An interesting aspect of this study is that the increased testosterone levels occurred in a group of competitive NCAA football players who were already strength-trained athletes.

Magnesium

Magnesium supplementation has been shown to increase protein synthesis and strength (Brilla and Haley 1992). The authors of another study concluded that insulin sensitivity could be improved by reduction of excess body weight, regular physical activity, and possibly by correcting a subclinical magnesium deficiency (Lefebvre and Scheen 1995).

Calcium

Calcium permits the contractile actin and myosin filaments of the muscle cell to associate and produce the force that generates movement. When the neuron innervating a muscle cell signals that cell to contract, calcium is released from the sarcoplasmic reticulum into the region of the contractile filaments, thereby permitting contraction to occur. In one study, supplemental calcium appeared effective in prolonging the time of onset of fatigue in striated muscle (Richardson et al. 1980).

Calcium can prevent muscle cramping during exercise. It is suspected that calcium may also increase growth hormone secretion during exercise. If you feel you need extra calcium, take 500 to 1,000 milligrams of calcium before working out and 500 to 1,000 milligrams during the workout. Calcium can be taken in the form of Rolaids and is especially useful in this format for those who may need an antacid as well. Vitamin D denotes a group of closely related chemicals that regulate absorption of ingested calcium by the intestine.

Chromium

Chromium is involved in carbohydrate and lipid metabolism. Because the need for chromium increases with exercise (Anderson et al. 1982), and since modern refined foods are low in chromium, athletes may need to incorporate chromium-rich foods or supplements into their diets. If you are engaged in a highly aggressive exercise program, chromium deficiency, even if just marginal, may become a concern (Lefavi et al. 1992).

Insufficient dietary chromium has been linked to maturity-onset diabetes and cardiovascular diseases, with supplemental chromium resulting in improvements of risk factors associated with these diseases (Anderson 1986).

Antioxidants

The focus of antioxidant use is on *free radicals*—highly reactive molecules that possess unpaired electrons. These free radicals play a sizable role in the normal metabolism of food and the use of energy resources during exercise.

It is also strongly suspected that they react with the components of body cells in a way that leads to molecular damage and cell death—and, eventually, to aging and death itself. Chemical reactions involving free radicals in the body have been implicated in causing or contributing to cancer, atherosclerosis (hardening of the arteries), hypertension, Alzheimer's disease, immune deficiency, arthritis, diabetes, Parkinson's disease, and various other diseases linked with the aging process. Antioxidants can significantly protect the body from the high free radical concentrations that may lead to these diseases (Packer and Landvik 1989).

A growing amount of data shows that heavy exercise can increase the formation of free radicals, which then leads to muscle fatigue, inflammation, and damage to muscle tissue (Reid et al. 1992). Exercise can also decrease the supply of antioxidants. Vitamin E levels, for instance, can decline severely with training, thus depleting the muscle of its most important antioxidant (Gohil et al. 1987).

Emotional stress can raise levels of free radicals just as effectively as does physical stress (as caused by exercise). During normal conditions, free radicals are generated at a low rate and neutralized by antioxidants in the liver, skeletal muscle, and other systems. But under stress, they greatly increase and can overwhelm the body's ability to neutralize them. Unchecked, they can cause premature aging and breakdown of the body.

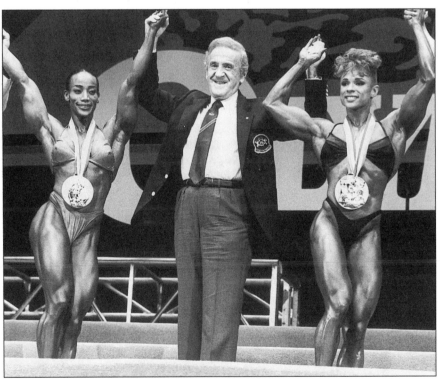

Lenda Murray and Laura Crevalle have always combined training, diet, and nutritional supplements to maintain championship physiques.

Though some recent studies have brought the overall role of antioxidants into some question, the preponderance of evidence still shows that antioxidants can help undo much of the dirty work done by free radicals. If you're involved with the Metabolic Diet, and especially if you are exercising as you should, you must make a place for antioxidants in your diet.

Use of Antioxidants by Athletes

Several studies have shown that bolstering antioxidant defenses may ameliorate exercise-induced damage (Packer 1997). For example, a recent study looked at the effects of resistance exercise on free radical production. Twelve recreationally weight-trained males were divided into two groups. The supplement group received 1,200 IUs of vitamin E once a day for a period of two weeks. The control group received placebos. The data indicated that high-intensity resistance exercise increased free radical production and that vitamin E supplementation may decrease muscle membrane disruption (Mcbride et al. 1998).

When used correctly, antioxidants can give an added edge in creating a healthy, fit, and attractive body. They are especially important for those who embark on an advanced, more demanding exercise program. If you are in such an advanced program, you may want to go beyond the minimum amounts provided by multivitamins and maximize the advantages antioxidants can bring.

While you can use antioxidants daily, you definitely should use them, in addition to your daily multivitamin, on days that you work out. We also recommend that people eat a lot of vegetables (especially broccoli, cabbage, lettuce, and leafy greens) and even drink a glass of red wine with their evening meal. With this combination we feel that anyone can cover their antioxidant needs.

Compounds With Potent Antioxidant Properties

Along with an ability to protect muscle tissue, vitamin E also seems to help limit arterial damage caused by aging and to help minimize adverse effects of harmful fats on the body (Yoshida and Kajimoto 1989). Vitamin C provides direct protection from free radical damage and also conserves vitamin E (Sies et al. 1992). They work together synergistically in controlling muscle breakdown.

Carotenes come naturally from plants like carrots, cantaloupes, sweet potatoes, and other green and yellow vegetables. Many of the carotenes are also called *provitamin A* because the body converts them into vitamin A. Beyond this, there is evidence that carotenes can also strengthen the immune system and protect against body tissue damage (Bendich 1989).

By far the most well known carotenoid is beta-carotene. What makes it especially compelling is its importance in oxidizing low-density lipoproteins (LDLs) (Lavy et al. 1993). Yet beta-carotene taken by itself can be counterproductive, reinforcing our feelings that antioxidants, or for that matter any vitamin or mineral, should not be used in large doses on their own.

Selenium plays a role in converting fats and protein into energy and provides antioxidant protection when taken with vitamin E. Note that vitamin E is not only an important force in its own right but is also important in enhancing the effects of other antioxidants.

Omega-3 Fatty Acids

Omega-3 fatty acids are long-chain polyunsaturated fatty acids that are converted to a number of active substances in the body such as prostaglandins and leukotrienes; they also are involved in a number of metabolic events. Linolenic acid is an essential omega-3 fatty acid, since the body cannot synthesize it. Other omega-3 fatty acids, however, are synthesized in the body from linolenic acid.

As discussed in chapter 5, the omega-3 fatty acids eicosapentaenoic acid (EPA) and docosahexaenoic acid (DHA) are found in fish oils, which we recommend. Omega-3 fatty acids may increase growth hormone secretion since they are involved in the formation of prostaglandin E1, which in turn is involved in release of growth hormone (GH) (Dray et al. 1980).

Conjugated Linolenic Acid (CLA)

Conjugated linoleic acid (CLA) is a mixture of positional and geometric isomers of linoleic acid (LA), which is found preferentially in dairy products and meat. CLA is present in cheese, milk, and yogurt that have undergone heat treatment, and in beef and venison. Supplementation with four ounces of cheddar cheese daily was found to increase the ratio of CLA to LA by 130 percent.

CLA appears to have beneficial properties beyond those of linoleic acid. It has shown potential as a powerful anticarcinogen (Ip, Scimeca, and Thompson 1994; Ip, Singh et al. 1994) and exhibits potent antioxidant activity (Pariza et al. 1991). CLA may be cytotoxic to human cancer cells in vivo (Shultz et al. 1992). Of importance for those wishing to maximize lean body mass, CLA has possible anticatabolic properties (Cook et al. 1993; Miller et al. 1994).

A team of Scandinavian researchers has found that CLA helped overweight and obese individuals mobilize fat from cells while revving up muscle metabolism (Blankson et al. 2000). Individuals taking CLA also saw reductions in total and LDL cholesterol. The authors of the study concluded that consumption of CLA appears to reduce body fat in overweight and moderately obese healthy people.

Caffeine and Ephedrine

While a number of studies have shown that caffeine may favorably affect long-term endurance performance (McNaughton 1986), data on high-intensity, short-term exercise have been mixed (Williams 1991). Still, it seems very likely from an analysis of the biochemical effects of caffeine that it has a beneficial effect on short-term fatigue and muscle fiber in high-intensity, short-term exercise like weightlifting (Dodd et al. 1993; Jacobson et al. 1992).

Ephedrine has mild amphetamine-like CNS effects and is used by athletes to enhance training and performance. Aspirin is widely used by athletes for several reasons. It is a common mild pain killer, has anti-inflammatory properties, and has some thermogenic effects. A combination of caffeine, ephedrine, and aspirin is

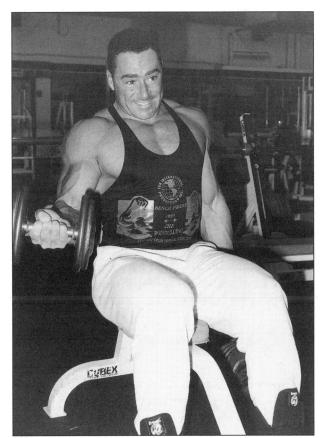

Vito Binetti pushing himself to the limit.

commonly used as a thermogenic cocktail to promote lipolysis while decreasing muscle breakdown. The result is increased ratio of lean body mass to fat.

The main hypothesis regarding adding aspirin and caffeine to ephedrine is that the synergism allows for reduced dosages of ephedrine without reducing efficacy. This results in a decrease of side effects, such as cardiac stimulation, from the ephedrine. Whether or not small amounts of aspirin have this effect is open to debate. Nevertheless aspirin is used widely with the other two compounds.

While the use of ephedrine and caffeine results in increased lipolysis, there is some doubt as to whether this lipolysis translates into fat loss. Some data indicate that ephedrine, while increasing lipolysis, does not increase the beta oxidation of fatty acids—the increased lipolysis simply results in increased reesterification of fatty acids and no net change in body fat. This is certainly the case with those adapted to higher-carbohydrate diets, but not with people adapted to higher-fat, low-carbohydrate diets where there is an increased use and oxidation of free fatty acids.

Anti-Cortisol Supplements

Any type of stress—including high levels of exercise, physical or emotional trauma, infections, or surgery—translates into hypothalamic and pituitary changes that result in increased cortisol secretion.

Exercise itself, while increasing cortisol, has compensatory anticatabolic effects. Short, intense training sessions tend to result in more moderate cortisol secretion. Well-conditioned athletes show less cortisol secretion during exercise compared to their out-of-shape peers. One measure of overtraining is the testosterone/cortisol ratio. Elevated cortisol in relation to testosterone is considered indicative of overtraining—that is, if you train properly, your testosterone will rise, while cortisol remains stable.

Vitamin C has some anticatabolic effects that likely involve decreasing exercise-induced cortisol but may also work through its antioxidant action. Conversely, some of the anticatabolic effects of antioxidants may be mediated through a decrease in cortisol. A gram or so of vitamin C, along with some vitamin E (400 IU), beta-carotene (20,000 IU), zinc (50 mg), and selenium (50 mcg) before workouts might be useful.

A supplement has recently been marketed that may decrease exercise-induced rises in cortisol. According to some studies, phosphatidylserine appears to blunt the pituitary-mediated cortisol response to exercise. Although more research needs to be done to see if the decrease in cortisol translates into increased gains, phosphatidylserine may be of benefit; you may want to include it in your supplement stack, taking one to two grams before each training session. One caveat: there may be an increase in training soreness, stiffness, and injuries secondary to the cortisol reduction. Consider the benefit-to-risk ratio when using these compounds.

L-Carnitine

L-carnitine appears to increase the body's use of free fatty acids and fatty tissue as an energy source. More fat becomes available for energy, thus saving protein in the muscle cells. Muscle breakdown may also be reduced. Athletes have used doses ranging from 100 to 3,000 milligrams or more per day before training with good effect. However, it seems that at least two grams or more per day (i.e., at least 2,000 milligrams) are needed for the desired effects.

On the other hand it does not appear that carnitine is a limiting factor in the transport and utilization of fatty acids. So while the jury is still out on the effectiveness of carnitine, it makes sense to use it especially at times when energy output is increased. If you're on an enhanced exercise program, you may at least want to try L-carnitine. Just be sure to look for the name "L-carnitine" on the label. Some manufacturers use a cheaper, less effective form.

Creatine Monohydrate

In the early 1980s, as anabolic steroids fell into disrepute, manufacturers began touting scores of products that were supposedly even "better than steroids," but that for the most part were fairly useless. Most athletes soon became skeptical that nutritional supplements really did anything at all to improve strength, muscle mass, or athletic performance.

But in the past several years the attitude of most athletes has turned from disbelief to amazement, because there are certain nutritional supplements that do work. One of the supplements that helped turn the tide is creatine monohydrate. While not as effective as high doses of anabolic steroids, creatine works—but it has none of the side effects associated with anabolic drugs. It helps increase muscle mass, provides greater levels of energy, and helps individuals recover more quickly after an exercise session. The basic mechanism of creatine's action is to help the cells convert ADP to ATP (the cells' basic energy source) at an accelerated pace.

Although it has been over six years since the creatine craze commenced, some athletes have used creatine for more than two decades. Now creatine is used by participants in all kinds of sports, including bodybuilders, Olympic athletes, football players, hockey players, soccer players, softball players, even tennis players. Potential side effects from overdosing are dehydration, overheating, and kidney damage.

Protein Supplementation

Athletes need higher levels of dietary protein than do sedentary people. Many athletes turn to protein supplements to augment their dietary protein intake.

Good sources of dietary protein include eggs, meat, fish, soy, and dairy products. Whole protein supplements are usually inexpensive and generally contain soybean, milk, and egg protein, hydrolyzed protein with variable amounts of di-, tri- and polypeptides, and amino-acid mixtures.

The consensus is that there are no valid scientific or medical studies to show that supplements of intact protein have an anabolic advantage over high-quality protein foods. Yet there do appear to be certain advantages to the use of whole protein supplements by some athletes, including the following:

- They are convenient to prepare and store and have a long shelf life.
- They are useful as a protein replacement for those wishing to decrease dietary fat (many protein-rich foods tend to contain fat).
- They enable individuals to raise their protein intake while minimizing caloric intake.

- They can increase dietary protein in people who cannot eat the volume of food necessary to insure adequate or increased protein intake.

- In some cases, the cost of protein supplements is lower than corresponding high-protein foods.

Protein supplements have other distinct advantages over whole food protein in hypocaloric, isocaloric, and hypercaloric diets. Many studies have shown that protein supplements, including milk and soy proteins, have ergogenic effects (Dragan et al. 1985; Dragan et al. 1988; Laricheva et al. 1977). These studies found that supplemental proteins significantly improved athletes' physiological condition, led to better sports performance, and resulted in significant increases of lean body mass and strength. Athletes who used dietary protein supplements experienced greater gain in muscle than those who simply took in the equivalent amount of calories. Moreover, protein supplements with other ingredients, such as creatine monohydrate, taurine, and L-glutamine, often enhance gains in lean body mass.

Meal replacement products (MRPs), whether for weight loss or weight gain, give you the standard macro- and micronutrients at different calorie levels. They may be convenient and either more or less costly than whole foods you can get at your supermarket. As an all-in-one package, they are usually more convenient and provide better nutrition than many people obtain with junk food meals and high-calorie but nutrient-deficient snacks. For certain effects, the engineered cutting-edge food supplements are better than whole food protein sources and can be safely and effectively used to increase dietary protein intake and as meal replacements for up to two meals a day. Nevertheless, if you are conscientious about what you buy and eat and are willing to put in the time and effort, you can do as well or better by just buying the whole foods and planning your own diet for weight gain or weight loss.

The best protein supplements are specific combinations of various high-quality proteins. Taking a combination of supplemental protein not only increases dietary protein—which should be even higher when you are trying to lose body fat and weight than at any other time—but will also give your metabolism, thyroid hormone levels, and metabolic rate a boost.

As mentioned previously, it is important to make sure you take in at least one gram of protein per pound of body weight every day. It's best to spread the intake out in intervals of no more than three hours while you are awake. Take some before bed and as soon as you get up to decrease the catabolic effects of the fast that you go through while sleeping. If you wake up during the night, that's a good time to take some more protein and even further decrease the muscle catabolism.

Amino Acids

Increased blood levels of amino acids, secondary to a high-protein meal, can cause insulin and growth hormone levels to rise. Increasing these hormones—while increasing amino-acid levels but at the same time decreasing muscle catabolism—leads to an enhanced anabolic response.

Studies have shown that ingestion of branched-chain amino acids modifies the hormonal milieu. There is also some information that amino acids (primarily methionine) and the dipeptides methionine-glutamine and tryptophan-isoleucine have a profound anabolic effect: they increase protein synthesis for reparative and

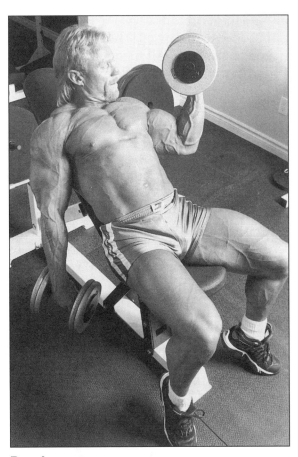

Repping out.

muscle wound healing. These substances could override or block the increase in glucocorticoid levels found in diabetic patients, but further research needs to be performed with diabetic patients to substantiate these findings.

Protein taken after training may increase both insulin and growth hormone and thus have anabolic effects. Increased amino-acid availability has been shown to directly influence protein synthesis, especially within a few hours after physical exercise. The rate of protein synthesis, protein catabolism, and amino-acid transport is normally increased after exercise and depends on amino-acid availability. If there is an increase in the availability of amino acids during this postexercise window, then catabolic processes are more than offset by increased anabolic processes, resulting in an overall increase in cellular contractile protein. Thus it is vital to increase the absorption of amino acids as quickly as possible after exercise.

Food intake can stimulate muscle protein synthesis secondary to increased insulin release, because insulin can directly stimulate muscle protein synthesis and, to at least some extent, decrease protein breakdown (Biolo et al. 1995); an improvement in energy balance may affect net muscle protein balance (Butterfield and Calloway 1984). However, the primary way in which one would expect food intake to stimulate muscle protein synthesis is through increased delivery of amino acids to the muscle.

Glutamine

Individual or selectively combined amino acids may also serve as performance supplements. An example is the amino acid glutamine. Glutamine is the most abundant amino acid in the body and makes up over 50 percent of the intracellular and extracellular amino acids. It plays a major role in liver function, serves as cellular fuel to muscle and other tissue in the body, and may regulate protein synthesis (Rennie et al. 1989).

Most important to the serious athlete and fitness enthusiast is glutamine's ability to increase production of protein (for muscle building) and decrease protein degradation (resulting in muscle breakdown). Both depend on the size of the glutamine pool in a muscle cell. If it is high, other amino acids won't be forced into glutamine production and will be available for protein synthesis. Skeletal muscle that might also be used to replace glutamine is also spared. Glutamine also acts to maintain amino-acid balance in the body, thus enabling the body to synthesize more protein and possibly decrease symptoms of overtraining.

Glutamine supplementation may offer a number of advantages to athletes. Exogenous glutamine can spare intramuscular glutamine and result in decreased proteolysis and potentially increased levels of muscle protein. Gastrointestinal and immune functions are maximized, and the morbidity secondary to overtraining is improved. Glutamine can efficiently lead to release of growth hormone and perhaps to higher levels of other anabolic hormones. All these factors strongly suggest that glutamine supplementation may play a major role in enhancing the effects of resistance training.

Branched-Chain Amino Acids: Isoleucine, Leucine, and Valine

The branched-chain amino acids (BCAAs) have a carbon chain that branches from the main linear carbon backbone. The BCAAs isoleucine, leucine, and valine have been investigated for their anticatabolic and anabolic effects. In heart and skeletal muscle in vitro, increasing the concentration of the three BCAAs or of leucine alone reproduces the effects of increasing the supply of all amino acids in stimulating protein synthesis and inhibiting protein degradation (May and Buse 1989).

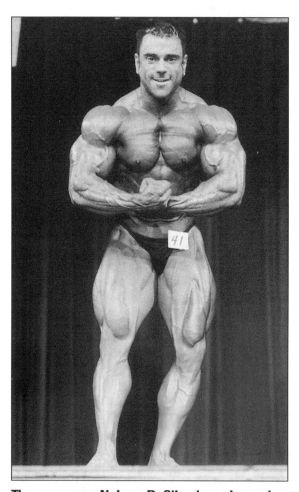

The awesome Nelson DaSilva has always believed that proper stacking, cycling, and timing of nutritional supplements plays a key role in peaking for an important event.

Maximizing Use of Supplements: Stacking, Cycling, and Timing

Nutritional supplements can be useful in many ways, providing they are appropriately targeted. Targeting nutritional supplements involves using a variety of supplements in tandem *(stacking)* in order to increase the effects of the supplements, using the supplements at the right time, and *cycling* some of the supplements. Cycling insures that the supplements will do the most good, and it also decreases any tolerance that might develop with long-term uninterrupted use.

Stacking

Nutritional supplements are used for various reasons, for example, to increase performance and to affect body composition. Since there are a large number of possible supplements, it is natural that certain ones will be used together to illicit certain effects, which is called stacking. Following are examples of different stacks for different situations.

Preworkout Stack

The purpose of a preworkout or pretraining stack is to maximize energy levels, minimize protein catabolism, increase protein synthesis, increase GH and testosterone levels, and decrease cortisol. An example of a preworkout stack is Resolve, a stack with ephedrine and yohimbine. It includes the following ingredients:

- Vitamin A
- Vitamin C
- Calcium (as calcium phosphate)
- Chromium
- White willow extract
- L-alanine
- Caffeine USP
- Cayenne (pepper)
- Cinnamon
- Cordycepic acid
- Ephedrine alkaloids
- Ginger
- Alpha-lipoic acid
- Yohimbine alkaloids
- Co-enzyme Q10
- N-acetyl cysteine
- Octacosanol
- Banaba extract
- Pyruvic acid
- Taurine
- Dimethylglycine
- Inosine
- Glutathione

Workout Stack

The combination of higher amino-acid levels at a time when blood flow is increased appears to maximize muscle protein synthesis.

An example of a workout stack to be used while training is a training drink. Concentrations of the drink's amino acids and other ingredients should vary depending on whether the training is for endurance or for muscle mass and power. In all cases the drink (1) should provide for rehydration, electrolyte replacement, energy replacement, and some of the preworkout functions—including increased protein synthesis and decreased muscle catabolism; and (2) should decrease overtraining effects and muscle injury.

A good training drink for power athletes should at least contain over 30 grams of whey protein isolate (a "fast" protein that results in high systemic amino-acid levels—over 25 percent of them branched). It also would do well to contain the following:

- Arginine
- Calcium

- Creatine
- Glutamine peptides
- Leucine
- Magnesium
- Phosphorus
- Potassium
- Ribose
- Sodium
- Taurine

Postworkout Stack

Intake of nutrients, protein, and individual amino acids (and, in particular, certain combinations of amino acids) after exercise can increase muscle glycogen and fat storage, protein synthesis, and the anabolic effects of exercise.

A proper combination of carbohydrate, protein, and some fat right after exercise appears able (1) to reverse the decreased protein synthesis seen with exercise, (2) to replenish muscle glycogen and intramuscular triglycerides, (3) to increase protein synthesis and decrease protein catabolism postexercise, (4) to raise levels of growth hormone and testosterone, and (5) to increase the efficiency of recuperation. This is especially true if you are following the Metabolic Diet and are fat adapted.

There are two distinct stages to consider: (1) immediately after training and (2) one to two hours later. Immediately after a workout, ingestion of a targeted mixture of amino acids that are absorbed almost immediately induces a strong and rapid increase of aminoacidemia, which in turn acutely stimulates protein synthesis and decreases muscle catabolism. Acute amino-acid intake and absorption stimulates the transport of amino acids into muscle, and there is a direct link between amino-acid inward transport and muscle protein synthesis (Wolfe 2000). It also appears that a number of amino acids may increase secretion of two powerful anabolic hormones, growth hormone and insulin (Bucci et al. 1990; Iwasaki et al. 1987).

Interestingly, the simultaneous ingestion of carbohydrates and protein decreases the absorption rate of amino acids (Mariotti et al. 2000). You therefore should limit your intake immediately postexercise to amino acids only—no carbohydrates.

An hour or two after training, you should ingest amino acids or whey protein powder in order to maximize protein synthesis, glycogen storage, and stores of intramuscular triglycerides.

ECA Stack

A combination of ephedra-caffeine-aspirin (ECA Stack is a proprietary product) is used to increase lipolysis and thermogenesis, increase both anaerobic and aerobic performance, and maintain protein synthesis. The net goal is increased lean body mass and less body fat. Many other compounds can be added to this stack to make it more effective for weight and fat loss and for maintaining muscle mass.

Cycling

Athletes cycle nutrient supplements for two reasons. First, they have increased need for certain supplements only at certain phases of training, and it is senseless to waste money on supplements when the supplements will do little good. Second, because the body adapts to certain supplements, they become less useful if they are taken for prolonged periods. Going off the supplements allows the body to return to normal so that it will once again get maximum results when the supplements are reintroduced.

The body sometimes adapts only to particular actions of supplements. For example, the ECA Stack gradually loses its effects on the CNS, but may not lose its ability to stimulate thermogenesis or to increase oxidation of free fatty acids during exercise. Athletes often cycle creatine, using it only during the most intensive training.

Just as training is most effective when periodized, nutritional supplements can be as well. If you are following a 12-week cycle of training, you might also vary your nutritional supplement intake according to the phase of training. At the beginning, in the first training cycle, you might use only a multivitamin-mineral tablet—or perhaps some antioxidants, some extra protein, or some meal replacement powders or bars. In the next, more intense phase of training, you may choose to introduce creatine, a pretraining stack, and a posttraining amino-acid mix. In the most intense phase of this training cycle, you might want to use some GH- and testosterone-boosting stacks and more comprehensive support in and around training.

We have included specific information on cycling both diet and nutritional supplements in the chapters describing the various training phases.

Timing

The timing of nutritional supplements can often determine whether a certain supplement stack is effective. There is almost always a best time to take supplements for maximum effects; there are ineffective times as well.

Timing differs according to the supplement.

- Not critical for some: multiple vitamin, creatine
- Critical for others: workout stack, GH stack
- Should not be used at certain times: ECA Stack before bedtime

The timing of supplement intake can be as important as the supplements taken. Ephedrine, caffeine, and certain amino acids, for example, are best taken within a half hour or so of training. A macronutrient mix works best when taken within a few hours of training. GH-boosting formulations work best before training and before sleep.

Timing can also maximize the use of protein supplements. For example, the best times for taking protein supplements are first thing in the morning to put an abrupt end to the catabolic effects of fasting while asleep; after training to take advantage of the increased protein synthesis that occurs after exercise; and immediately before bed to make use of the increased growth hormone secretion during the night and to put off the nighttime catabolic response. In conclusion, there are optimal times to use certain nutritional supplements, including proteins and amino acids, fat burners and thermogenics, growth hormone enhancers, prohormones, and creatine.

Summary and Recommendations

For maximum effects from the use of nutritional supplements, use products in which a number of ingredients have been stacked together synergistically, and that are designed for use at specific times and training cycles.

Use of nutritional supplements is both an art and a science. Even with the scientific information in hand, individuals must experiment to determine how each supplement interacts with their unique metabolism and with their specific needs and goals. Only you can work out which supplements work best for you and when to use them.

Athletes must determine the usefulness of supplements by rationally evaluating any perceived ergogenic effects—keeping an open but critical mind as to the benefits they receive from using a supplement, and determining if they are making progress beyond what they would ordinarily expect from their diet and training. Is there an objective increase in any measurable parameters such as stamina, strength, or lean body mass? If there is an increase, is it a result of the supplement or of increased training intensity and enthusiasm?

Despite the potential benefits of many of the nutritional supplements (especially protein and amino acids) for increasing lean body mass and athletic performance, the use of nutritional supplements needs to be more systematically investigated. We need more empirical evidence to fine-tune the use of supplements in order to maximize the anabolic effects of exercise.

PART II

MAXIMUM
STIMULATION
EXERCISES

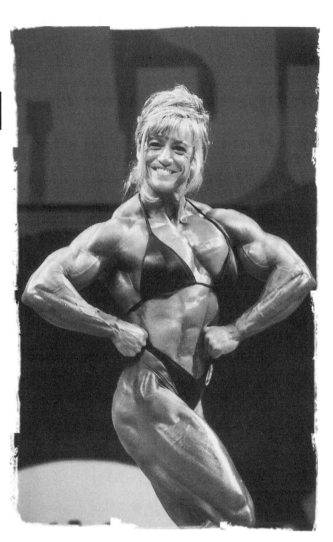

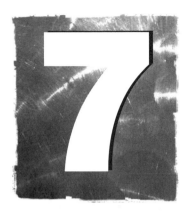

CHOOSING THE BEST EXERCISES

Unlike in strength training, very little research has been done in the area of bodybuilding. Much of the "knowledge" put forth by self-proclaimed experts in the industry is primarily the product of trial-and-error, scientifically void observations, with the passing on of belief systems from one generation to the next. Tradition, unsupported by scientific information, has validated and perpetuated a number of myths in the world of bodybuilding and even in that of strength training. In the interest of safety, and for the development of our sport, we took to the laboratory in order to test some of these myths.

Electromyographical (EMG) Research

Electromyography (EMG) has become an essential research tool, allowing physiologists and medical experts to determine the role of muscles during specific movements (Melo and Cararelli 1994-5). Electromyography measures the level of excitation (electrical signal) of a muscle group. Muscle contraction is initiated by electrical charges that travel across the membrane of muscle fibers, and this movement of ion flow can be measured at the skin by a *surface electromyogram* (SEMG) (Kobayashi Matsui 1983; Moritani et al. 1986). An SEMG is representative of the entire electrical activity of the motor units and the frequency of their firing rates for each muscle being examined (DeLuca et al. 1982; Moritani and deVries 1987).

The purpose of our series of studies was to find, through EMG recordings, which exercises cause the greatest amount of stimulation within each muscle group and, consequently, to determine which exercises will produce the greatest gains in mass and strength. Figure 7.1 shows the EMG activity during a standing barbell biceps curl.

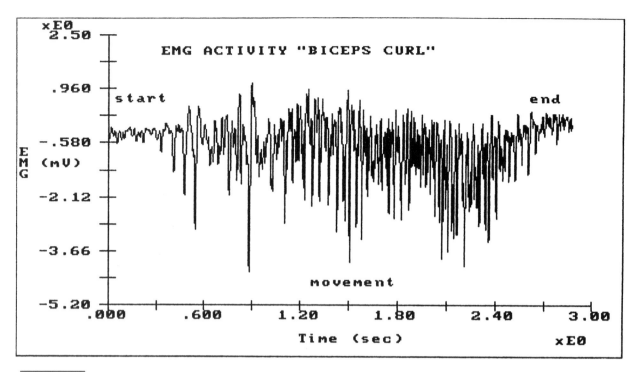

Figure 7.1 EMG activity during a standing barbell biceps curl.

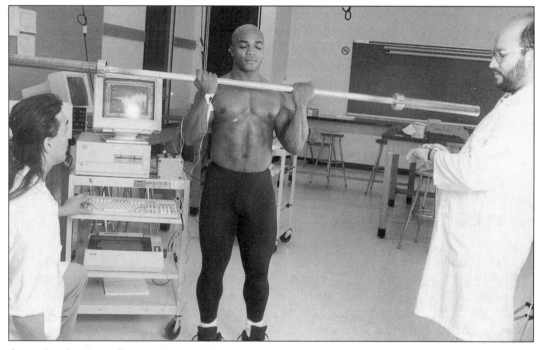

Coauthor Lorenzo Cornacchia (left) with exercise physiologist Louis Melo (right) determining the electromyographical activity during a biceps curl.

Methods

For each study, we used both male and female bodybuilders/strength trainers who were free of neuromuscular disease, had at least two years of bodybuilding experience, and had been free of performance-enhancing drugs for at least two years.

We performed the testing on two separate days. On the first day, 1RM was determined for all exercises. Each subject underwent a warm-up of 10 reps at 50 percent 1RM, 5 reps at 80 percent 1RM, and 2 reps at 90 percent 1RM, with a five-minute rest interval between sets; 1RM was then performed three times, with a five-minute rest interval between each repetition. On the second day, the subjects performed 80 percent 1RM five times, with three-minute rest intervals.

We measured electromyographical activity (EMG) during all exercises, spacing electrodes four centimeters apart over the belly of the muscle group being examined. All EMG data were rectified and integrated (IEMG) for one second. For each muscle, the exercise that yielded the highest IEMG determined at 1RM was designated as "IEMG max" for the specified muscle. We determined IEMG at 80 percent 1RM by taking the average of the five 80 percent 1RM trials.

We analyzed the data using two one-way repeated-measures analyses of variance, to determine which exercise yielded the greatest percent IEMG max for each muscle. We determined differences between exercises with the Newman-Keuls post hoc test.

Results of EMG Research

The results of our EMG studies show which exercise produces the greatest amount of stimulation within each target muscle group.

In order to comprehend the scientific validity of electromyographical research, it is important to understand the basis for recruitment of muscle fibers and motor units. Entire muscles contain many motor units; each contains a single motoneuron and all of the muscle fibers that it innervates. The number of muscle fibers belonging to a single motor unit can be described as the *innervation ratio*. The number of muscle fibers and the number of motor units vary widely from muscle to muscle. For example, the lateral gastrocnemius muscle has an innervation of approximately 2,500 to 5,000. The significance of the innervation ratio is largely related to the tension generated in each motor unit (Alway 1997).

Recruitment of muscle fibers within each motor unit begins in the brain, and the signal is sent to the cell bodies in the spinal cord and then finally to the neuromuscular junction. The neuromuscular junction does not provide a true direct connection between the muscle and nerve, but rather an indirect connection. It is similar to a spark plug in a car, where there is a small gap (synaptic cleft) that the electrical signal must "jump" in order to ignite the engine's performance. However, unlike the spark plug analogy, the electrical signal that is passed down the axon does not actually jump the synaptic cleft. Rather, once the electrical signal reaches the end of the axon at the neuromuscular junction, it causes small vesicles to open and flood the synaptic cleft with a neurotransmitter chemical (a substance that transmits the signal from the nerve to the other side of the synaptic cleft) called acetylcholine (Alway 1997).

Acetylcholine crosses the synaptic cleft and binds to receptors in the muscle membrane, and this causes a new electrical impulse to be generated on the membrane surrounding the muscle fiber (sarcolemma). Once the electrical signal (action potential) is generated on the muscle sarcolemma, it travels along this membrane and inside the muscle fiber at each of the open tubes, called transverse tubules, along the sarcolemma. The transverse tubules connect to calcium-containing sacs called the sarcoplasmic reticulum (SR). Once the electrical signal passes from the transverse tubule to the SR, calcium floods the myofibrils, which then set in motion a series of events leading to muscle fiber (sarcomere portions in each fiber) shortening. After the action potential has stopped (the electrical signal from the nerve has ceased), calcium returns to the SR and waits for the next electrical impulse. The more frequently action potentials are sent down the nerve, the more frequently action potentials are formed on the muscle sarcolemmas; and the greater the signal to initiate release of calcium from the SR, the greater the force that will be generated (Alway 1997).

In bodybuilding, muscle hypertrophy correlates directly with tension (force output = high intensity). High-intensity training induces growth when done carefully and correctly. Many bodybuilders shy away from high intensity; or they stop most of their sets before the action becomes quite uncomfortable, choosing to compensate by simply doing more.

Unfortunately, the "more is better" logic is wrong, especially when you are trying to build maximum muscle size as rapidly as possible. When it comes to gaining size and strength, intensity is the bottom line. The harder you work a muscle, the more it is forced to adapt (grow). Lengthening your workouts will have little or no effect on muscle growth; and in most cases adding sets will only cause problems, such as overtraining and muscle atrophy.

The effectiveness of a program is strongly related to its intensity and the exercises performed. Exercises that provide the greatest amount of electrical activity during muscle contraction will produce the highest levels of muscle hypertrophy and strength. The exercises contained in this book are recognized for their potential to increase muscular strength and size. It is important for everyone to understand, however, that the best program is the one that suits their individual goals. Electromyographic studies have demonstrated that the way in which a muscle responds to an exercise differs among athletes. Many bodybuilders keep plodding along, hoping to make gains using another person's routine or recommendations. They expect to get the same results that he or she got. This is a mistake.

Tables 7.1 and 7.2 (pages 109-110) display the results of the EMG studies. Refer to figure 7.2 (page 111) for anterior and posterior views of the human muscular system.

Individualizing a Training Regimen

After you lay the foundation within an all-around routine of basic, gradually progressive exercises (anatomical adaptation), only your personal judgment (or one of a professional trainer) can guide you to outstanding gains. Your body is unique. If our book gives you nothing else but the confidence and independence to listen to your instincts in determining what works best for you, then you will be better off in the end.

Table 7.1 IEMG Max Motor-Unit Activation

Exercise	% IEMG max	Exercise	% IEMG max
Study 1: Pectoralis major		**Study 7: Triceps brachii (outer head)**	
(Decline dumbbell bench press	93	Decline triceps extension (Olympic bar)	92
Decline bench press (Olympic bar)	90	Triceps press-down (angled bar)	90
Push-up between benches	88	Triceps dip between benches	87
Flat dumbbell bench press	87	One-arm cable triceps extension (reverse grip)	85
Flat bench press (Olympic bar)	85	Overhead rope triceps extension	84
Flat dumbbell fly	84	Seated one-arm dumbbell triceps extension (neutral grip)	82
Study 2: Pectoralis minor		Close-grip bench press (Olympic bar)	72
Incline dumbbell bench press	91	**Study 8: Latissimus dorsi**	
Incline bench press (Olympic bar)	85	Bent-over barbell row	93
Incline dumbbell fly	83	One-arm dumbbell row (alternate)	91
Incline bench press (Smith machine)	81	T-bar row	89
Study 3: Medial deltoids		Lat pull-down to the front	86
Incline dumbbell side lateral	66	Seated pulley row	83
Standing dumbbell side lateral	63	**Study 9: Rectus femoris (quadriceps)**	
Seated dumbbell side lateral	62	Safety squat (90-degree angle, shoulder-width stance)	88
Cable side lateral	47	Seated leg extension (toes straight)	86
Study 4: Posterior deltoids		Hack squat (90-degree angle, shoulder-width stance)	78
Standing dumbbell bent lateral	85	Leg press (110-degree angle)	76
Seated dumbbell bent lateral	83	Smith machine squat (90-degree angle, shoulder-width stance)	60
Standing cable bent lateral	77	**Study 10: Biceps femoris (hamstring)**	
Study 5: Anterior deltoids		Standing leg curl	82
Seated front dumbbell press	79	Lying leg curl	71
Standing front dumbbell press	73	Seated leg curl	58
Seated front barbell press	61	Modified hamstring dead-lift	56
Study 6: Biceps brachii (long head)		**Study 11: Semitendinosus (hamstring)**	
Biceps preacher curl (Olympic bar)	90	Seated leg curl	88
Incline seated dumbbell curl (alternate)	88	Standing leg curl	79
Standing biceps curl (Olympic bar/narrow grip)	86	Lying leg curl	70
Standing dumbbell curl (alternate)	84	Modified hamstring dead-lift	63
Concentration dumbbell curl	80	**Study 12: Gastrocnemius (calf muscle)**	
Standing biceps curl (Olympic bar/wide grip)	63	Donkey calf raise	80
Standing E-Z biceps curl (wide grip)	61	Standing one-leg calf raise	79
		Standing two-leg calf raise	68
		Seated calf raise	61

Note: Studies performed in 1998 and documented in *Serious Strength Training*. Copied with permission from Bompa and Cornacchia 1998.

Table 7.2	IEMG Max Motor-Unit Activation		

Exercise	% IEMG max	Exercise	% IEMG max
Study 1: Biceps brachii (long head)		**Study 4: Rectus abdominis**	
Standing dumbbell curl with arm blaster	87	Weighted incline crunch	81
Incline seated dumbbell curl (palms up/ lateral rotation)	86	Ab bench crunch	80
		Weighted crunch	80
Incline seated dumbbell curl (palms up)	84	Ab rocker crunch	72
Study 2: Rectus femoris		Nautilus crunch	69
Safety squat	90	Pulley crunch	68
Hip belt squat	85	**Study 5: Eccentric vs. concentric biceps femoris**	
Leg extension (toes straight)	85	Concentric standing hamstring curl	79
Squat (90 degrees)	80	Eccentric standing hamstring curl	72
Study 3: Trapezius		**Study 6: Eccentric vs. concentric latissimus dorsi**	
Behind-the-back barbell shrug	59	Concentric chin-up	79
Front barbell shrug	54	Eccentric chin-up	72
Press behind the neck	41		

Note: Studies performed in 2001. Data provided by authors (unpublished).

The routines you see in muscle magazines are basically worthless. Sure, it is interesting to know how Mr. Olympia prepared for victory; yet his training regimen probably would not work for you. Those articles should be of academic interest only. Many trainees tend to imitate others rather than pay attention to their bodies' responses to various exercises. When bodybuilders discover that a certain exercise or variation works best for them, then they should use it. Follow our training programs; but your ultimate goal should be to maximally build your physique, while using your own self-determined training regimen.

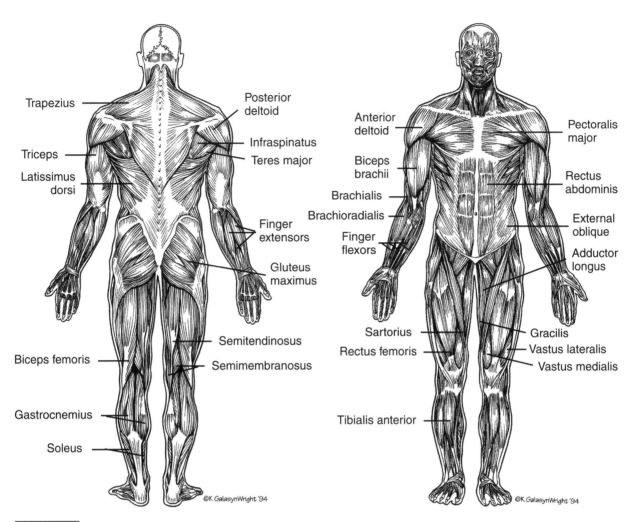

Trapezius

Posterior deltoid

Triceps

Infraspinatus

Teres major

Latissimus dorsi

Finger extensors

Gluteus maximus

Semitendinosus

Semimembranosus

Biceps femoris

Gastrocnemius

Soleus

©K. Galasyn Wright '94

Anterior deltoid

Pectoralis major

Biceps brachii

Rectus abdominis

Brachialis

Brachioradialis

External oblique

Finger flexors

Adductor longus

Sartorius

Gracilis

Rectus femoris

Vastus lateralis

Vastus medialis

Tibialis anterior

©K. Galasyn Wright '94

Figure 7.2 **The posterior and anterior views of the human skeletal musculature.**

© K. Galasyn-Wright, Champaign, IL 1994.

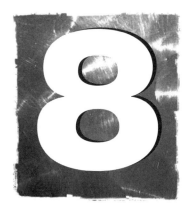

LOWER BODY EXERCISES

This chapter presents exercises to work the muscles of the lower body:

- Abdominals
- Thighs, hips, and gluteals
- Hamstrings
- Calves

Abdominals

The muscle groups that give complete development to the midsection are among the most important, in part because they contribute to the health and integrity of an individual's lower back and abdomen. Many lower back injuries result from weak abdominal muscles rather than underdeveloped spinal erectors.

The abdominal muscles are very important to a competitive bodybuilder's physique. A tightly packed midsection is a characteristic all panel judges look for. A bodybuilder who enters a competitive stage with great abdominals creates a psychological impact that the evaluating judges and audience cannot overlook. Abdominals that are thickly muscled and tightly defined create a good first impression, resulting in a favorable response throughout the rest of the prejudging and show.

Today men who are competing at 260 to 270 pounds and women who are competing at 160 to 180 pounds must have total abdominal development. They should have thick ridges of muscle in the front abdominals, obliques, and intercostals, with deep grooves between the major abdominal groups.

Nautilus Crunches

Primary Muscles Worked
• Rectus abdominis (upper part)

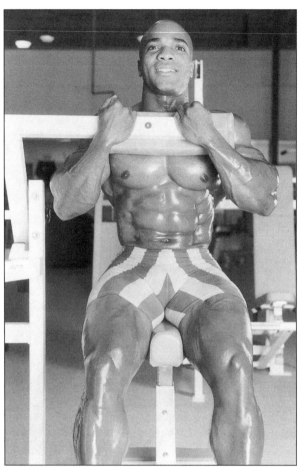

Starting Position

1. Sit on the seat of the crunch machine.
2. At this point, a chest pad should be resting firmly against the chest.
3. Place hands across the back of the chest padding for support.

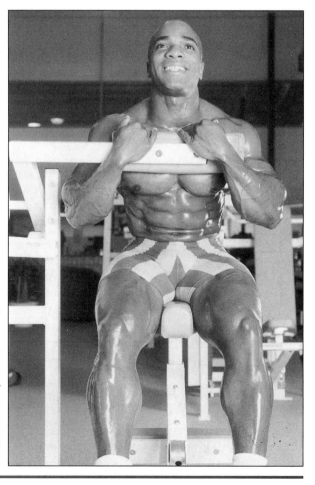

Exercise Technique

1. Bend your torso forward until your abdominals are maximally contracted.
2. Blow all the air out of your lungs as the movement is performed.
3. Slowly return to the starting position, never letting the weighted plates make contact (removes tension from the working muscles).
4. Repeat until the desired number of repetitions is completed.

Primary Muscles Worked

- Rectus abdominis (upper part)
- Serratus anterior and intercostals

Pulley Crunches

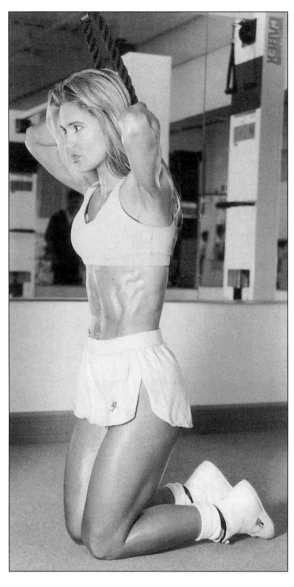

Starting Position

1. Attach a rope handle to an overhead pulley and grasp the rope handles with an overhand grip.
2. Hold the rope behind your neck and kneel down (approximately 1 foot from the pulley machine).

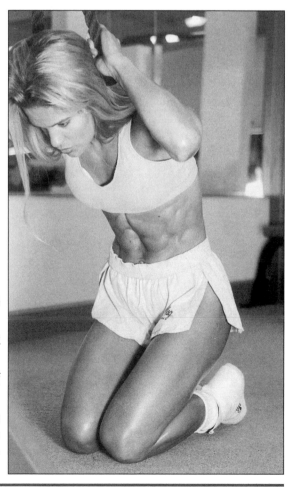

Exercise Technique

1. Bend over at the waist until your abdominals are maximally contracted.
2. Blow all the air out of your lungs as the movement is performed.
3. Repeat the movement until the desired number of repetitions is completed.
4. The objective is to perform the exercise in a controlled manner and to maintain the tension on the working muscles throughout the entire movement.

Knee-Ups
(Flat Bench)

Primary Muscles Worked
• Rectus abdominis (mainly lower)

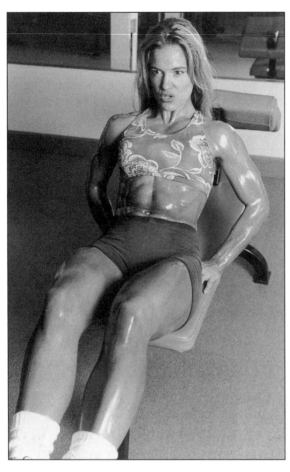

Starting Position

1. Sit on the end of a flat bench and place your hands behind your buttocks to support your body.
2. Lean back until your torso is approximately at a 45-degree angle to the bench.
3. Extend your legs until they are almost straightened.

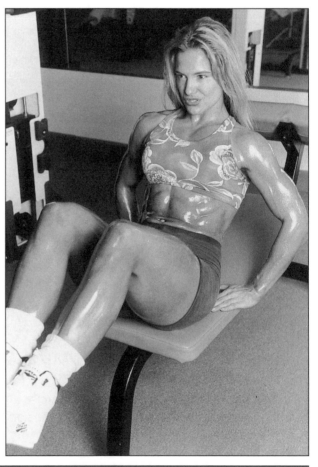

Exercise Technique

1. Pull your knees toward your chest.
2. As your knees approach your chest, flex your neck, allowing your head to curl toward your knees (this will ensure maximal abdominal contraction).
3. Return to the starting position.
4. Repeat the movement until the desired number of repetitions is completed.

Primary Muscles Worked
• Rectus abdominis (mainly upper)

Crunches
(Flat Abdominal Bench)

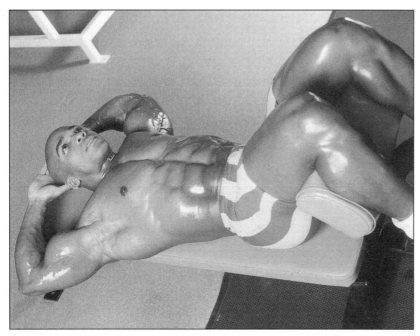

Starting Position

1. Lie flat on an abdominal bench with knees bent and feet locked under the ankle pads.
2. Place hands and arms behind your head.

Exercise Technique

1. Use upper abdominal strength to raise your head and shoulders from the abdominal bench.
2. When rectus abdominis muscles are maximally contracted, pause briefly and return to the starting position.
3. To keep tension on your working muscles, do not allow your torso (upper trapezius and shoulders) to make contact with the bench.
4. Repeat the movement until the desired number of repetitions is completed.

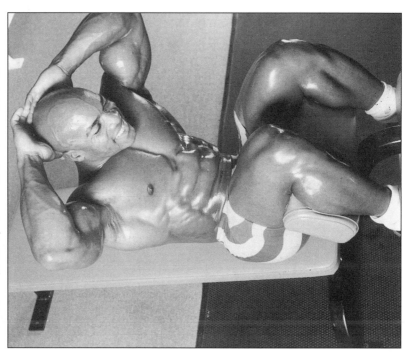

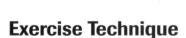

Hanging Leg Raises

Primary Muscles Worked

- Rectus abdominis (mainly lower)
- Serratus anterior and intercostals

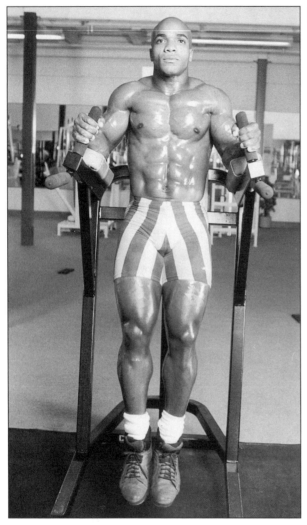

Starting Position

1. Grasp handles and support your body weight with your arms.
2. Allow your torso to hang down in a straight vertical line.
3. Keep your knees slightly bent throughout the entire movement to remove any unnecessary stress from your lower back.

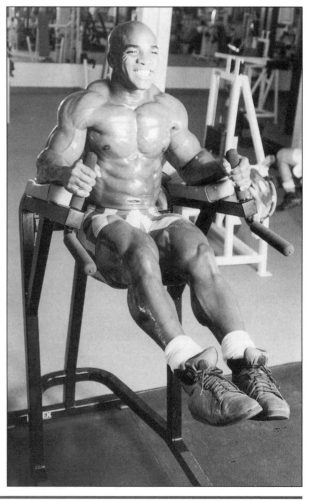

Exercise Technique

1. Using abdominal strength, slowly raise your legs to the level of your hips.
2. Hold the contraction for a moment, then slowly lower your legs to the starting position.
3. Repeat the movement until the desired number of repetitions is completed.

Primary Muscles Worked

• Serratus anterior   • Rectus abdominis   • Intercostals
                        (mainly upper)

Diagonal Curl-Ups

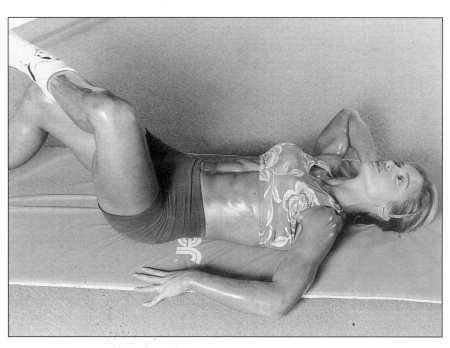

Starting Position

1. Lie down on an abdominal board or floor mat with knees bent and feet on the floor.
2. Place your left ankle across your right knee.
3. A triangle should form from their contact.
4. Place your right hand behind your head and place your left hand on the mat for support.

Exercise Technique

1. Curl your torso diagonally, bringing your right shoulder up toward your left knee.
2. Once you have reached maximum contraction, pause briefly.
3. Return to the starting position and repeat until the desired number of repetitions has been completed.
4. Reverse body position and repeat for the other side.

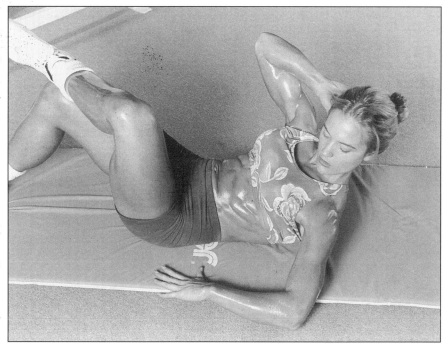

Thighs, Hips, and Gluteals

"Massively carved, ripped, chiseled, and separated." In bodybuilding these words describe the perfect pair of thighs. As the foundation of human muscularity, the thighs are clearly the most powerful muscles of the physique.

Squatting can be an excellent exercise for strengthening numerous muscles, bones, ligaments, and tendinous insertion points within the lower body. In fact, for years the squat has been considered the quintessential leg exercise. Unfortunately, due to the occurrence of injuries to the lumbar spine and knees that frequently accompany this exercise, many professional and amateur bodybuilders have reluctantly eliminated conventional squats (with the Olympic bar) from their training routines. Due to the substantial gains made while squatting, however, most strength trainers and coaches were not prepared to witness its extinction; and so much research was done to develop other, safer squatting methods and equipment.

For maximum quad, hip, and glute development, safety squats should be a part of all quad (rectus femoris) programs. The leg extension is an excellent vastus medialis (quads) exercise.

Primary Muscles Worked

- Vastus lateralis
- Vastus medialis
- Rectus femoris
- Vastus intermedius
- Gluteals

Safety Squats

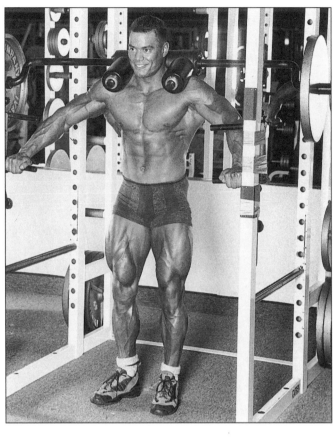

Starting Position

1. Rest the pads of the safety squat bar on your trapezius muscles, and lift the safety squat bar off the squatting holders.
2. Feet should be parallel and shoulder-width apart, with knees slightly bent.
3. Keep the safety squat bar steady on your shoulders and place your hands on the rack handles.

Exercise Technique

1. Keeping your hands on the rack handles throughout the entire movement, slowly lower your glutes toward the floor by bending the knees.
2. When an approximate angle of 90 degrees is reached, push upward with your quadriceps muscles, allowing them maximal muscle activation.
3. Repeat until the desired number of repetitions is completed.

CUE

Using your hands during the safety squat helps to balance and maintain strict squatting form, actually allowing you to spot yourself through your sticking point. This will help you to work with heavier loads without fear of sustaining injuries when exerting force through your weakest point.

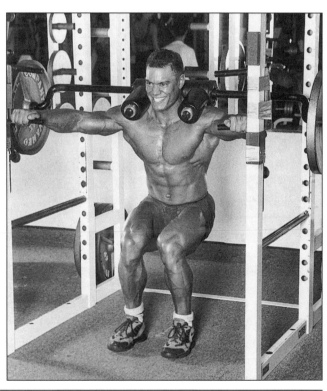

Seated Leg Extensions
(Toes Straight)

Primary Muscles Worked
- Vastus lateralis
- Vastus medialis
- Rectus femoris
- Vastus intermedius

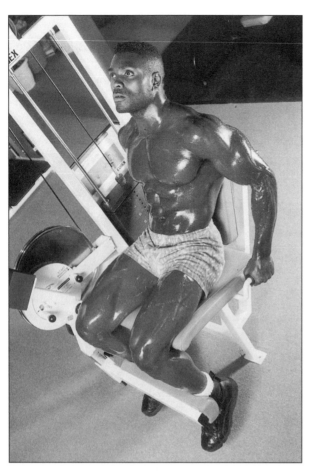

Starting Position

1. Sit on a leg extension machine and press the back of your knees firmly against the edge of the seat.
2. Place the front of your ankles under the foot pad and grasp the handles at the sides of the machine.

Exercise Technique

1. Moving only your lower legs, lift the desired weight until your quadriceps muscles are fully extended.
2. Hold this position for one second, allowing peak quadriceps contraction to occur.
3. Lower the weight slowly to the starting position and repeat the movement until the desired number of repetitions is completed.

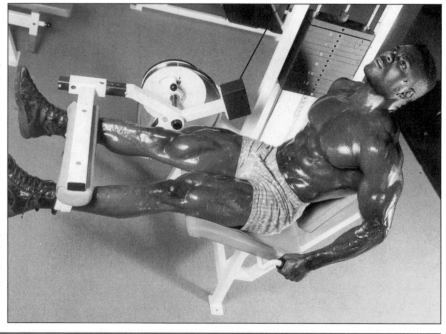

Primary Muscles Worked

- Vastus lateralis
- Vastus medialis
- Rectus femoris
- Vastus intermedius
- Gluteals

Hack Squats

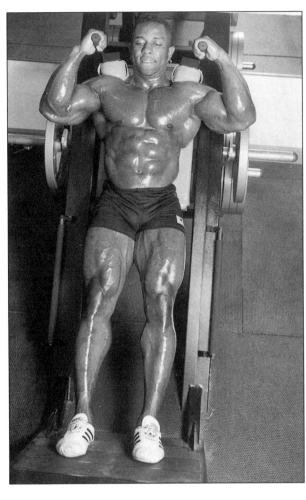

Starting Position

1. Position your body on the hack squat machine with trapezius muscles under the shoulder pads, and back pressed firmly against the back rest.

2. Place your feet on the angled foot rest, with heels approximately 8 inches apart (varies depending on the individual), and toes angled slightly outward.

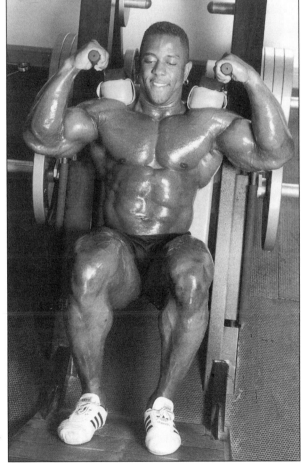

Exercise Technique

1. Slowly bend at the knees, bringing your torso down toward your heels.

2. When your knees are lowered to an approximate 90-degree angle, push upward to return to the starting position.

3. Repeat the movement until the desired number of repetitions is completed.

Leg Press

Primary Muscles Worked
- Vastus lateralis
- Vastus medialis
- Vastus intermedius
- Rectus femoris

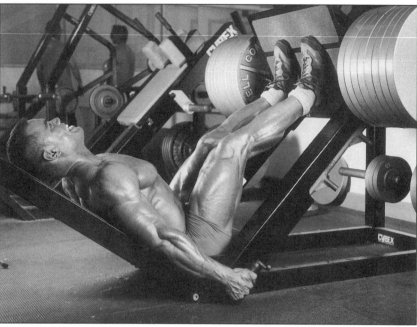

Starting Position

1. Lie on the leg press machine with your buttocks supported on the seat and your back pressed firmly against the back rest pad.

2. Place your feet flat on the platform with a shoulder-width stance and toes slightly angled outward.

3. Grasp the handles and unlock the weight in preparation to perform the leg press.

Exercise Technique

1. Slowly bend your legs, allowing your knees to travel toward your chest.

2. When your knees have reached an angle slightly greater than 90 degrees (110-115 degrees), slowly straighten your legs to return to the starting position (do not lock your knees at top of movement).

3. Repeat the movement until the desired number of repetitions is completed.

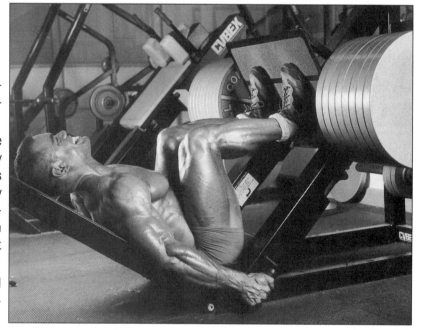

Primary Muscles Worked
- Vastus lateralis
- Vastus medialis
- Vastus intermedius
- Rectus femoris

Smith Machine Squats

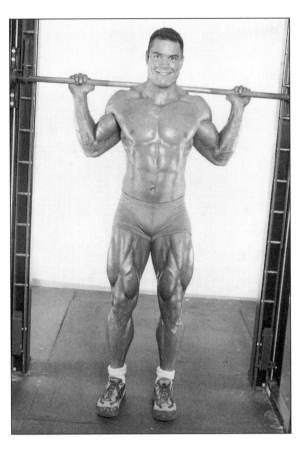

Starting Position
1. Position your body underneath the Olympic bar attached to the Smith machine.
2. Grasp the bar with an overhand grip with hands slightly wider than shoulder-width apart.
3. At this point, the bar is resting comfortably on your trapezius muscles and your feet are apart in a shoulder-width stance.
4. Unhook the bar from the standards and step forward slightly with both feet.
5. Remember to keep your back erect and look forward throughout the entire movement.

Exercise Technique
1. Slowly bend your legs until your knees reach a 90-degree angle.
2. Without bouncing at the bottom of the movement, slowly straighten your legs and return to the starting position.
3. Repeat the movement until the desired number of repetitions is completed.

CUE
Squatting is an exercise in which technique and balance are of the utmost importance. Squatting inside the Nautilus Smith Machine removes the element of balance because the Olympic bar is attached to the apparatus. Despite being considered a revolutionary development in the squatting world, Nautilus Smith Machine squats may produce too much strain on the lower back and knees.

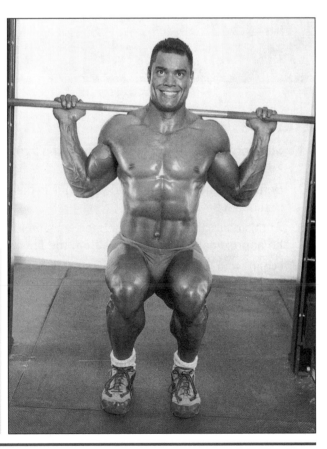

Lunges
(Dumbbells)

Primary Muscles Worked

• Quadriceps   • Gluteals   • Hamstrings

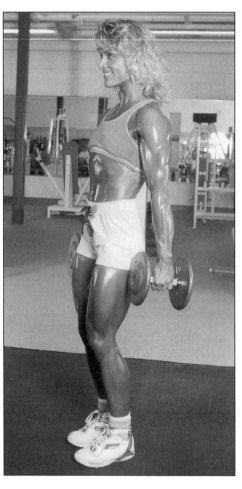

Starting Position

1. Grasp a dumbbell with each hand.
2. Hold the dumbbells at the sides of your body, with arms fully extended (palms facing your torso).

Exercise Technique

1. Step forward with your lead leg (stepping leg), keeping your back erect.
2. Bend the knee of your lead leg until it has reached a 90-degree angle.
3. At this point, the knee of your back leg should be approximately 2 to 3 inches from the floor.
4. When your back leg is fully lowered, push forcefully with your lead leg and return to the starting position.
5. Repeat the exercise with your other leg, and continue to alternate until the desired number of repetitions is completed.
6. Remember that a shorter lead step allows more emphasis to be placed on the quadriceps muscles, and a larger step places more emphasis on the gluteal and hamstring muscles.

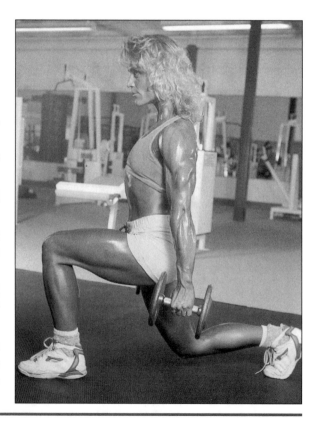

Primary Muscles Worked

• Quadriceps • Gluteals • Hamstrings

Lunges
(Olympic Bar)

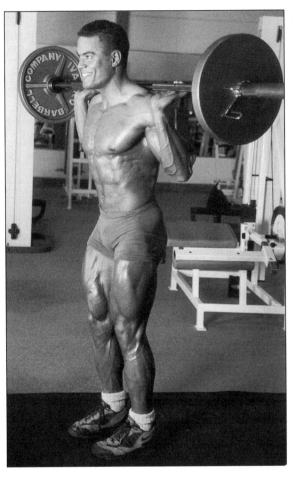

Starting Position

1. Position your body underneath the Olympic bar and lift it from the standards.

2. The bar should be resting on your trapezius muscles, with your hands grasping the bar slightly wider than shoulder-width apart.

3. Take several steps backward, giving enough clear space to lunge forward.

Exercise Technique

1. Step forward with your lead leg (stepping leg), keeping your back erect.

2. Bend the knee of your lead leg until it reaches a 90-degree angle.

3. At this point, the knee of your back leg should be approximately 2 to 3 inches from the floor.

4. When your back leg is fully lowered, push forcefully with your lead leg and return to the starting position.

5. Repeat with the other leg, and continue to alternate until the desired number of repetitions is completed.

6. Remember that a shorter lead step allows more emphasis to be placed on the quadriceps muscles, and a larger step places more emphasis on the gluteal and hamstring muscles.

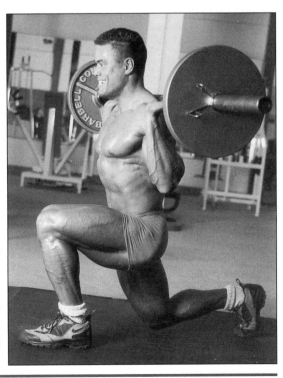

Hamstrings

Few people ever talk about the hamstring muscles. Even if you constantly read bodybuilding magazines, very rarely will you encounter professional bodybuilders who discuss hamstrings like they discuss pec training, back blasting, or arm blitzing. However, all bodybuilders will tell you how important the hamstring muscles are to overall leg development. Nothing is more impressive than a bodybuilder who turns to the side to reveal the belly of the hamstring as a massive rounded mound of flesh.

Standing, seated, and lying hamstring curls seem to be the best hamstring exercises.

Primary Muscles Worked

- Biceps femoris
- Semitendinosus
- Semimembranosus

Standing Leg Curls

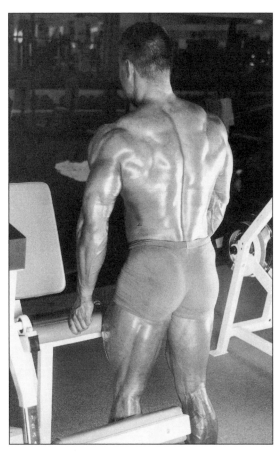

Starting Position

1. Standing on the right side of the machine, place your left quad against the thigh pad, and your left heel (calf) under the rectangular ankle pad.
2. With your left hand grasp the pad directly in front, and lean your torso slightly forward.

Exercise Technique

1. Slowly raise your foot toward your buttocks.
2. Go as far upward as possible to allow for maximal contraction.
3. Once the top of the movement is reached, slowly lower your leg while resisting against the weight (do not let your foot touch the floor).
4. Repeat until the desired number of repetitions is completed.
5. Reverse your body position and repeat exercise for the other leg.

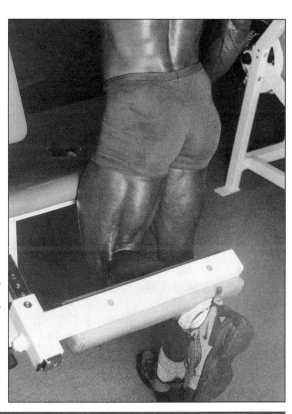

Lying Leg Curls

Primary Muscles Worked
- Biceps femoris
- Semitendinosus
- Semimembranosus

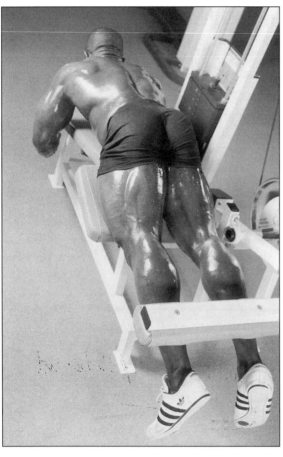

Starting Position

1. Lie facedown on the hamstring curl machine.
2. Slide your ankles underneath the ankle pads and place your knees at the edge of the bench.
3. Grasp the handles at the top of the machine to keep your body stabilized while performing the set.

Exercise Technique

1. Raise your heels, bringing them toward your buttocks.
2. Go as far upward as possible to allow for maximal contraction.
3. Once the top of the movement is reached, slowly lower your leg while resisting against the weight (do not let the plates touch—keep tension on the working muscles).
4. Repeat until the desired number of repetitions is completed.

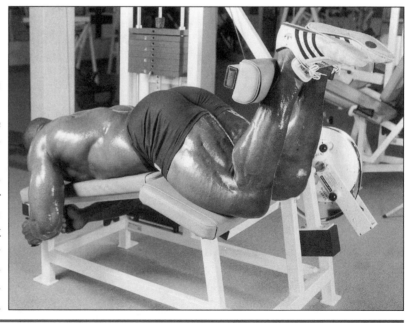

Primary Muscles Worked
- Biceps femoris
- Semitendinosus
- Semimembranosus

Seated Leg Curls

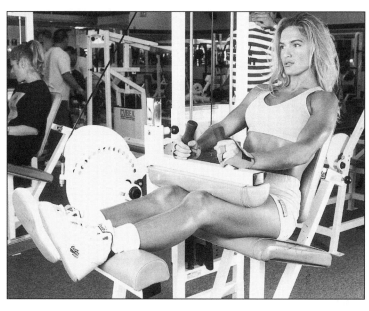

Starting Position

1. Sit on the hamstring curl machine with ankles on top of the ankle pads.
2. Adjust the thigh pad and lock it down comfortably across your thighs.
3. Keep back pressed firmly against the back support.

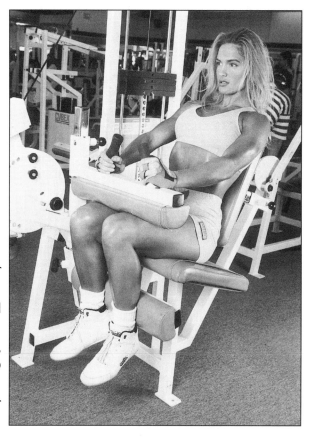

Exercise Technique

1. Bend your knees, bringing the heels under your body and toward your buttocks.
2. Go as far back as possible to allow for maximal contraction.
3. Once your hamstrings are maximally contracted, and while resisting slowly, allow the weight to bring your body back to the starting position.
4. Repeat the movement until the desired number of repetitions is completed.

Modified Hamstring Dead-Lifts

Primary Muscles Worked
- Biceps femoris
- Semimembranosus
- Semitendinosus

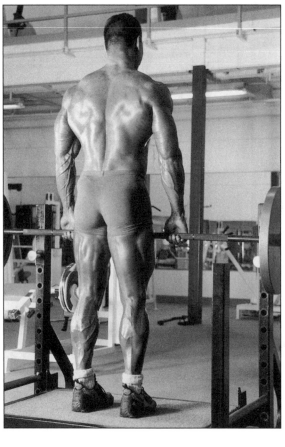

Starting Position

1. Grasp an Olympic bar with hands slightly wider than shoulder-width apart.
2. Hold the bar with arms fully extended at thigh level.

Exercise Technique

1. Keep back flat, buttocks out, and knees slightly bent.
2. Slowly lower the bar past your knees (2-3 inches).
3. At this point, you should feel a stretch in your glutes and hamstrings.
4. Slowly raise the bar by contracting your glutes and hamstrings and by straightening your torso.
5. Repeat until the desired number of repetitions is completed.

CUE
Most lifters perform this exercise incorrectly by bending too far over. Once the hip muscles are fully flexed, the only way to further lower the bar to the shoes is to hyperflex the spine. When this occurs, the lifter places the lumbar spine in a very vulnerable position (career-ending injury or serious complications).

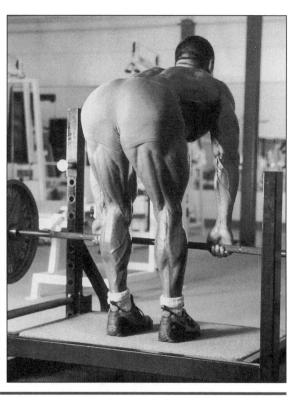

Primary Muscles Worked
- Gluteus maximus muscle group
- Upper hamstring area

Cable Kick-Back

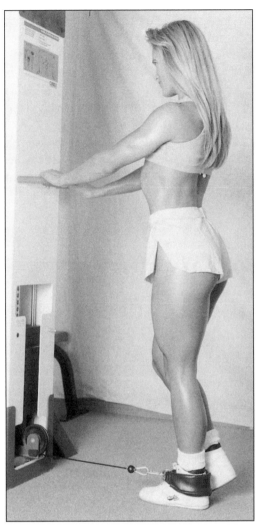

Starting Position

1. Attach an ankle strap to the low cable pulley.
2. Facing the pulley, slip your left ankle into the strap and take two steps backwards.
3. Grasp the support bar with both hands to stabilize your torso throughout the entire movement.

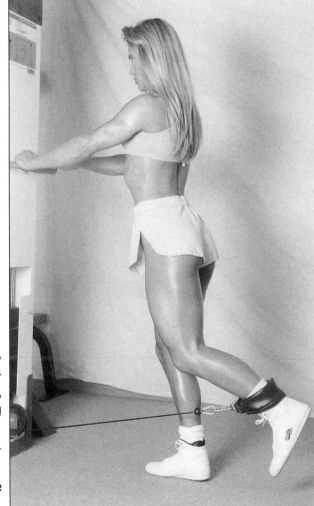

Exercise Technique

1. Keeping your supporting leg slightly flexed, slowly kick your left leg back from the hips.
2. Hold this contracted position for a moment, and then return your foot to the starting position.
3. Repeat the movement until the desired number of repetitions is completed.
4. Reverse body position and repeat with the right leg.

Calves

All of the really great bodybuilders have awesome calves. Some of the greatest bodybuilders with unparalleled calf development are Arnold Schwarzenegger, Tom Platz, and Gary Strydom. Many bodybuilders believe that the calves are virtually impossible to build because their size is genetically determined. But persistence is the hallmark of every champion, especially with stubborn muscles like the calves. Arnold Schwarzenegger is a prime example of an individual with no genetically-gifted calf development. He therefore prioritized calf development and used heavy training to develop huge diamond-shaped calves.

If your calves lack width, you should concentrate your efforts on seated calf raises. Seated calf raises are also excellent for carving deep cuts in the outer sides of your calves. To enlarge your gastrocnemius muscles you must do plenty of donkey calf, standing calf, and one-legged calf raises.

Primary Muscles Worked
- Gastrocnemius
- Soleus

Donkey
Calf Raises

Starting Position

1. Stand with toes on the edge of a calf board (approximately 3-5 inches in height).

2. Bend forward at the hips until your torso is parallel to the floor, and stabilize your body by holding onto a piece of equipment (e.g., squat rack).

3. At this point, a partner climbs onto your back and straddles your hips.

4. Allow your heels to drop as far as comfortably possible below the level of your toes.

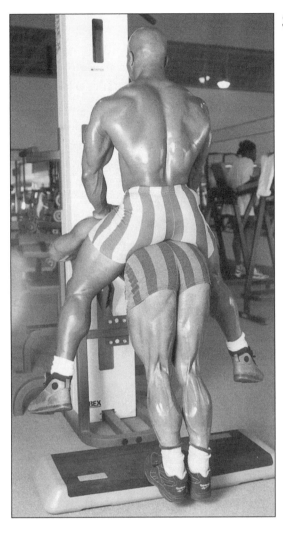

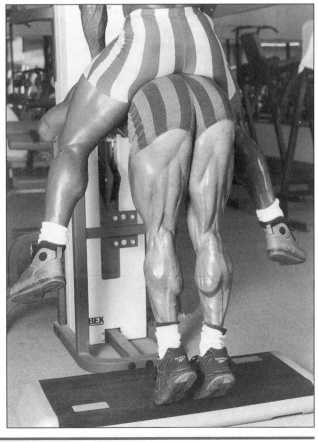

Exercise Technique

1. Raise your torso as high as possible on the balls of your feet.

2. Once the top of the movement is reached, slowly lower your heels as far below the level of your toes as possible, returning to the starting position.

3. Repeat the movement until the desired number of repetitions is completed.

Standing One-Legged Calf Raises

Primary Muscles Worked
• Gastrocnemius • Soleus

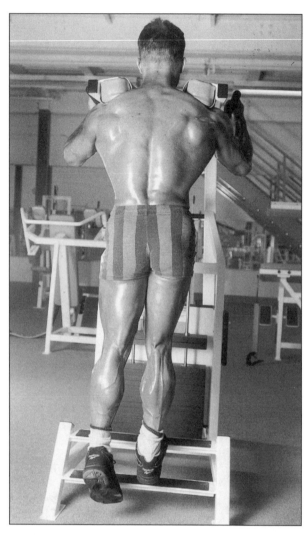

Starting Position

1. Stand on a calf machine, with the ball of your right foot at the edge of the platform.
2. Allow your heel to drop as far below the level of your toes as possible.
3. Place your hands on top of the shoulder pads to stabilize your body.

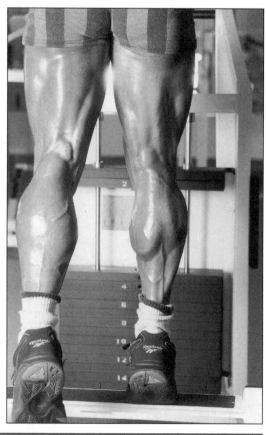

Exercise Technique

1. Raise your torso as high as possible on the ball of your foot and toes.
2. Once the top of the movement is reached, slowly lower your heel as far below the level of your toes as possible, returning to the starting position.
3. Repeat the movement until the desired number of repetitions is completed.
4. Repeat for the left foot.

Primary Muscles Worked
- Gastrocnemius
- Soleus

Standing Calf Raises

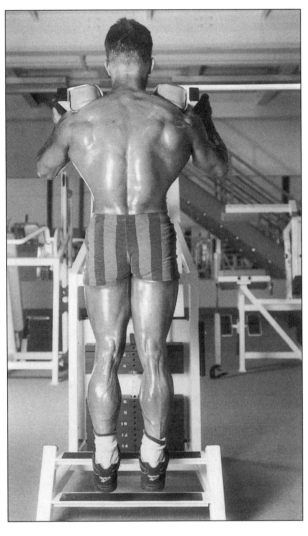

Starting Position

1. Stand on a calf machine with the balls of your feet at the edge of the platform.
2. Allow your heels to drop as far below the level of your toes as possible.
3. Place your hands on top of the shoulder pads to stabilize your body.

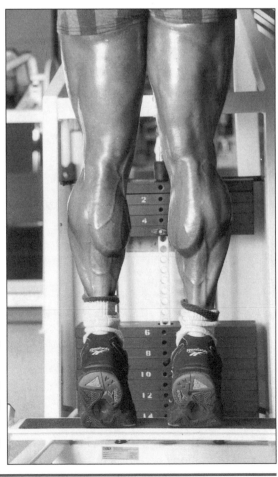

Exercise Technique

1. Raise your torso as high as possible on the balls of your feet and toes.
2. Once the top of the movement is reached, slowly lower your heels as far below the level of the toes as possible, returning to the starting position.
3. Repeat until the desired number of repetitions is completed.

Seated
Calf Raises

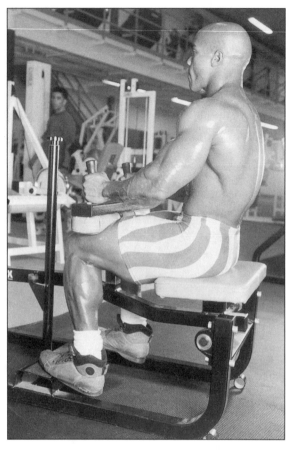

Starting Position

1. Sit on the calf machine with the balls of your feet on the edge of the platform.
2. Hook your knees underneath the pads and grasp the handles to stabilize your body.
3. Unhook the safeguard for the weight.
4. Allow your heels to drop as far below the level of your toes as possible.

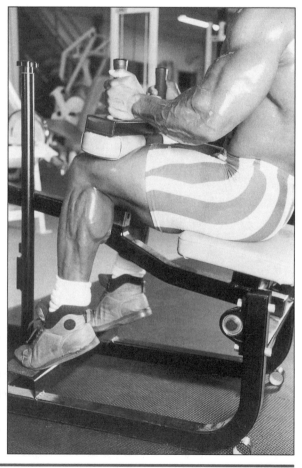

Exercise Technique

1. Raise your heels until your calves are fully contracted.
2. Once the top of the movement is reached, slowly lower your heels as far below your toes as possible, returning to the starting position.
3. Repeat the movement until the desired number of repetitions is completed.

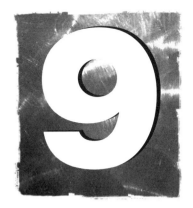

UPPER BODY EXERCISES

This chapter presents exercises to work the muscles of the upper body:

- Chest
- Back
- Deltoids
- Triceps
- Biceps
- Forearms

Chest

There is nothing more impressive in the sport of bodybuilding than a pair of striated, slab-like pectoral muscles. When you look at Arnold Schwarzenegger and Lee Haney, you undoubtedly will conclude that you must beef up your chest if you are ever to win a big bodybuilding title. When these bodybuilders stand relaxed, their chests look twice as thick as their waists from the side.

Many professional bodybuilders look great from the front because they have good pecs; yet from the side view they clearly lack deep rib cages—their chests and waists appear to have about the same thickness. Fully expanding the rib cage is one of the essential factors in developing an impressive chest. The bigger the foundation on which the pectoral muscles are set, the greater the level of development and impressiveness they will achieve.

The pecs should be worked from all angles. Certain basic exercises—like incline flat dumbbell bench presses, or incline flat and decline barbell bench presses—build muscles on your chest. Flys and pulley crossovers are more effective for shaping and striating the pectoral region. Complete pectoral development results from working all four regions of the muscles: upper, lower, outside, and inside.

Primary Muscles Worked

• Pectoralis major   • Anterior deltoids
(lower chest)

Decline Dumbbell Bench Press

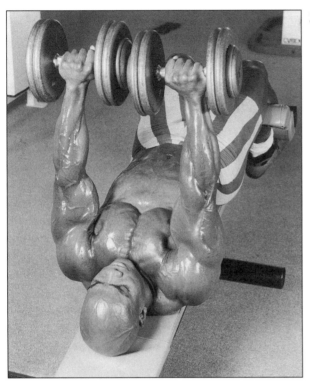

Starting Position

1. Grasp two dumbbells using an overhand grip, while sitting at the high end of a decline bench.
2. Secure ankles and feet underneath the pads.
3. Rest the dumbbells in an upright position on your knees.
4. Lie on the decline bench, simultaneously bringing the dumbbells to the sides of your torso at chest level.
5. Raise the dumbbells to a position of straight arms' length (elbows not locked), with palms facing forward.
6. At this point the dumbbells are positioned directly over your chest in contact with each other.

Exercise Technique

1. Slowly bend your arms and lower the dumbbells until they are at either side of your chest.
2. Dumbbells are lowered to a position where a comfortable but maximum stretch is achieved.
3. Raise the dumbbells from the sides of your chest to the starting position.
4. Perform the desired number of repetitions while keeping the movement fluent, slow, and controlled.

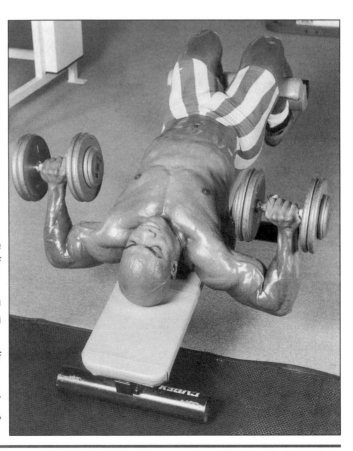

Decline Bench Press
(Olympic Bar)

Primary Muscles Worked
- Pectoralis major (lower chest)
- Anterior deltoids

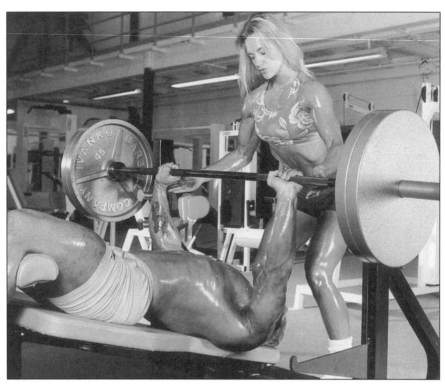

Starting Position

1. Lie down on a decline bench with back pressed firmly against the padding and feet and ankles secured underneath the pads.

2. Grasp the Olympic bar using an overhand grip with hands 3 to 5 inches wider than shoulder-width apart, and lift the bar from the standards.

3. Arms should be fully extended (not locked) as the bar is held over your chest area.

Exercise Technique

1. Slowly lower the bar to touch the nipple line of your chest.

2. Once the bar lightly touches your chest, push it upward to the starting position.

3. Remember never to lock your elbows during this movement. This will allow continuous tension to remain on the working muscles.

4. Perform the desired number of repetitions while keeping the movement fluent, slow, and controlled.

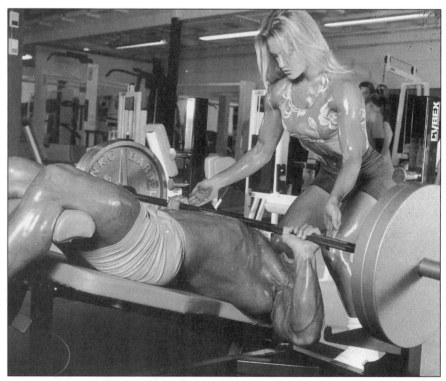

Primary Muscles Worked

- Pectoralis major (midchest)
- Anterior deltoids

Push-Ups Between Benches

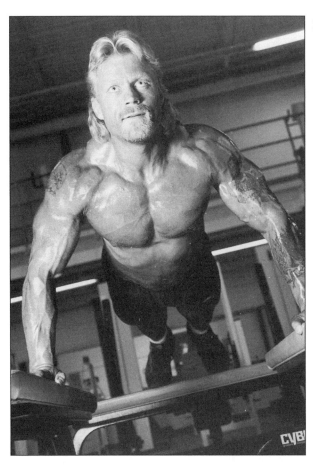

Starting Position

1. Arrange three benches—two parallel to each other and slightly wider than chest-width apart, and one perpendicular to and behind the other two benches.

2. Place both feet on the rear bench, and one hand on each of the parallel benches.

3. At this point you are in a supported position ready to perform push-ups.

Exercise Technique

1. Lower your body as far down between the benches as possible until a comfortable stretch (midchest area) is achieved.

2. Then push your body upward to the starting position.

3. Perform the desired number of repetitions while keeping the movement fluent, slow, and controlled.

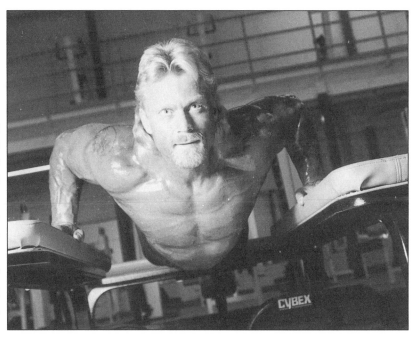

Flat Dumbbell Bench Press

Primary Muscles Worked

• Pectoralis major (midchest)   • Anterior deltoids

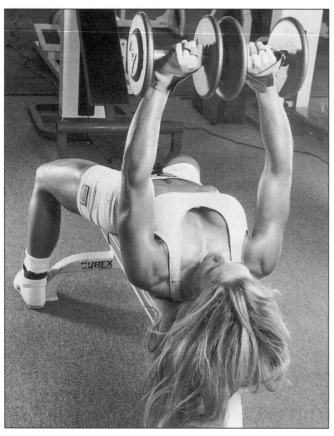

Starting Position

1. Grasp two dumbbells using an overhand grip, while sitting at the edge of the flat bench.
2. Rest the dumbbells in an upright position on your knees.
3. Lie on the flat bench, simultaneously bringing the dumbbells to the sides of your torso at chest level.
4. Raise the dumbbells to a position of straight arms' length (elbows not locked).
5. At this point the dumbbells are held directly over your chest area, in contact with each other, with palms facing forward.

Exercise Technique

1. Slowly bend your arms and lower the dumbbells until they are at either side of your chest.
2. Lower the dumbbells to a position where a comfortable but maximum stretch is achieved.
3. Raise the dumbbells from the sides of your chest to the starting position.
4. Perform the desired number of repetitions while keeping the movement fluent, slow, and controlled.

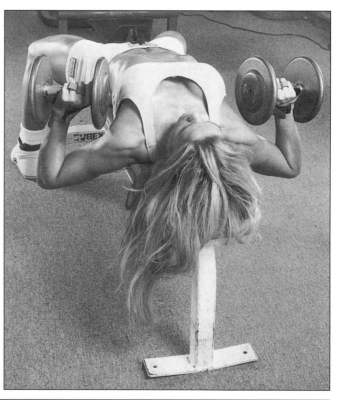

Primary Muscles Worked
- Pectoralis major (midchest)
- Anterior deltoids

Flat Bench Press
(Olympic Bar)

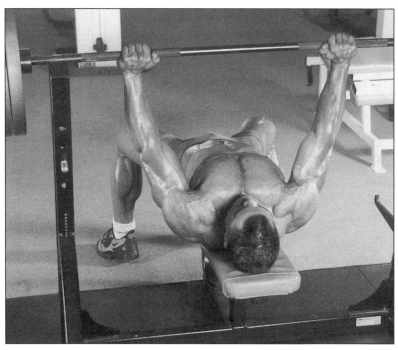

Starting Position

1. Lie on the flat bench, with back pressed firmly against the padding and feet flat on the floor.

2. Grasp the bar using an overhand grip, with hands 3 to 5 inches wider than shoulder-width apart, and lift the bar from the standards.

3. Arms should be fully extended (not locked) as the bar is held over the chest area.

Exercise Technique

1. Slowly lower the barbell to touch the nipple line of your chest.

2. Once the bar lightly touches your chest, push it upward to the starting position.

3. Repeat the movement until the desired number of repetitions is completed, keeping the movement fluent, slow, and controlled.

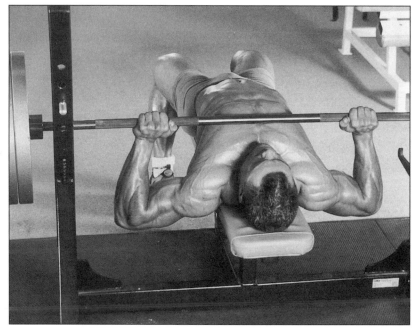

Flat Dumbbell Flys

Primary Muscles Worked

• Pectoralis major   • Anterior deltoids
(midchest)

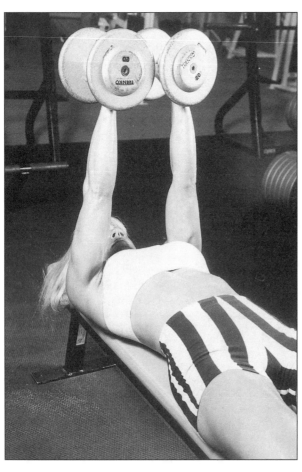

Starting Position

1. Grasp the dumbbells using an overhand grip, while sitting at the end of the flat bench.
2. Rest the dumbbells in an upright position on your knees.
3. Lie on the flat bench, simultaneously bringing the dumbbells to the sides of your torso at chest level.
4. Raise the dumbbells to a position of straight arms' length.
5. At this point the dumbbells are held directly over your chest, in contact with each other, while your palms are facing inward.
6. Elbows must remain flexed throughout the entire movement.

Exercise Technique

1. Slowly lower the dumbbells in an arc-like motion toward the floor until your chest is comfortably stretched (visualize opening a book).
2. Once this stretch is reached (dumbbells at either side of your chest), return the dumbbells to the starting position, using the same arc-like motion.
3. Perform the desired number of repetitions while keeping the movement fluent, slow, and controlled.

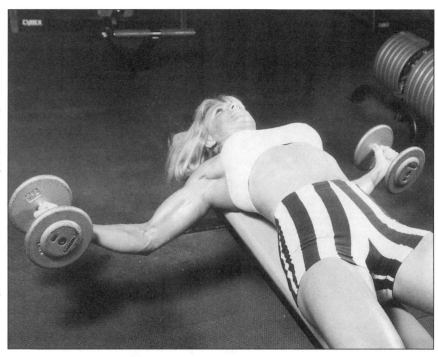

Primary Muscles Worked
• Pectoralis major   • Anterior deltoids
(upper chest)

Incline Dumbbell Bench Press

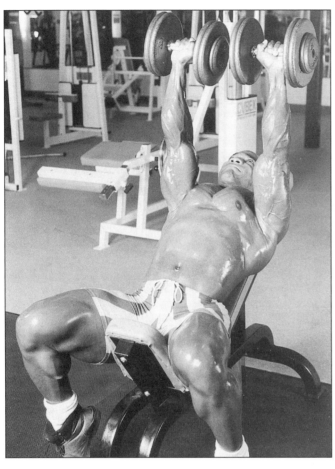

Starting Position

1. Grasp the dumbbells using an overhand grip, while sitting at the edge of the incline bench.
2. Rest the dumbbells in an upright position on your knees.
3. Lie on the incline bench, simultaneously bringing the dumbbells to the sides of your torso at chest level.
4. Raise the dumbbells to a position of straight arms' length (elbows not locked).
5. At this point the dumbbells are held directly over your upper chest, in contact with each other, while your palms are facing forward.

Exercise Technique

1. Slowly bend your arms and lower the dumbbells until they are at either side of your chest.
2. Lower dumbbells to a position where a comfortable stretch is achieved.
3. Raise the dumbbells from the sides of your chest to the starting position.
4. Perform the desired number of repetitions while keeping the movement fluent, slow, and controlled.

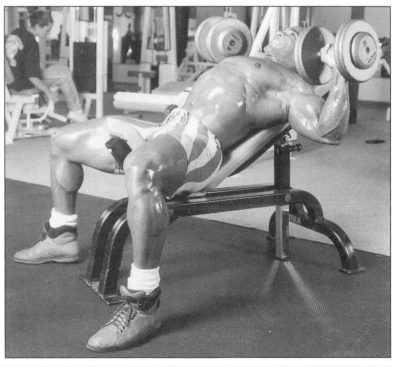

Incline Bench Press
(Olympic Bar)

Primary Muscles Worked

• Pectoralis major   • Anterior deltoids
(upper chest)

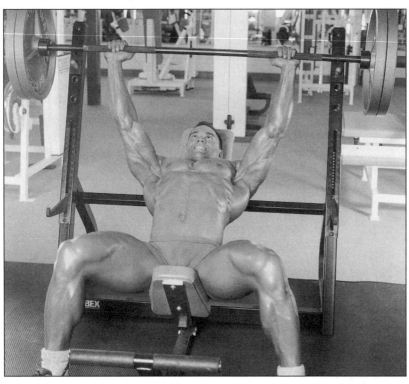

Starting Position

1. Lie down on an incline bench with back pressed firmly against the padding and feet placed flat on the floor.

2. Grasp the Olympic bar using an overhand grip, with hands slightly wider than shoulder-width apart, and lift the bar from the standards.

3. Arms should be fully extended (not locked) as the bar is held over your chest area.

Exercise Technique

1. Slowly lower the Olympic bar to touch your upper pectoral area.

2. Once the bar lightly touches your upper chest, push it upward to the starting position.

3. Remember: never lock your elbows. This will allow the tension to remain on the upper chest area.

4. Repeat the movement until the desired number of repetitions is completed, keeping the movement fluent, slow, and controlled.

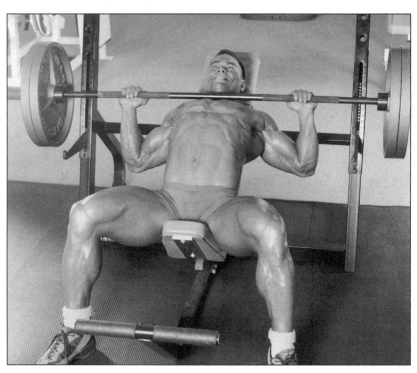

Primary Muscles Worked
- Pectoralis major (upper chest)
- Anterior deltoids

Incline
Dumbbell Flys

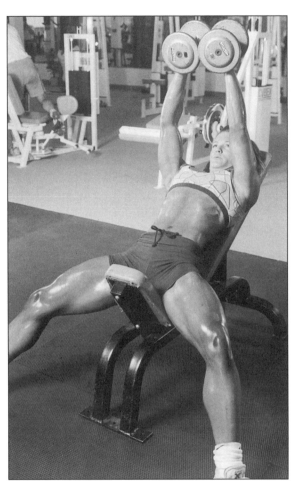

Starting Position

1. Grasp the dumbbells using an overhand grip, while sitting on an incline bench.
2. Rest the dumbbells in an upright position on your knees.
3. Lie on the incline bench, simultaneously bringing the dumbbells to the sides of your torso at chest level.
4. Raise the dumbbells to a position of straight arms' length.
5. At this point the dumbbells are held directly over your upper chest, in contact with each other, while your palms are facing inward.
6. Elbows must remain flexed throughout the entire movement.

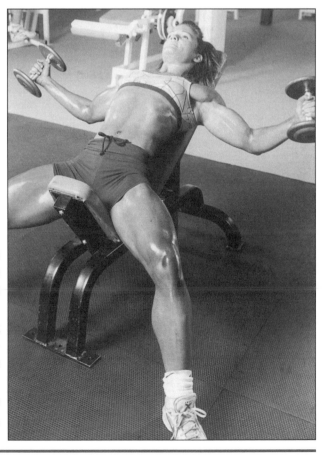

Exercise Technique

1. Slowly lower the dumbbells in an arc-like motion toward the floor until your chest is comfortably stretched (visualize opening a book).
2. Once this stretch is reached (dumbbells at either side of your chest), return the dumbbells to the starting position, using the same arc-like motion.
3. Perform the desired number of repetitions while keeping the movement fluent, slow, and controlled.

Incline Bench Press: Smith Machine

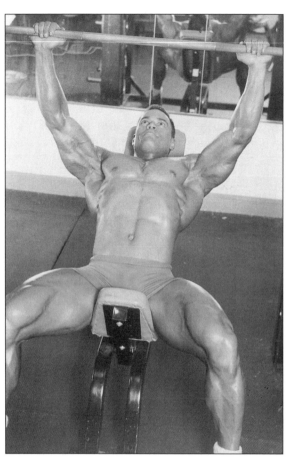

Starting Position

1. Lie down on an incline bench (inside Smith machine work station) with back pressed firmly against the padding and feet placed flat on the floor.
2. Grasp the Olympic bar using an overhand grip, with hands 3 to 5 inches wider than shoulder-width apart, and unlock the bar from the safety standards.
3. Arms should be fully extended (not locked) as the bar is held over your upper chest area.

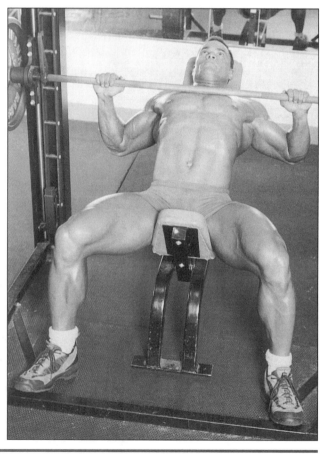

Exercise Technique

1. Slowly lower the Olympic bar (Smith machine) to lightly touch your upper pectoral area.
2. Once the bar lightly touches your upper chest, push it upward to the starting position.
3. Remember: never lock your elbows. This will allow the tension to remain on the upper chest area.
4. Repeat the movement until the desired number of repetitions is completed, keeping the movement fluent, slow, and controlled.

Primary Muscles Worked

- Pectoralis major (lower and midchest)
- Anterior deltoids

Cable Crossovers

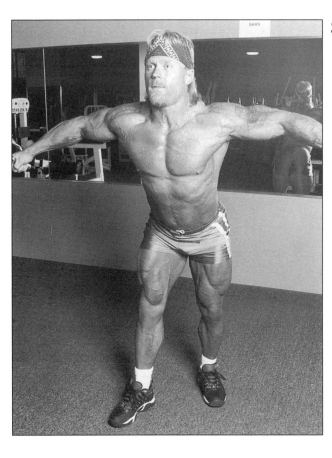

Starting Position

1. Grasp each cable using an overhand grip with palms facing inward.
2. Stand in the middle of the cable machine, with feet slightly wider than shoulder-width apart, or with one foot slightly in front of the other (use whatever stance you are comfortable with).
3. Keep back erect and elbows slightly bent throughout the entire motion.
4. To begin exercise, extend the cables to the point where your chest is completely stretched (arms wide open).

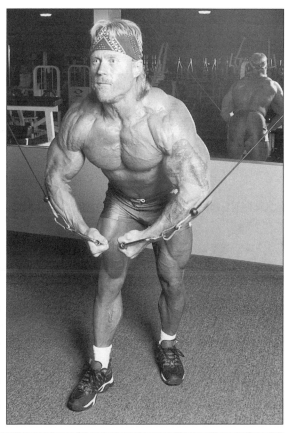

Exercise Technique

1. Move the cables in a downward arcing motion until hands make contact (6-8 inches from front aspect of pelvis).
2. Hold this position for approximately 1 to 2 seconds to fully contract your pectoral muscles.
3. Slowly resist as the cables are returned to their starting position.
4. Repeat the movement until the desired number of repetitions is completed, keeping the movement fluent, slow, and controlled.

Parallel Bar Dip

Primary Muscles Worked
- Pectoralis major and minor
- Anterior deltoids

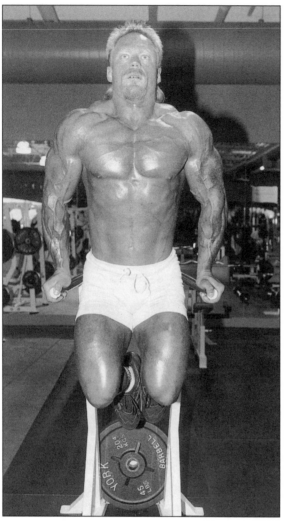

Starting Position

1. Support your body at straight arms' length with your chin down.
2. Keep knees flexed, feet behind you, and torso erect at starting position.

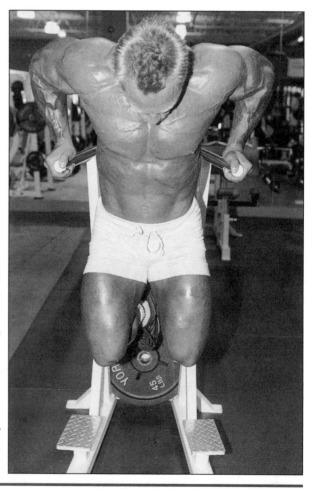

Exercise Technique

1. Bend your arms, allowing your elbows to travel slightly out to your sides while your torso inclines forward.
2. Lower your body to a point where a comfortable stretch is achieved.
3. When this occurs, slowly push your torso upward to the starting position.
4. Remember: never lock your elbows.
5. Repeat the movement until the desired number of repetitions is completed, keeping the movement fluent, slow, and controlled.

Back

In the sport of bodybuilding, nothing is more impressive than a front or back lat spread. Those wide thick wings look like they are ready for flight. All top professional bodybuilders have thick, well-developed latissimus dorsi muscles, and their erector spinae muscles look like huge mounds of flesh.

Back routines are structured around exercises for width, such as lat machine pull-downs or wide-grip chin-ups, and mass exercises, such as bent-over barbell rows, T-bar rows, and one-arm dumbbell rows.

Bent-Over Barbell Rows

(Olympic Bar)

Primary Muscles Worked
- Latissimus dorsi
- Trapezius (mid)
- Biceps, brachialis

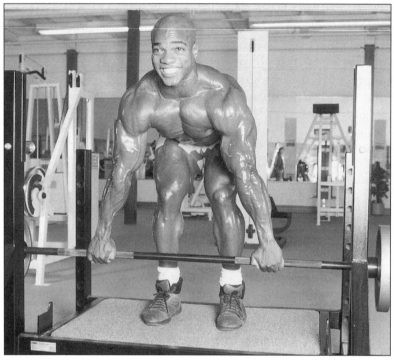

Starting Position

1. Grasp the bar using an overhand grip, with hands approximately 4 to 6 inches wider than shoulder-width apart, and remove the bar from the standards.

2. Take a shoulder-width stance, and keep feet flat on the ground.

3. Slowly bend forward at the hips, keeping back flat and allowing for a slight bend in the knees.

4. At this point, your torso should be parallel to the ground, with arms fully extended, holding the bar.

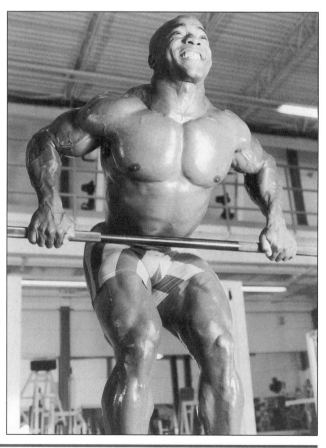

Exercise Technique

1. Moving only your arms, slowly pull the bar upward, allowing it to touch the lower part of your rib cage (torso should not move upward more than 2-4 inches).

2. Lower the weight slowly to the starting position. Repeat the movement until the desired number of repetitions is completed.

Primary Muscles Worked
- Latissimus dorsi
- Trapezius (mid)
- Biceps, brachialis

One-Arm Dumbbell Rows
(Alternate)

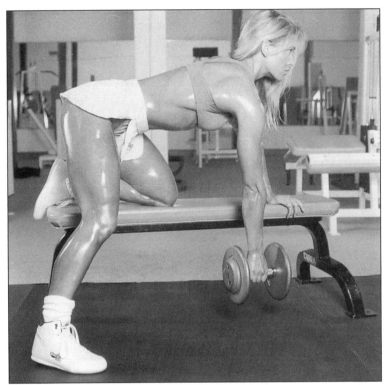

Starting Position

1. Grasp a dumbbell with your right hand, using an overhand grip (palms facing your body).
2. Rest your left knee on a flat bench. Right leg should be flexed, with your foot flat on the floor.
3. Bend forward at the hips and stabilize your body with a straightened left arm.
4. At this point, your torso should be nearly parallel to the floor.
5. The dumbbell in your right hand is held at full arms' length.

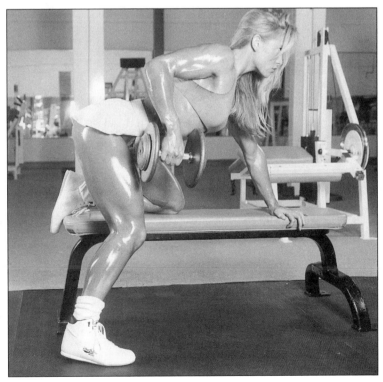

Exercise Technique

1. Keeping your elbow close to your torso, pull the dumbbell upward in a straight vertical line, allowing it to lightly touch your ribcage.
2. Slowly lower the dumbbell to the starting position. Repeat the movement until the desired number of repetitions is completed.
3. Repeat for the left hand.

T-Bar Rows

Primary Muscles Worked
- Latissimus dorsi
- Erector spinae
- Rhomboids
- Biceps, brachialis

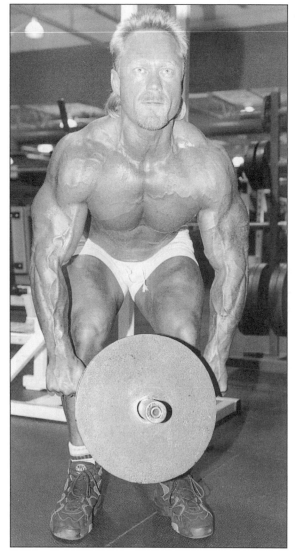

Starting Position

1. Bend forward at the hips, keeping your back flat and knees bent.
2. Grasp the T-bar handles using an overhand grip (palms facing backward).
3. Raise your torso to a position where it is parallel to the floor.
4. Arms should be fully extended.

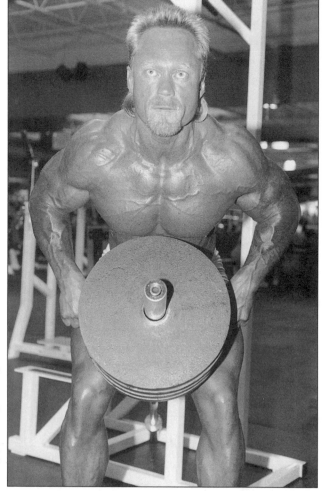

Exercise Technique

1. Pull hands upward until the weight touches your chest.
2. Your torso should not move upward more than 2 to 4 inches.
3. Slowly return to the starting position. Repeat the movement until the desired number of repetitions is completed.

Primary Muscles Worked
- Latissimus dorsi
- Rhomboids
- Posterior deltoids
- Biceps, brachialis

Lat Pull-Downs to the Front

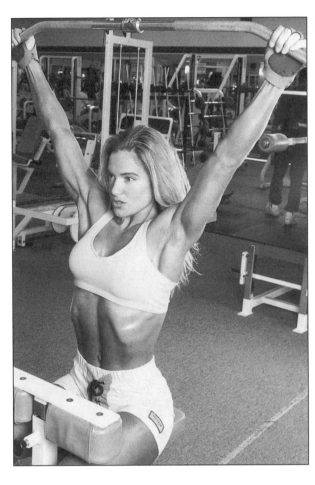

Starting Position

1. Stand in front of the lat pull-down machine and grasp the bar, using an overhand grip (wide).
2. Sit down with feet flat on the floor, back straight, and thighs secured underneath thigh pads.
3. Arch your torso and lean backward at a 45-degree angle.
4. Your torso remains rigid throughout the entire movement.
5. At this point, your arms are fully extended holding the lat bar overhead.

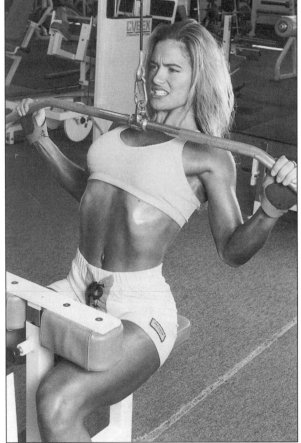

Exercise Technique

1. Initiate the movement by pulling your elbows downward and backward.
2. Bring the bar in front of your head until it touches the upper part of your chest, and pause.
3. Slowly bring the bar back to the starting position and repeat the movement until the desired number of repetitions is completed.

Seated Pulley Row

Primary Muscles Worked
- Latissimus dorsi
- Rhomboids
- Trapezius muscles
- Erector spinae

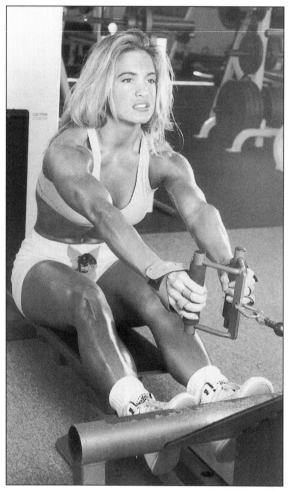

Starting Position
1. Grasp the seated pulley handle with palms facing inward.
2. Straighten your arms, sit on the padding, and place feet on the floor rests at the front end of the machine.
3. Keep a slight bend in your knees throughout the movement.
4. Lean forward, allowing your head to lower between your arms (excellent prestretch for the lats) and keeping your back flat.

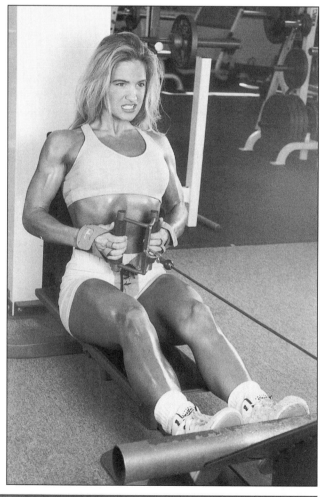

Exercise Technique
1. Bring your torso to an erect position, pulling the handle toward your abdominals.
2. Remember to slightly arch your back and keep your elbows close to your torso while pulling the handle toward the abdominals, to maximally contract your lats.
3. Return to the starting position. Repeat the movement until the desired number of repetitions is completed.

Primary Muscles Worked
- Latissimus dorsi
- Biceps brachii, brachialis
- Upper trapezius

Front Chin-Ups

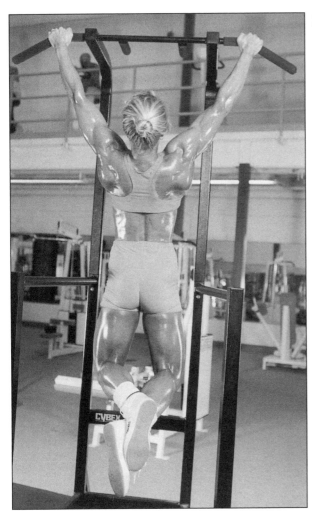

Starting Position
1. Grasp a chin-up bar with an overhand grip approximately 3 to 5 inches wider than shoulder-width apart.
2. Knees are flexed at a 90-degree angle so that your ankles can cross over each other.

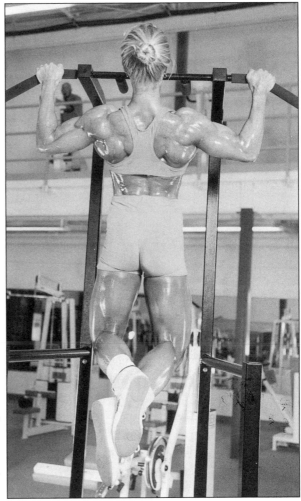

Exercise Technique
1. Pull your body up in a vertical line until your chin is parallel to the chin-up bar.
2. Slowly lower your body to the starting position. Repeat the movement until the desired number of repetitions is completed.

Lat Pull-Downs Behind the Neck

Primary Muscles Worked
- Latissimus dorsi
- Upper trapezius
- Posterior deltoids
- Biceps brachii, brachialis

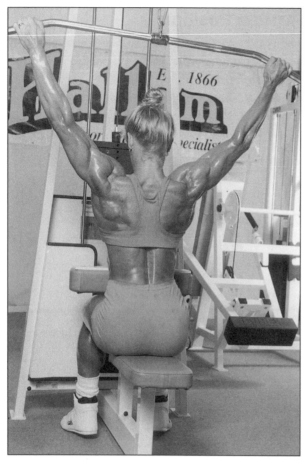

Starting Position

1. Stand in front of the lat pull-down machine and grasp the bar with an overhand grip (wide).
2. Sit down with feet flat on the floor, back straight, and thighs secured underneath the thigh pads.
3. At this point arms are fully extended, holding the bar overhead.

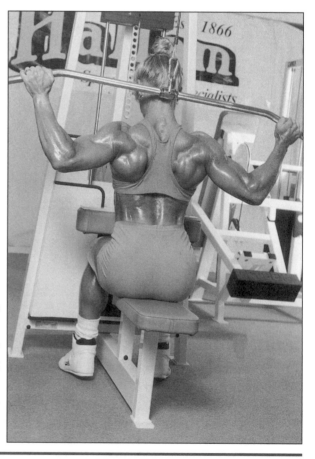

Exercise Technique

1. Initiate the movement by pulling your elbows downward and backward.
2. As the bar approaches your head, lean slightly forward, allowing the bar to touch the top part of your neck.
3. Slowly bring the bar back to the starting position. Repeat the movement until the desired number of repetitions is completed.

Primary Muscles Worked
- Erector spinae
- Gluteals

Back Extensions

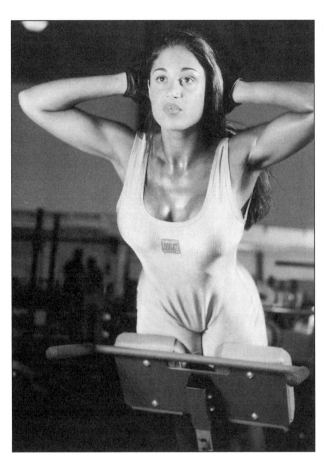

Starting Position

1. Holding the handles of the back extension machine, secure your ankles underneath the small pads and lower your hips onto the larger pads at the front of the apparatus.
2. Keep your legs straight and arms crossed behind your head throughout the entire movement.
3. At this point, your torso should be almost parallel to the floor.

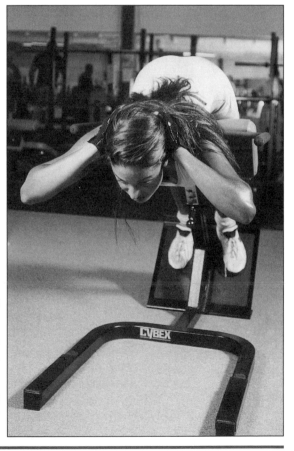

Exercise Technique

1. Lower your torso until it is almost perpendicular to the floor.
2. Slowly bring your torso back to the starting position. Repeat the movement until the desired number of repetitions is completed.
3. Remember not to arch upward excessively, for this can cause compression of the vertebrae in your spine.

Deltoids

The whole idea behind bodybuilding is to make your physique stand out above the rest. Combine a wide shoulder structure with well-developed deltoids and a thin waistline and you can potentially build the type of symmetry and size that wins bodybuilding titles and competitions. No one with weak deltoids has ever won a major bodybuilding title or competition. In fact, no one with even average deltoids will ever win a major bodybuilding show, because the deltoids are such a key muscle group. Why are the deltoids so important to bodybuilders? Because they are visible from every angle during a pose—therefore weak deltoids can be detected from every angle. Have you ever seen a competitive bodybuilder turn to his or her back side to perform the back double biceps pose—and that huge mound of flesh that creates the rear deltoid is lacking? It is an unfavorable attribute.

For teens who are starting to train, clavicle widening movements can be very effective. Your ligaments, tendons, and cartilage are still soft, and your epiphyseal plates have not yet closed (your bones have not stopped growing). Therefore, further bone growth is still possible; in fact, the skeletal frame and fascia tissues can still stretch. Although most bodybuilders are not in their teens and their bone plates have stopped growing, they can still widen their clavicles through a thickening of the cartilage; and by building a lot of mass on their medial deltoid, they can give the illusion that their shoulders are wider than they really are.

Exercises such as ultra-wide chin-ups and wide-grip lat machine pull-downs can stretch the clavicles and widen the shoulder blades. Ultra-wide chin-ups must not be confused with wide-grip chin-ups for the lats. Your hands must be placed as wide as physically possible. For clavicle stretching to occur, you must perform the reps slowly and fully and at the bottom of each rep hang and feel the stretching and widening of your shoulder blades. It is as if you were trying to dislocate your scapulae (without actually doing it). If you are not strong enough to perform the ultra-wide chin-ups, use wide-grip lat machine pull-downs for clavicle stretch and superset it with wide-grip chin-up hangs. Your aim in wide-grip chin-up hangs is to hold the widened position as long as you can without actually dislocating your clavicles. Remember that pain and discomfort are normal with these exercises, because you are stretching and pulling the clavicles apart. Understand also these exercises are not performed for lat development.

Mass exercises—such as seated-front dumbbell press, or standing dumbbell side and bent laterals—will definitely put size on all three deltoid heads, especially the medial deltoids (standing dumbbell side laterals).

Trapezius

Bodybuilders are easily visible in a large crowd. Many critics have written how bodybuilders actually "wear their sport." No part of the human body is more visible year-round than the neck.

The trapezius muscles are large muscles in the upper back area. They form a star. The points of the star are situated at the base of the skull (upper points), near the points of the shoulders, and about halfway down the spine (lower point). The primary function of the trapezius muscles is to pull the shoulders upward and backward. They also contract to help arch the lower back.

When performing a lot of back exercises and deltoid exercises, you place primary stress on the trapezius muscles. According to our research, behind-the-back barbell shrugs produce the highest levels of electrical activation for the trapezius muscles.

Primary Muscles Worked

• Medial deltoids

Standing Dumbbell Side Laterals

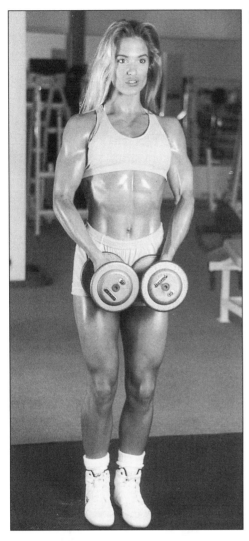

Starting Position

1. Stand with back straight, knees slightly bent, and feet slightly less than shoulder-width apart.
2. Keep back erect and elbows slightly flexed throughout the entire movement.
3. Grasp the dumbbells using an overhand grip, with palms facing each other.
4. Press dumbbells together approximately 4 to 6 inches in front of your hips.

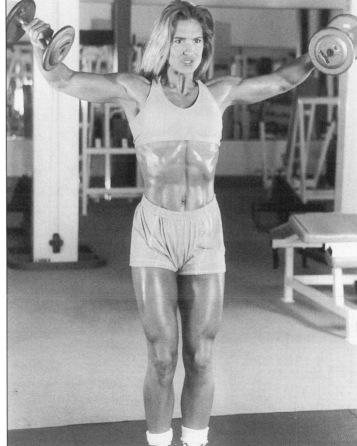

Exercise Technique

1. Keeping elbows slightly bent, raise the dumbbells laterally, in an arc toward the ceiling, until arms are parallel to the floor, and hold briefly.
2. Slowly lower the dumbbells to the starting position. Repeat the movement until the desired number of repetitions is completed.

Standing Dumbbell Bent Laterals

Primary Muscles Worked
- Posterior deltoids
- Medial deltoids
- Upper trapezius

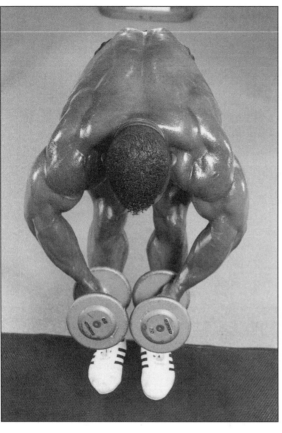

Starting Position

1. Stand with back straight, knees bent, and feet shoulder-width apart.
2. Grasp the dumbbells using an overhand grip, with palms facing each other.
3. Bend at the hips until back is parallel to the floor and arms are hanging down in an extended position (arms perpendicular to the floor).

Exercise Technique

1. Keeping elbows slightly bent, raise the dumbbells laterally in an arc-like motion until arms are parallel to the floor.
2. Slowly lower the dumbbells to the starting position. Repeat the movement until the desired number of repetitions is completed.

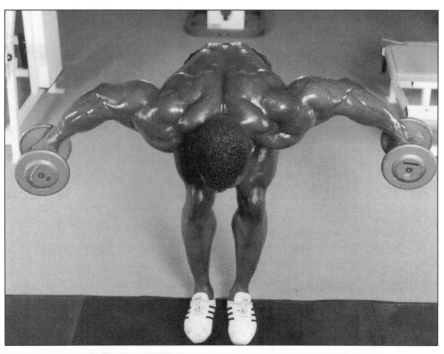

Primary Muscles Worked
  • Anterior deltoids

Seated Front Dumbbell Press

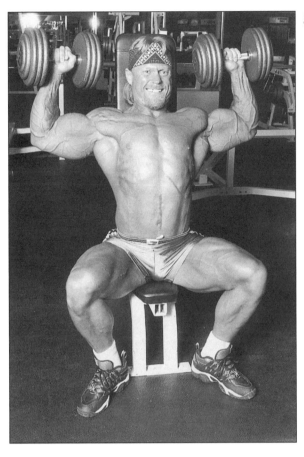

Starting Position

1. Grasp two dumbbells using an overhand grip, and sit down on an upright bench.
2. Lift the dumbbells to shoulder level.
3. Rotate palms so they are facing forward.

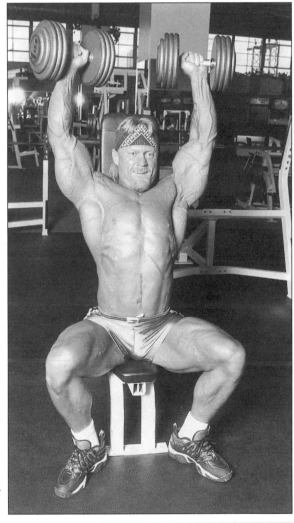

Exercise Technique

1. Slowly push the dumbbells directly upward until they touch each other at straight arms' length, and slowly return the dumbbells to the starting position.
2. Remember never to lock your elbows at the top of the movement.
3. Repeat the movement until the desired number of repetitions is completed.

Standing Front Dumbbell Raises

Primary Muscles Worked
• Anterior deltoids

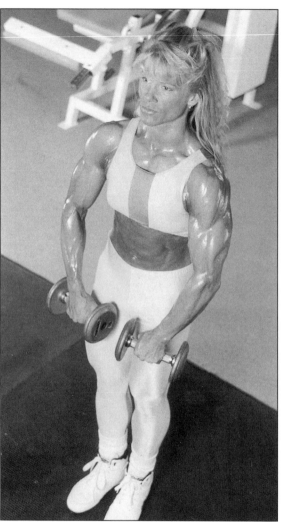

Starting Position

1. Stand with back straight, knees slightly bent, and feet slightly less than shoulder-width apart.
2. Grasp the dumbbells using an overhand grip, with palms facing downward.
3. Let arms hang straight down at your sides, holding the dumbbells approximately 2 to 4 inches from upper thigh level.

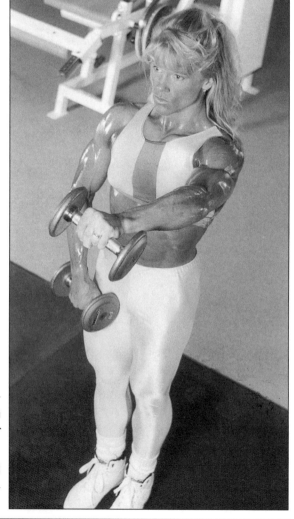

Exercise Technique

1. Keeping elbows slightly bent throughout the entire movement, raise the right dumbbell from upper thigh level to eye level, and slowly lower dumbbell to starting position.
2. Repeat the movement with the left dumbbell, and continue alternating right and left until the desired number of repetitions is completed.

Primary Muscles Worked
• Anterior deltoids

Seated Front Barbell Press

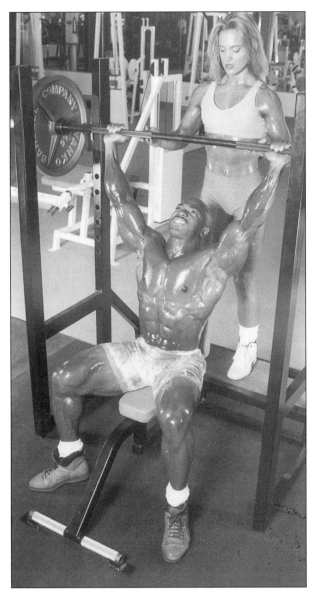

Starting Position

1. Sit on the bench with back pressed firmly against the padding for support.
2. Grasp the barbell using an overhand grip, with hands approximately 3 to 5 inches wider than shoulder-width apart.
3. Have a spotter help you lift the Olympic bar from the standards.
4. At this point the Olympic bar is held straight above your head, with elbows slightly flexed.

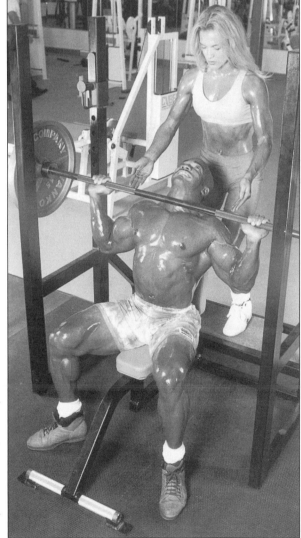

Exercise Technique

1. Slowly lower the weight down to your anterior deltoids (in front of head), and without bouncing the barbell at the bottom of the movement push it upward to the starting position.
2. Never lock your elbows at the top of the movement.
3. Repeat the movement until the desired number of repetitions is completed.

DELTOIDS AND TRAPEZIUS

Shrugs
(Olympic Bar)

Primary Muscles Worked
• Upper trapezius   • Rhomboids

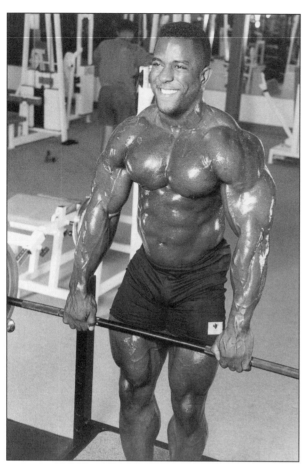

Starting Position

1. Keep back erect, knees slightly bent, and a shoulder-width stance throughout the movement.

2. Grasp the Olympic bar using an overhand grip with hands slightly wider than shoulder-width apart.

3. At this point the barbell is held at straight arms' length, with a slight bend in your elbows.

4. The Olympic bar is resting across your upper thighs.

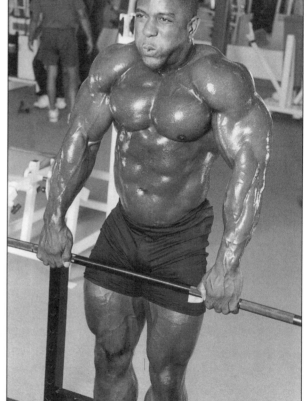

Exercise Technique

1. To initiate the movement, lift your shoulders toward your ears and hold the contraction for a moment.

2. When the contraction is complete, slowly lower the bar to a point where a comfortable stretch is felt in the working muscles (facilitates maximum range of motion).

3. Repeat the movement until the desired number of repetitions is completed.

Primary Muscles Worked

• Trapezius muscles   • Anterior and medial deltoids

Upright Rows
(Olympic Bar)

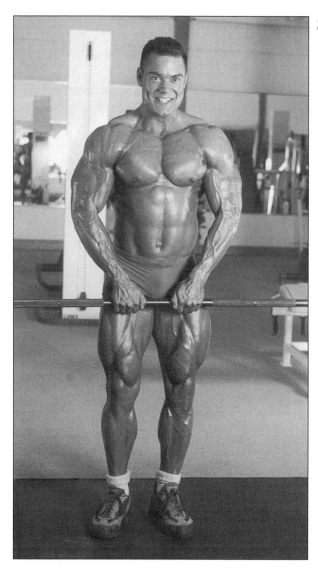

Starting Position

1. Keep back erect, knees slightly bent, and a shoulder-width stance throughout the movement.

2. Grasp barbell with an overhand grip, with hands approximately two thumb-widths apart.

3. At this point the barbell is held at straight arms' length, with a slight bend in your elbows.

4. The Olympic bar is resting across the upper thighs.

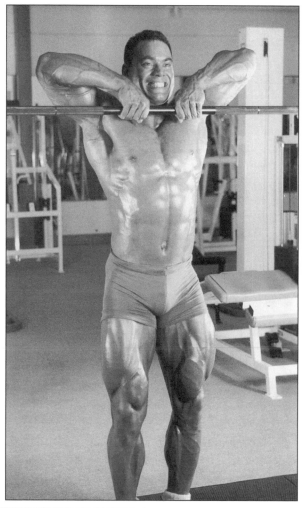

Exercise Technique

1. Raise the bar from the extended position to the point where it reaches your chin (raise elbows high), and slowly lower the bar to the starting position.

2. Repeat the movement until the desired number of repetitions is completed.

Press Behind Neck
(Olympic Bar)

Primary Muscles Worked
• Posterior deltoid   • Upper trapezius

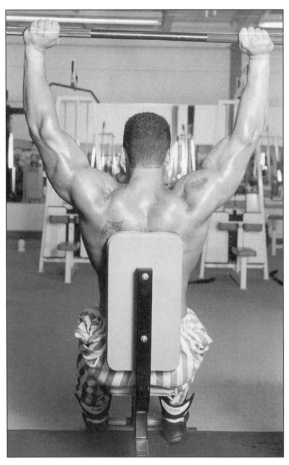

Starting Position

1. Sit on the bench with back pressed firmly against the padding for support.
2. Grasp the Olympic bar using an overhand grip, with hands placed 3 to 5 inches wider than shoulder-width apart.
3. Lift the Olympic bar from the standards and hold it directly above your head, with elbows slightly flexed.

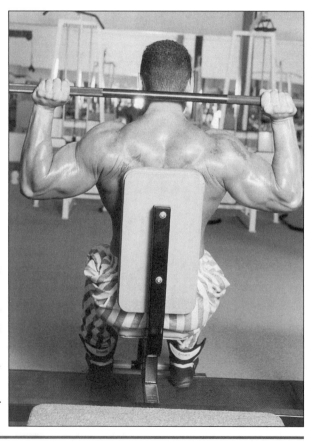

Exercise Technique

1. Slowly lower the Olympic bar behind your head to a level slightly below your ears.
2. Without bouncing at the bottom of the movement, push the bar upward to the starting position.
3. Never lock your elbows at the top of the movement.
4. Repeat the movement until the desired number of repetitions is completed.

Triceps

Although today's bodybuilders do plenty of isolation exercises in their triceps workouts, much of triceps mass development comes from pressing exercises. Whenever bodybuilders do bench presses for the pectorals—whether incline or decline and dips—they also place serious stress on the triceps. By performing overhead presses for deltoids, you are also placing intense stress on the triceps muscles. As a result, the potential for overtraining the triceps muscles is high.

How many sets of triceps work should you be doing in a workout? At the beginner level, do no more than 3 to 5 sets of total triceps training. With three to six months of steady training, you can probably increase this total to 5 to 7 sets. An advanced bodybuilder will probably need 8 to 12 sets for the triceps.

Decline Triceps Extension (Olympic Bar)

Primary Muscles Worked
• Outer and medial heads of triceps

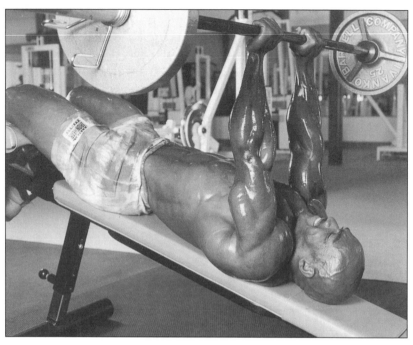

Starting Position

1. Grasp the Olympic bar using an overhand grip (palms facing downward), with hands less than shoulder-width apart.

2. Sit on the edge of the decline bench and secure feet and ankles underneath pads.

3. Lie on the decline bench, simultaneously bringing the Olympic bar to a position where you simulate a bench press movement.

4. Once your arms are extended and palms are facing upward, the Olympic bar is held directly over eye level.

Exercise Technique

1. Keeping your upper arms fixed, slowly flex your elbows and lower the bar to your forehead.

2. Once the bar almost touches your forehead, use your triceps muscle to push your arms back to full extension.

3. Repeat the movement until the desired number of repetitions is completed.

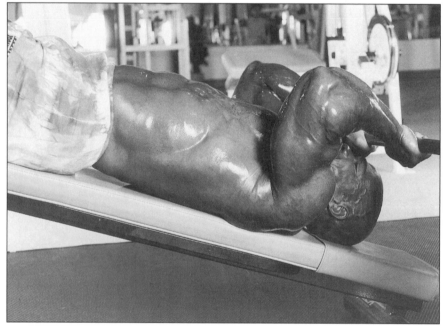

Primary Muscles Worked
  • Outer and medial heads
    of triceps

Triceps Press-Down
(Angled Bar)

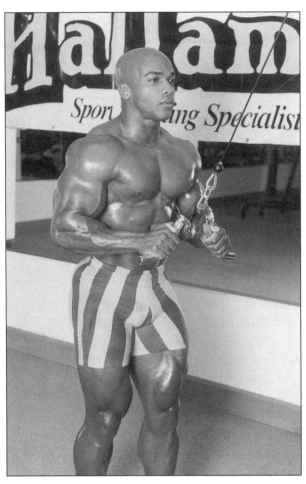

Starting Position

1. Attach the angled bar to the overhead pulley.
2. Keep your knees slightly bent, back erect, and feet shoulder-width apart.
3. Facing the overhead pulley, grasp the angled bar using an overhand grip.
4. Pull the bar down far enough to allow your upper arms to rest against the sides of your torso.
5. Your elbows should be flexed.

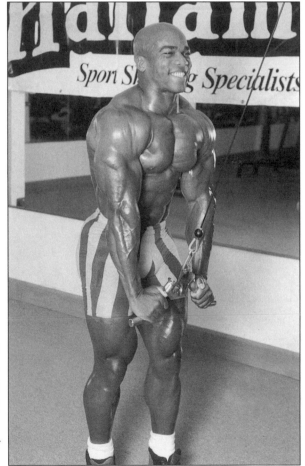

Exercise Technique

1. Moving only your lower arms, slowly press down on the bar until arms are fully extended.
2. Hold the extended position for a moment and then resist as lower arms return to the starting position.
3. Repeat the movement until the desired number of repetitions is completed.

Triceps Dip
Between Benches

Primary Muscles Worked
• Outer and medial heads
of triceps

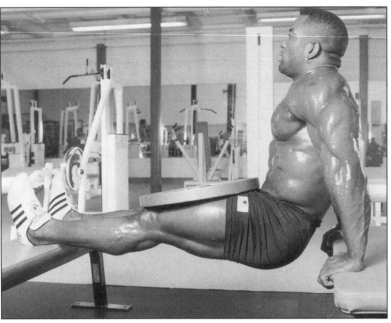

Starting Position

1. Stand between two flat benches that are approximately 3 feet apart (varies depending on size of person).

2. Place your hands on the edge of one bench, shoulder-width apart, and place your heels on the other bench.

3. Extend your arms completely and hold this position.

Exercise Technique

1. Initiate the movement by slowly bending your arms until your body is lowered between the benches.

2. Slowly push back up to the starting position by straightening your arms, and repeat the movement until the desired number of repetitions is completed.

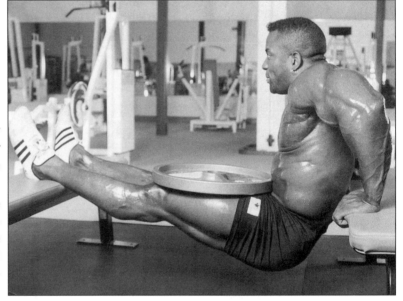

Primary Muscles Worked
  • Outer head of triceps

One-Arm Cable Triceps Extensions

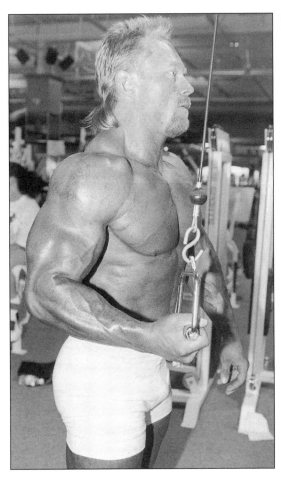

Starting Position

1. Attach a loop handle to the overhead cable pulley.
2. Facing the pulley, grasp the loop handle in your right hand with an underhanded grip and step approximately one foot back from the pulley.
3. Pull the handle down far enough to allow your upper arm to rest firmly against the side of your torso.
4. Your elbows should be flexed.

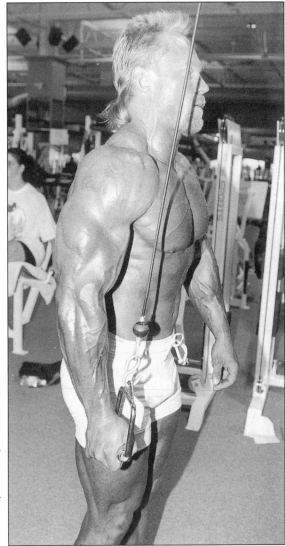

Exercise Technique

1. Moving only your lower arm, slowly pull the handle back and downward until your arm is fully extended.
2. Hold the position in full extension for a moment and then resist as your lower arm returns to the starting position.
3. Repeat the movement until the desired number of repetitions is completed.
4. Repeat for the other hand.

Overhead Rope Triceps Extensions

Primary Muscles Worked
• All heads of triceps

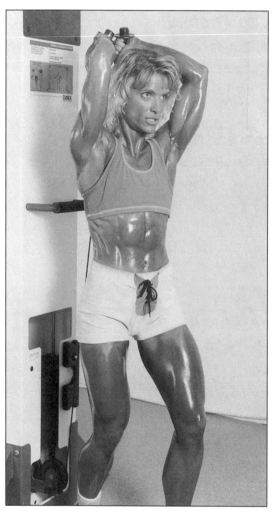

Starting Position

1. Attach the rope to the overhead pulley.
2. Stand with back facing the pulley machine.
3. With feet staggered (one leg in front of the other), place your forward foot flat on the floor. Flex your back foot, with only the ball of your foot touching the ground.
4. Grasp the rope with an overhand grip (palms facing each other), and bend slightly forward at the waist.
5. In the starting position, your upper arms follow your ear line.
6. Your elbows are completely flexed and the rope is behind your neck.

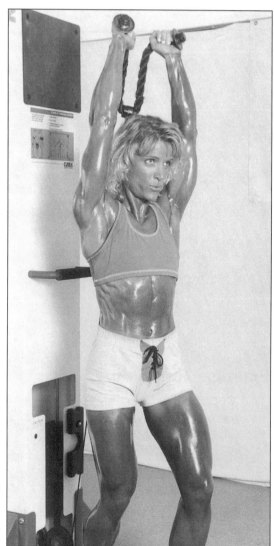

Exercise Technique

1. Initiate the movement by slowly extending the lower part of your arms.
2. Hold the fully extended position for a moment.
3. Slowly bring your arms back to the starting position.
4. Repeat the movement until the desired number of repetitions is completed.
5. Bending occurs only at your elbows—your upper arms remain motionless.

Primary Muscles Worked
- Inner and medial heads of triceps

Seated One-Arm Triceps Extensions (Neutral Grip)

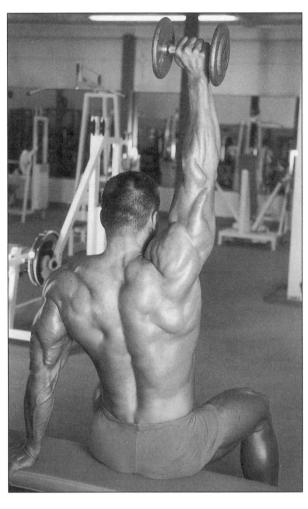

Starting Position

1. Sit on a flat bench with feet flat on the floor.
2. Grasp a dumbbell with an overhand grip (palm faces forward throughout the movement).
3. Hold the dumbbell overhead, with your arm fully extended.

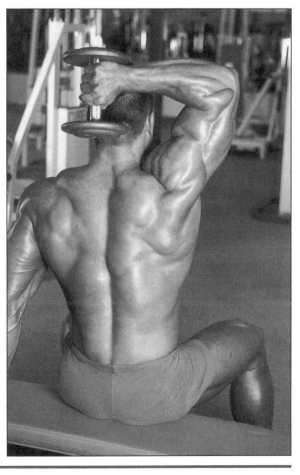

Exercise Technique

1. Lower the dumbbell until your forearm is parallel to the floor.
2. At this point the dumbbell is positioned behind your neck (finish of movement).
3. Without bouncing the weight at the bottom of the movement, slowly extend the dumbbell to the starting position. Repeat the movement until the desired number of repetitions is completed.
4. Repeat for the other hand.

Close-Grip
Bench Press (Olympic Bar)

Primary Muscles Worked

- All heads of triceps
- Anterior deltoids
- Pectoralis major (mid and lower chest)

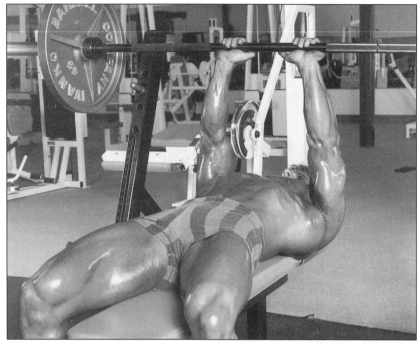

Starting Position

1. Lie on a flat bench, with back pressed firmly against the padding and feet on the floor.

2. Grasp the bar using an overhand grip with hands approximately two thumb-widths apart, and lift bar from the standards.

3. Arms should be fully extended (not locked) and palms facing forward as the bar is held.

Exercise Technique

1. Bend at the elbows, lowering the bar to the midpoint of your chest.

2. Without bouncing the weight off your chest, use your triceps muscles to press it back to the starting position.

3. Repeat the movement until the desired number of repetitions is completed.

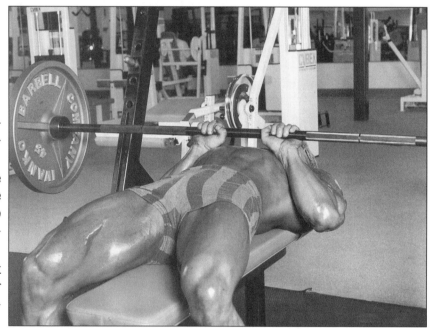

Primary Muscles Worked
- Outer and medial heads of triceps

Dumbbell or Cable Kickbacks

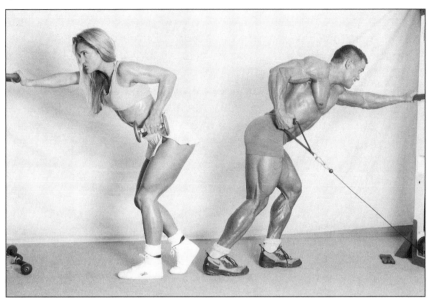

Starting Position

1. Grasp a dumbbell or loop handle on the low pulley cable, using an overhand grip (palm facing body with dumbbell, palm facing downward with loop handle).

2. Bend forward at hips and grasp the support handle on the pulley with your nonworking arm.

3. Press your upper working arm firmly against the side of your torso (upper arm is now parallel to the floor, and lower arm is perpendicular to the floor).

4. Feet should be staggered, one in front of the other.

Exercise Technique

1. Initiate the movement by slowly extending your arm fully.

2. Once your arm is fully extended, hold the position for a moment, and then lower the weight to the starting position.

3. Repeat the movement until the desired number of repetitions is completed.

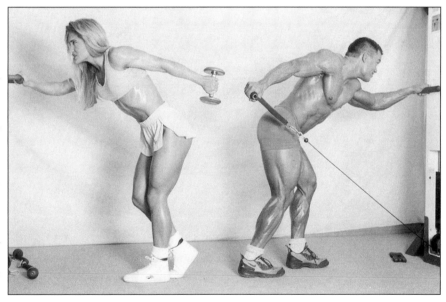

Biceps

The biceps are most bodybuilders' favorite muscles to train. Despite the biceps' relatively small size compared to the muscles of the thighs, back, and chest, our love affair with the biceps no doubt arises from our culture's association of big biceps with strength and masculinity. Every great champion in the past six decades has had huge arms and biceps.

Use biceps preacher curls, standing dumbbell curls, and incline dumbbell curls to pack mass and peak your biceps. Movements such as dumbbell or cable-concentration curls are better for adding height to the peak of your biceps muscles.

Primary Muscles Worked
• Biceps brachii   • Brachialis

Biceps Preacher Curls
(Olympic Bar)

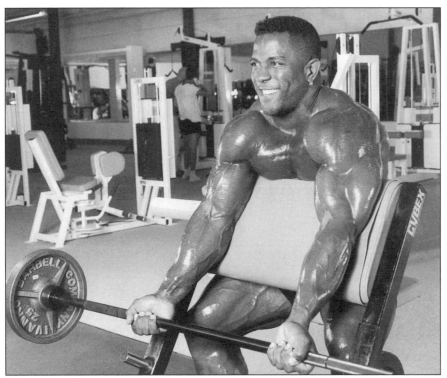

Starting Position

1. Sit on the preacher curl bench.
2. Grasp the Olympic bar using an underhanded grip (palms facing upward), with hands shoulder-width apart.
3. Arms are extended (not locked) as triceps are resting over the angled surface of the preacher bench.

Exercise Technique

1. Initiate the movement by flexing at the elbow and curling the bar upward toward the shoulders.
2. Triceps always maintain direct contact with the angled surface of the preacher bench.
3. Bar is then slowly lowered to the starting position. The movement is repeated until the desired number of repetitions is completed.

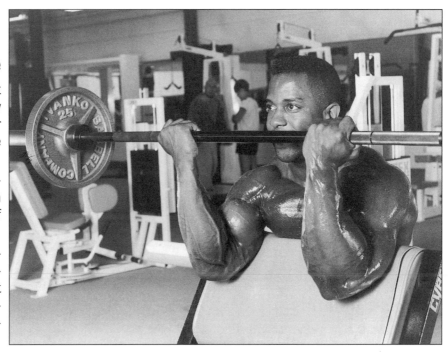

Standing Biceps Curl
(Olympic Bar/Narrow Grip)

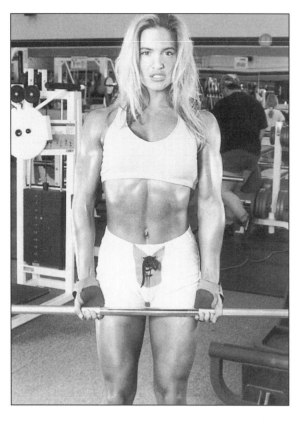

Starting Position

1. Grasp the barbell using an underhanded grip (palms facing forward), with hands slightly less than shoulder-width apart.
2. Stand with back erect, knees slightly bent, and feet shoulder-width apart throughout the movement.
3. Arms are fully extended and pressed firmly against your torso.
4. At this point the bar is resting across your upper thighs.

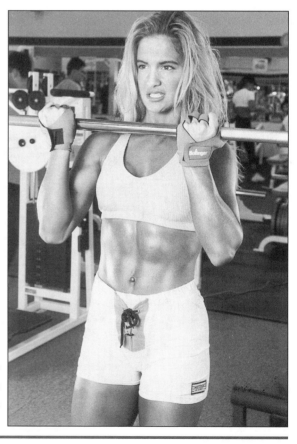

Exercise Technique

1. Initiate the movement by flexing at the elbows, curling the bar toward your shoulders.
2. When your biceps are maximally contracted, slowly lower the bar to the starting position. Repeat the movement until the desired number of repetitions is completed.

Primary Muscles Worked
• Biceps brachii

Incline Seated
Dumbbell Curl (Alternate)

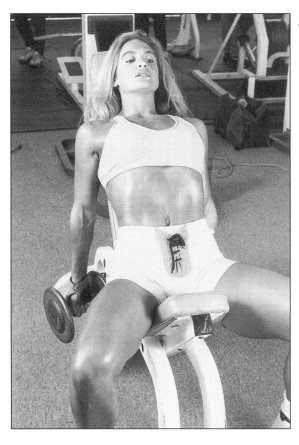

Starting Position

1. Lie on an incline bench, with back pressed firmly against the padding and feet flat on the floor.
2. Hang arms down at your sides, holding the dumbbells with an underhanded grip (palms facing upward).

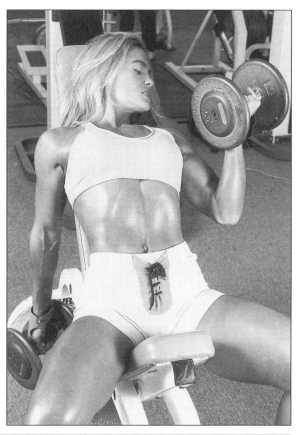

Exercise Technique

1. Slowly curl the right dumbbell toward your right shoulder.
2. When maximum biceps contraction occurs, slowly lower the dumbbell to the starting position and repeat the movement with the left arm.
3. Continue alternating right and left arms until the desired number of repetitions is completed.

Standing Dumbbell Curl
(Alternate)

Primary Muscles Worked
• Biceps brachii

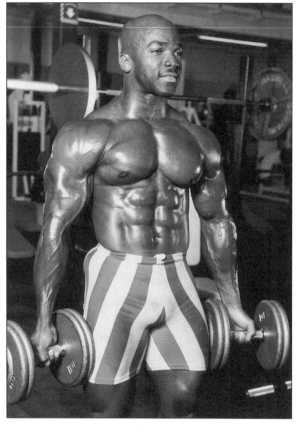

Starting Position

1. Grasp the dumbbells using an underhanded grip (palms facing forward).
2. Stand with back erect, knees slightly bent, and feet shoulder-width apart throughout the movement.
3. Arms are fully extended, and the dumbbells are hanging straight down at your sides.

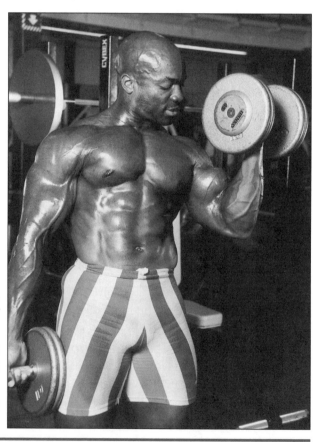

Exercise Technique

1. Initiate the movement by flexing at the elbow, curling the right dumbbell up toward your shoulder.
2. The dumbbell is then slowly lowered to the starting position, and the movement repeated with the left arm.
3. Continue alternating arms until the desired number of repetitions is completed.

Primary Muscles Worked
• Biceps brachii

Concentration Dumbbell Curl

Starting Position

1. Grasp the dumbbell with your right hand, using an underhanded grip (palms facing upward), and sit on a flat bench.

2. Legs are spread wide apart.

3. Lean forward at the waist and rest your right elbow on the inside of your right thigh, with your arm in full extension.

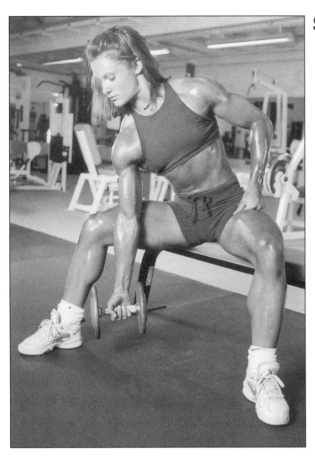

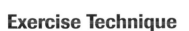

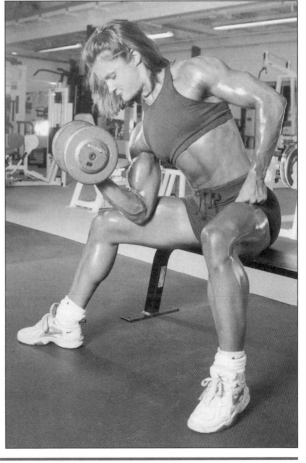

Exercise Technique

1. With your elbow resting on the inside of your thigh, slowly curl the dumbbell toward your shoulder.

2. When maximum biceps contraction occurs, slowly lower the dumbbell to the starting position. Repeat the movement until the desired number of repetitions is completed.

3. Repeat for the left hand.

Standing Biceps Curl
(Olympic Bar/Wide Grip)

Primary Muscles Worked
- Biceps brachii
- Brachialis

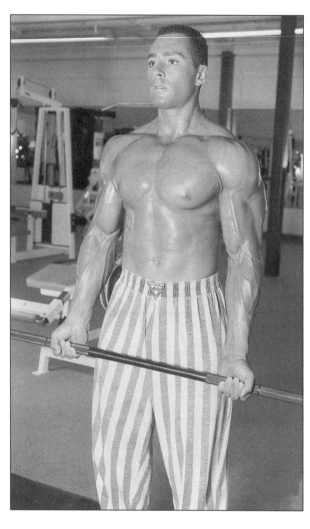

Starting Position

1. Grasp the barbell using an underhanded grip (palms facing upward), with hands 2 to 3 inches wider than shoulder-width apart.

2. Stand with back erect, knees slightly bent, and feet slightly wider than shoulder-width apart throughout the movement.

3. At this point arms are fully extended, with the bar resting across your upper thighs.

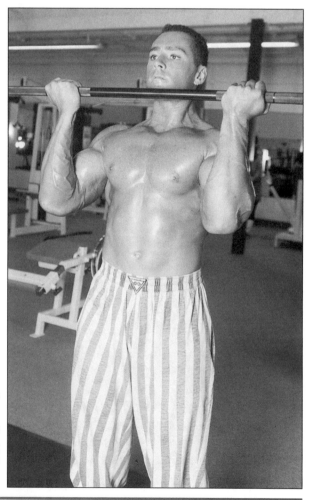

Exercise Technique

1. Initiate the movement by flexing at the elbow, curling the bar up toward your shoulder.

2. When biceps are maximally contracted, slowly lower the bar to the starting position. Repeat the movement until the desired number of repetitions is completed.

Primary Muscles Worked
• Biceps brachii   • Brachialis

Standing EZ Biceps Curl
(Wide Grip)

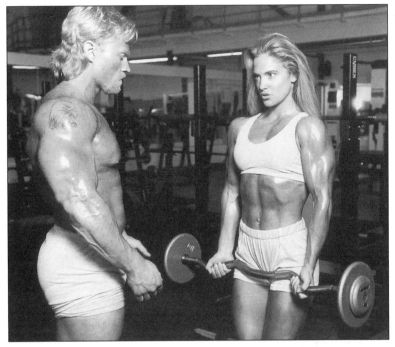

Starting Position

1. Stand with back straight, knees slightly bent and feet slightly less than shoulder-width apart throughout the entire movement.

2. Grasp the EZ curl bar using an underhanded grip (palms facing forward), with hands slightly wider than shoulder-width apart.

3. Arms are fully extended and pressed against the sides of your torso.

Exercise Technique

1. Initiate the movement by flexing at the elbows and curling the bar up toward your shoulders.

2. When your biceps are maximally contracted, slowly lower the bar to the starting position. Repeat the movement until the desired number of repetitions is completed.

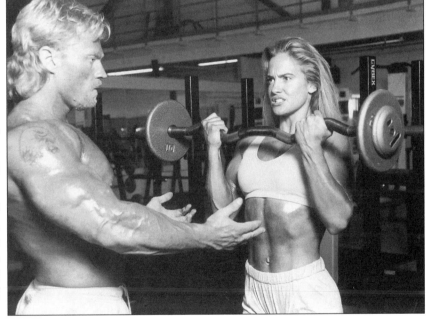

Forearm

Some bodybuilders have genetically gifted forearms without even directly training the muscle group. Others are less fortunate: regardless of how hard they work, they never have fantastic forearms.

Now all great pro and amateur bodybuilders at the national and international level have exceptional forearms. If you are lucky enough to have optimum genetics for fabulous forearm development, good for you. If you are average or below average in forearm development, here are some pointers: save your forearms for the end of your workout; train your forearms two or three times a week; finally, train them hard and do not get discouraged—gains are slow in coming, but they will come.

Wrist Curls
(Olympic Bar)

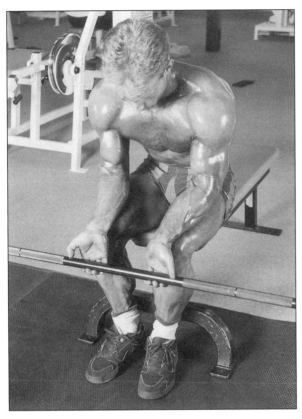

Starting Position

1. Grasp the bar with an underhanded grip (palms facing upward), and sit on the end of a flat bench.

2. Place feet flat on the floor, slightly wider than shoulder-width apart.

3. Leaning your torso forward, run your forearms down your thighs until your wrists and hands hang over the ends of your knees.

4. Allow the weight to be lowered until the bar is rolled onto your fingers.

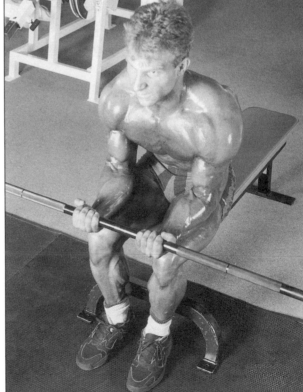

Exercise Technique

1. Using your forearm muscles, raise the bar by flexing your fingers and curling your wrists to as high a position as possible.

2. Slowly lower the weight to the starting position. Repeat the movement until the desired number of repetitions is completed.

Wrist Extensions
(Olympic Bar)

Primary Muscles Worked
• Forearm flexors

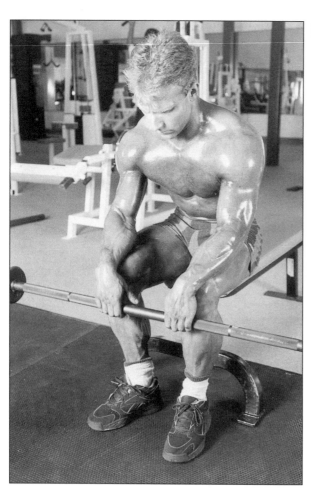

Starting Position

1. Grasp the bar with an overhand grip (palms facing downward), and sit on the end of a flat bench.
2. Place feet flat on the floor, slightly closer than shoulder-width apart.
3. Leaning your torso forward, run your forearms down your thighs until your wrists and hands hang over the ends of your knees.
4. Allow the weight to be lowered until the barbell is rolled onto your fingers.

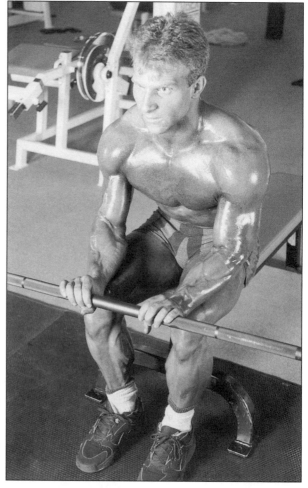

Exercise Technique

1. Using your forearm muscles, raise the bar by extending your wrists to as high a position as possible.
2. Slowly lower the weight to the starting position. Repeat the movement until the desired number of repetitions is completed.

PART III

THE SIX PHASES OF TRAINING

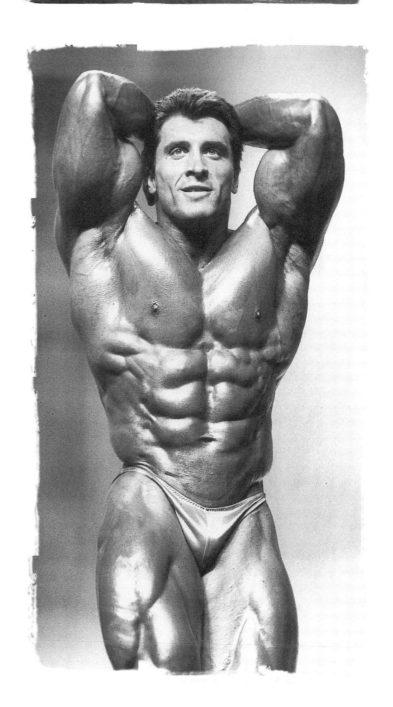

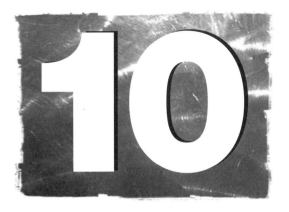

ANATOMICAL ADAPTATION (AA)

Most bodybuilders at the beginner level start rigorous training programs without being ready for it. Many times such rigorous programs immediately focus either on increasing muscle size (hypertrophy), or on increasing muscle density and strength through use of heavy loads.

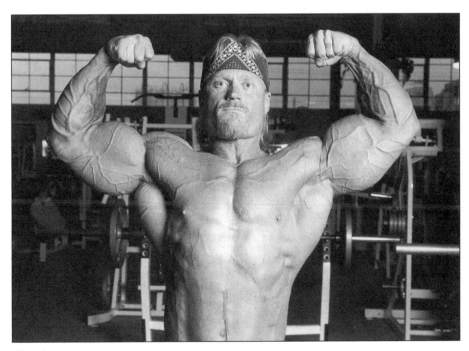

Absolute power.

Yet the body needs time to progressively adapt to a new and more demanding training stimulus without incurring injury along the way. Individuals must develop anatomical readiness (muscles, ligaments, and tendons) for strenuous training; and they must understand that vigorous strength or bodybuilding training places high stress on ligaments and tendons, potentially leading to injury. Training programs that follow long interruptions, therefore, must begin with *anatomical adaptation* (AA). Between three and six weeks of progressive training can activate the main parts of the body, helping to create a foundation for more difficult programs to follow.

Scope of AA Training

• Activates all of the muscles, ligaments, and tendons of the body so they will better cope with the heavy loads of subsequent training phases.

• Brings all of the body parts into balance—that is, begins to develop previously neglected muscles or body parts and to restore symmetry.

• Prevents injuries through progressive adaptation to heavy loads.

• Progressively increases the athlete's cardiorespiratory endurance.

Duration and Frequency of AA Training

Entry-level bodybuilders and strength trainers need 6 to 12 weeks to train their tendons and ligaments. Although the AA program is not a stressful one, some beginners might experience an increase in muscle size. A lengthy AA phase gives novices time to improve their lifting skills before introducing heavy loads. Six weeks are sufficient for recreational bodybuilders and strength trainers with 2 to 3 years of training. Advanced bodybuilders and strength trainers can make do with 3 to 6 weeks of training. Any longer than 6 weeks will not produce a training effect—at that point the body has nothing to adapt to.

Training frequency depends on one's training background and overall commitment to training. Two to three sessions per week are expected for entry-level and recreational bodybuilders, while four to five sessions per week are appropriate for advanced and elite bodybuilders.

Training Method for AA Phase

As previously mentioned, the purpose of the AA phase is to progressively adapt the body to work—to develop the muscles as well their attachments to the bones. The best training method for the AA phase is *circuit training* (CT), mainly because it alternates muscle groups and involves most or all of the body parts and muscles.

Circuit Training

The first variant of circuit training was proposed by Morgan and Adamson (1959) from Leeds University, and was used as a method to develop general fitness. Initially, CT used several stations

Scott Milnes engaging in AA training to prepare for upcoming rigorous training.

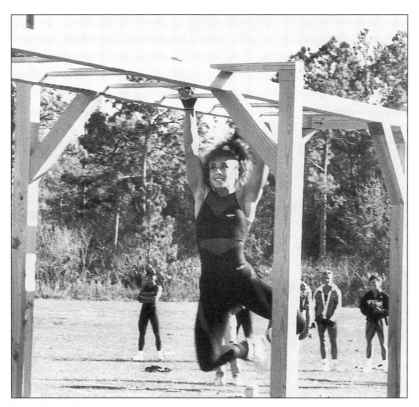

Exercises that use one's own bodyweight are perfect for AA training.

arranged in a circle, hence the name "circuit training." The exercises were organized so that the muscle groups used were constantly alternating from station to station.

A huge variety of exercises are appropriate for CT programs, including those that use a person's own body weight (such as dips and pull-ups) and those that require dumbbells, barbells, or strength-training machines (such as leg extensions, bench presses, etc.).

A circuit may be repeated several times—depending on the number of exercises involved, number of repetitions per station, the load used, and the individual's work tolerance and fitness level. Select CT exercises to *alternate muscle groups,* thus facilitating a better and faster recovery between stations. The rest interval (RI) should be 60 to 90 seconds between stations, and one to three minutes between circuits. Most gyms offer many different apparatuses that make it possible to create circuits that involve most or all of the muscle groups and that continually challenge athletes' skills and maintain their interest.

Strength and Cardiovascular Circuit Training

For individuals whose goal is both strength training for a better AA phase and creation of a good cardiovascular base, we offer the following combination:

- 10 to 15 minutes of cardiovascular training
- 3 to 4 strength training exercises
- 10 minutes cardiovascular exercise
- 3 to 4 strength exercises
- 10 minutes of cardiovascular exercise

Such a program can last 45 to 60 minutes. To make it longer, you may either repeat the circuit or add another segment of 3 to 4 exercises, ending with more cardiovascular work.

Program Design for the AA Phase

From the first week of training, athletes must plan their workouts based on objective data. This means testing your 1RM for at least the main exercises or prime movers, so that you can objectively calculate your training loads as a percentage of maximum (see chapter 3).

During the first one to two weeks, it is normal to experience some muscle soreness and fatigue—especially in people who have not been very active in the past. Once the muscles become accustomed to working again, these problems quickly disappear. As the program continues, you will begin to feel good and the program will seem easy! The best thing you can do for yourself is to continue to train as per the original plan.

ADAPTATION CUE

Resist the temptation to increase the load! There will be plenty of time to do that in the next phase. Remember that even though your muscles feel as if they have adapted, your tendons and ligaments need more time.

The total physical demand per circuit must be progressively and individually increased. Figure 10.1 demonstrates how load patterns differ between entry-level and advanced bodybuilders. Because entry-level bodybuilders need a more gradual adaptation, their load remains the same for two weeks (two microcycles) before increasing the demand. Advanced bodybuilders can change their load every microcycle. Use these guidelines when creating your own plan.

To better monitor improvements in training and be constantly able to calculate the load, we suggest testing for 1RM at the beginning of weeks 1 and 4, and at the beginning of week 1 of the next training phase.

As figure 10.1 illustrates, toward the end of the AA phase the load reaches a percentage of maximum that allows you to immediately make the transition to the H phase. Use the guidelines in table 10.1 to create your own AA phase.

This chapter suggests several types of AA training programs. To perform the circuit, follow the exercises from the top down, performing only one set before moving to the next station. This approach facilitates recovery for each muscle group, since the groups are constantly alternated. If too many bodybuilders are competing for the same equipment, however, or you have to wait too long between sets, then perform all the sets at one station before moving to the next. See tables 10.2 to 10.5 on pages 201-202 for the programs.

If you are doing a large number of exercises per session, you can follow a split routine in which you train the same muscle groups every second day. If you are doing a small number of exercises, you can perform all of them in one day and repeat them as many times as you train per week.

Table 10.1 Guidelines for Creating an Individual Anatomical Adaptation Plan

	Bodybuilder's classification		
	Entry-level	**Recreational**	**Advanced**
Duration of AA phase (weeks)	6-12	6	3-6
Number of stations	9-12	9	9
Number of sets/training sessions	2	3	3-4
RI between sets (minutes)	2-3	2	2
Frequency/week	2-3	3-4	3-5
Aerobic training sessions/week	1	1-2	2

Reprinted from Bompa 1996.

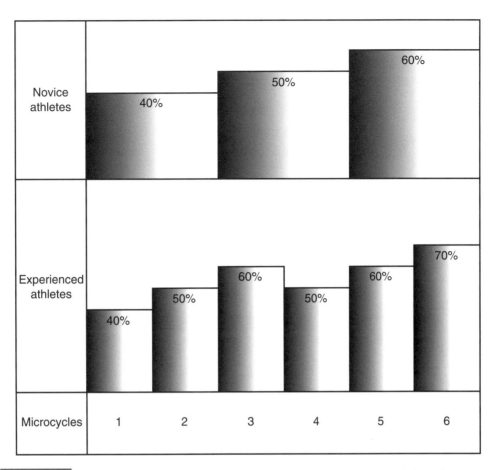

Figure 10.1 A suggested pattern of load increments for circuit training, for entry-level and advanced bodybuilders and strength trainers.

Reprinted from Bompa 1996.

ANATOMICAL ADAPTATION CUES

- Other exercises may be selected.
- Test for 1RM early in week 1 and at the end of weeks 4 and 7 (first week of the next phase).
- Progression over the 6 weeks occurs in the form of increased load, and more sets and repetitions.
- Load increments for leg curls start at a lower load and have a slower progression, because the hamstring muscles are easier to injure. Go slowly on hams!
- Do 20 to 25 minutes of aerobic work as part of your warm-up.
- Remember that 40/15 $\times$ 3 means load/# of repetitions $\times$ sets (in this example, three sets of 15 repetitions using a load equal to 40 percent of 1RM).

Nutrition for the Anatomical Adaptation Phase

We will assume that you are beginning the Metabolic Diet during this phase. Our assumption may not necessarily be the case, but following that plan makes the most sense for anyone wanting to follow our Periodization plan.

During most of your time on the Metabolic Diet, you won't often find yourself restricting calories. In fact, some people find they have a problem getting enough calories, especially in the hypertrophy phase. Even in other phases, many athletes find that with increased training and exercise they can take in huge amounts of food without any negative consequences. The only phase that usually requires a gradual reduction in calories is the definition phase.

At the beginning, you should make the dietary switch gradually. Don't jump right in at a low calorie level. Often the fatigue and discomfort you may feel are simply from a lack of food rather than a lack of carbohydrates. And if some of this discomfort is from the actual metabolic switch, it is compounded if you are starving. We also don't want you to feel bloated or to suffer from the constipation and diarrhea that you may have as a result of the sometimes radical change in your macronutrient intake. Dieting per se often affects the bowels and can compound any effect that may come from starting on the Metabolic Diet.

Your starting point for daily calories on this diet should be 18 times your bodyweight. If you weigh 200 pounds, this would call for 200 $\times$ 18, or 3,600, calories a day during the weekday portion of the diet. This intake level creates a static phase where you lose some body fat, gain some muscle mass, and maintain about the same weight. This is a phase in which you'll be changing the ratio of internal masses to some degree, but most of what you're trying to do is allow your body its easiest path toward adapting to the diet.

As you continue in this phase, you should experiment with the above formula to find your precise maintenance level for calories. This will let you know from what point you need to add or subtract calories for gains or losses in other parts of the diet. It's also not a bad idea to keep a two- to three-day diary of what you're eating and then have someone who has some expertise in diets look at it. That way you will get numbers and foods you can best work with and figure what you need precisely for maintenance.

One result of the Metabolic Diet is that the bowels must readjust to large amounts of meat; and since the fats can act as a stool softener, you may experience some diarrhea. You'll need to firm them up with a fiber supplement. The radical change in diet can also cause constipation.

Most of the problems we've found with people initiating the diet stem from their failure to take the fiber necessary to soften stools or push processed food through the eliminative tract. Although you may be able

Understanding nutrition was one of Bruneau's strong points for acquiring a perfectly muscled and symmetrical physique.

to get away with just eating bran, there is a good chance you will need a supplement to get through this period with minimum discomfort.

The nutritional supplement line we formulated for the Metabolic Diet includes Regulate, a multi-ingredient low-carbohydrate supplement (none of the fiber is absorbed) meant to regulate the bowels and keep the whole intestinal tract healthy. Its combination of ingredients, including several soluble and insoluble fibers, is very effective.

If you use a common commercial fiber product, check the carbohydrate count on the package before purchasing it—refined carbohydrates are often added to make such products taste better.

You will probably have to take the fiber supplement for the first few weeks to a month of the diet. In most cases, your body will have fully adapted to the diet by that time or at least within a few months. If not, it's a good idea to stay on a fiber supplement on a regular or on an as-needed basis.

Some bodybuilders have found that eating a meal high in fiber in the middle of the day provides sufficient fiber. A Caesar salad, for example, provides about 7-1/2 grams of carbohydrates and, as long as you stick close to overall carbohydrate limits, should not present any problem—especially after you have been on the diet for a while.

The "Sweet Tooth" Society

The anatomical adaptation phase will run more smoothly and get you in gear more quickly if you remember that refined carbohydrates are hidden in almost everything you find on supermarket shelves. Seasoning, ketchup, mustard, salad dressings, nuts, BBQ sauce, breaded or processed meats, gourmet coffee, and sausages can all present a problem. These foods are renowned for hidden carbohydrates, and you must check the labels to know what you're getting.

Likewise, restaurants sometimes use a watery sugar on their vegetables. Our society has a sweet tooth that you will encounter at every turn during the weekdays. You will have to be especially careful during this start-up phase as you get used to the diet and learn where the trouble spots are.

Don't Mix Diets

You may be strongly tempted to mix diets, combining the Metabolic Diet with parts of other diets such as high-carbohydrate or low-fat diets. Please resist the temptation!

Many people go on the Metabolic Diet but try to be true to their old high-carbohydrate master. They eat meat, but it's all fish, chicken, and turkey—and while these foods may be

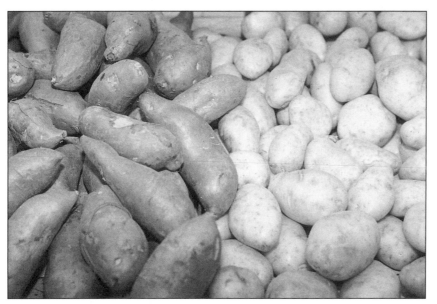
Yams and potatoes are both good sources of complex carbohydrates.

quite nutritious and beneficial, even when used in the Metabolic Diet, they can't be used as a total replacement for red meat. They just don't have enough fat.

What you end up doing with the turkey, chicken, and fish approach is going on a high-protein, low-carbohydrate, low-*fat* diet. Along with being even harder to stay on than the Metabolic Diet, this diet will not provide the advantages you are seeking from the Metabolic Diet. You won't burn the fat like you should. You won't have the energy. You won't build the mass.

You need some red meat, and the more the better. You need the fat it provides. And you need to supplement your diet with other fats, such as the healthy omega-3 fatty acids found in flax and fish oils. Don't shortchange yourself by trying to avoid fat (and certainly don't cut out healthy amounts of the essential fatty acids), as many do when on low-fat diets in some misled effort to stay true to forces in society who have labeled meat some kind of monster. This is simply not true.

Supplements for the Anatomical Adaptation Phase

In the anatomical adaptation phase you should concentrate on making the metabolic shift, keeping everything else basically the same. Besides fiber supplements and perhaps a daily vitamin and mineral tablet, you generally won't need anything else in this phase. If you are used to taking certain supplements on a regular basis, you may want to continue doing so. But this phase is designed to get you into the Metabolic Diet and to make that all-important shift from using carbohydrates to using fats as your primary fuel—therefore it's best to concentrate on making this shift and keeping other changes to a minimum.

Supplements you could use include MVM, Antiox, and EFA+. Also useful is Regulate. Regulate is an effective blend of natural soluble and insoluble fibers formulated to deal with occasional constipation and frequent bowel movements. The various soluble fibers and other compounds contained in Regulate have also been found useful in maintaining cholesterol levels that are already within normal range; supporting a healthy heart; and increasing natural insulin sensitivity.

If you are having a hard time adjusting to the low carbohydrates, before you adjust your carbohydrate levels, try using Metabolic and Creatine Advantage to help get you through the rough spots.

Nelson DaSilva demonstrates what happens when diet, supplements, and training come together perfectly.

KEYS TO SUCCESS
IN THE ANATOMICAL ADAPTATION PHASE

- Find the *maintenance level* of calories that maintains your body weight (18 × your present body weight is a good starting point).
- Take a fiber supplement.
- Watch for hidden carbohydrates.
- Don't mix diets.
- The first week is the toughest; stick it out.

Table 10.2	Example of a Six-Week AA Phase for Recreational Bodybuilders and Strength Trainers						
No.	**Exercise**	**Week 1**	**Week 2**	**Week 3**	**Week 4**	**Week 5**	**Week 6**
1	Leg extension	40/15 × 3	50/12 × 3	60/8 × 3	50/15 × 4	60/12 × 4	70/10 × 4
2	Flat bench press	40/15 × 3	50/12 × 3	60/8 × 3	50/15 × 4	60/12 × 4	70/10 × 4
3	Seated pulley row	40/15 × 3	50/12 × 3	60/8 × 3	50/15 × 4	60/12 × 4	70/10 × 4
4	Back extension	40/15 × 3	50/12 × 3	60/8 × 3	50/15 × 4	60/12 × 4	70/10 × 4
5	Standing leg curl	40/12 × 3	40/15 × 3	50/12 × 3	40/15 × 3	50/12 × 4	50/12 × 4
6	Donkey calf raise	40/15 × 3	50/12 × 3	60/8 × 3	50/15 × 4	60/12 × 4	70/10 × 4
7	Nautilus crunch	3 × 12	3 × 15	3 × 15	4 × 12	4 × 15	4 × 15

Note: You may select exercises other than the above, as per your needs, individual development, and desire to balance muscles or parts of your body; 40/15 × 3 means load/# of repetitions × sets (in this example, 3 sets of 15 repetitions using weight equal to 40 percent of 1RM).

Table 10.3	A Three-Week AA Phase for Advanced Bodybuilders, Recreational Bodybuilders, and Strength Trainers			
No.	**Exercise**	**Week 1**	**Week 2**	**Week 3**
1	Bench press	50/15 × 3	60/12 × 4	70/10 × 4
2	Leg extension	50/15 × 3	60/12 × 4	70/10 × 4
3	Leg curl	40/8 × 3	50/10 × 3	60/12 × 4
4	Standing calf raise	50/15 × 3	60/12 × 4	70/10 × 4
5	Lat pull-down	50/15 × 3	60/12 × 4	70/10 × 4
6	Preacher curl	50/15 × 3	60/12 × 4	70/10 × 4
7	Military press	50/15 × 3	60/12 × 4	70/10 × 4
8	Abdominal crunch	To maximum exhaustion	
9	Back extension	To maximum exhaustion	

Note: Add/change exercises as per your own needs; 50/15 × 3 means load/# of repetitions × sets (in this example, 3 sets of 15 repetitions using weight equal to 50 percent of 1RM).

Table 10.4	A Six-Week AA Phase for an Entry-Level or Recreational Bodybuilder With a Strength and Cardiovascular Component						
No.	Exercise	Week 1	Week 2	Week 3	Week 4	Week 5	Week 6
1	Cardio minutes	10	10	10	15	15	15
2	Leg extension	40/15	40/15	50/12	50/12	60/10	60/12
3	Flat bench press	40/15	40/15	50/12	50/12	60/10	60/12
4	Preacher curl	40/15	40/15	50/12	50/12	60/10	60/12
5	Cardio minutes	10	10	10	10	10	10
6	Back extension	To minimum exhaustion					
7	Standing calf raise	40/15	50/15	50/18	60/15	60/18	60/20
8	Leg curl	40/10	40/12	50/12	50/15	60/12	60/15
9	Cardio minutes	10	10	10	15	15	15

- 40/15 refers to load/# of repetitions.
- Perform the first 5 exercises nonstop.
- Take 1 minute rest, and do the balance (exercises 6-9).
- As you have just finished an entire circuit, take a 2-minute rest interval.
- Try the second circuit, especially after you have reached a decent level of adaptation.

Table 10.5	A Three-Week AA Phase for Advanced Bodybuilders With a Strength and Cardiovascular Component			
No.	Exercise	Week 1	Week 2	Week 3
1	Cardio minutes	10	12	15
2	Bench press	50/12	60/12	70/10
3	Leg extension	50/12	60/12	70/10
4	Leg curl	50/8	60/10	60/12
5	Lat pull-down	50/10	60/12	70/8-10
6	Cardio minutes	10	10	10
7	Military press	50/12	60/12	70/12
8	Preacher curl	50/15	60/12	70/12
9	Abdominal crunch	To maximum exhaustion		
10	Back extension	To maximum exhaustion		
11	Cardio minutes	10	12	15

- 50/12 refers to load/# of repetitions.
- You may change some exercises as per your needs.
- Perform a circuit nonstop from the top to the bottom.
- No RI between stations.
- Take a 2-minute RI after the circuit.
- Repeat circuit once.

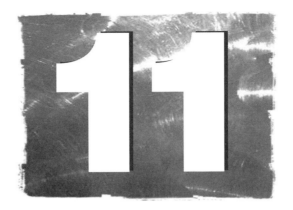

11

HYPERTROPHY (H)

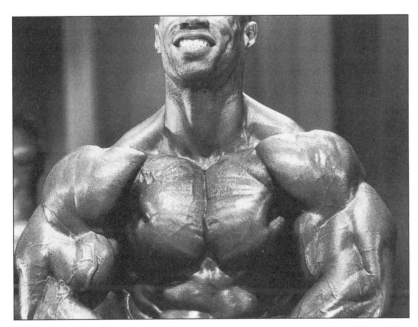

These fabulous delts and pecs belong to none other than the awesome Kevin Levrone.

The standard Periodization model (figure 2.1 on page 23) calls for two six-week hypertrophy phases (H1 and H2) to provide sufficient time for you to address your own needs for improving muscle size and refinement. Between these two H phases we recommend a one-week transition phase during which the volume and intensity of training are significantly reduced. This week of lower-intensity training helps to remove the fatigue accumulated during the first H phase and gives the body a chance to fully replenish its energy stores before commencing the next H phase.

Similar short transition phases are prescribed between all of the training phases of the basic model of Periodization.

Duration of H Training

The duration of H training depends on several factors, including the athlete's classification, training background, specific body goals (e.g., increased size vs. density, or perhaps muscle definition), and the type of Periodization being followed. To learn how to customize your plan, refer to chapter 3.

To achieve substantial gains in muscle size, athletes should plan at least one or, better yet, two six-week H phases. During this time, the athletes must apply the training methods that best suit them. They should carefully select the variations of training methods (see later in this chapter) that will achieve their planned training goals.

The RI between sets is perhaps the most important element of training if hypertrophy is to be stimulated. The RI must be calculated in such a way that it brings the body to exhaustion after each set, as well as at the end of a workout. It is necessary to plan such exhaustion days mostly during the second, and especially during the third step, as per the step-type loading method (see figures 3.5-3.6 on pages 43-44).

Hypertrophy Training Methods

The main objective of bodybuilding is to provoke significant chemical changes in the muscles necessary for the development of mass. For some bodybuilders, unfortunately, increased muscle size often results from increased fluid/plasma within the muscles rather than enlarged contractile elements within the muscle fibers (the myosin filaments). In other words, the enlargement of the muscles may be due to a shift of body fluids to the worked muscle, as opposed to an actual increase in muscle fiber size. This is why the strength of some bodybuilders is not always proportional to their size—a problem that can be corrected by applying the Periodization concept of training.

Hypertrophy training employs submaximal loads in order to avoid provoking maximum tension within the muscles. The training objective with submaximal loads is to contract muscles to exhaustion in an effort to recruit *all* of the muscle fibers. As you "rep-out" to exhaustion, muscle fiber recruitment increases: as some fibers begin to fatigue, others start to function, and so on, until exhaustion is reached.

In order to achieve optimum training benefits, an athlete must perform the greatest number of repetitions possible during each set. Bodybuilders should always reach the state of local muscular exhaustion that prevents them from performing one more repetition, even when applying maximum force. If the individual sets are not performed to exhaustion, muscle hypertrophy will not reach the expected level because the first repetitions do not produce the stimulus necessary to increase muscle mass. *The key element in hypertrophy training is the cumulative effect of exhaustion over the total number of sets, and not just exhaustion per set.* This cumulative exhaustion stimulates the chemical reactions and protein metabolism responsible for optimal muscle hypertrophy.

Bodybuilding/hypertrophy training mostly uses the fuels specific to the anaerobic system (ATP/CP). Training should be designed to exhaust or deplete these energy stores, thereby

Scope of H Training

- Increase muscle size to the desired level by constantly taxing the ATP/CP stores.
- Refine all the muscle groups of the body.
- Improve the proportions among all the muscles of the body, especially between arms and legs, back and chest, leg flexors and extensors.

threatening the energy available for the working muscle. This depletion can be achieved by taking shorter RIs between sets (30-45 seconds)—for when the body has only a limited amount of rest, the muscles have less time to restore the ATP/CP energy reserves. As an exhaustive set depletes ATP/CP stores, and the short RI does not allow for its complete restoration, the body is forced to adapt by increasing its energy transport capacity, which in turn stimulates muscle growth.

Variations of Training Methods for Hypertrophy

Because repetitions to exhaustion represent the main element of success in bodybuilding and strength training, we present below several variations of the original method. Each of the variations has the same objective—to achieve two or three more repetitions *after* you reach exhaustion. The result is increased muscle growth and hypertrophy.

Assisted repetitions: Once you have performed a set to temporary exhaustion of the neuromuscular system, a partner gives you sufficient support to enable you to perform two or three more repetitions.

Resisted repetitions: Once you perform a set to temporary exhaustion, a partner helps you execute two or three more repetitions concentrically, and provides resistance for the eccentric segments of contraction—hence the term *resisted repetitions*. During these last two or three reps, the eccentric part of the contraction is twice as long as the concentric part, thereby overloading the muscles beyond the standard level.

Note that the longer active muscle fibers are held in tension, the higher the nervous tension and energy expenditure becomes. If a normal contraction is two to four seconds long, a repetition performed against resistance can be six to eight seconds long, consuming 20 to 40 percent more energy. The longer the muscles remain in tension, the more strongly activated the muscles' metabolism becomes, stimulating muscle growth to new highs.

Superset: You perform a set for the agonistic muscles of a given joint, followed *without a rest period* by a set for the antagonistic muscles. For example, you do an elbow flexion or biceps preacher curl, followed immediately by an elbow extension or decline triceps extension.

Variation of the superset: You perform a set to exhaustion followed, after 20 to 30 seconds, by another set for the same muscle group. For example, you perform triceps extensions and then dips. Of course, due to exhaustion, you may not be able to perform the same number of repetitions in the second set as in the first set.

Cheated repetitions: Athletes normally resort to this technique when there is no spotter available. When you are unable to perform another repetition with proper form through the entire range of motion, complement the action by jerking another segment of the body toward the performing limb. For example, perform elbow flexions to exhaustion, then jerk the trunk toward the forearm to trick, or "cheat," the body into performing additional reps. This sustains the crucial tension in the exhausted muscle. This method is limited to certain limbs and exercises, and should be attempted only by athletes with a sound training base.

Helpful Tips for the Hypertrophy Method

Even with the split-routine method, hypertrophy workouts are very exhausting to those who might perform perhaps 75 to 160 repetitions per training session. Such high muscle loading requires a long recovery period after a session. The type

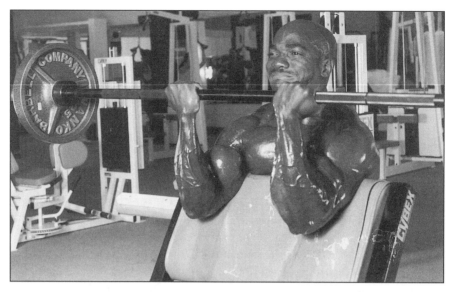

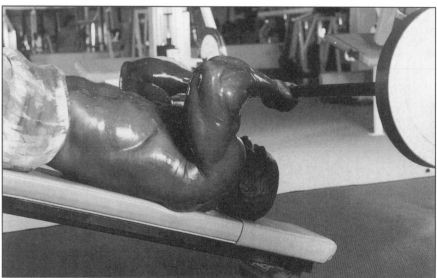

Wesley Mohammed performing a superset with biceps preacher curls followed immediately by decline triceps extensions.

of training specific to this phase exhausts most if not all of the ATP/CP and glycogen stores during a demanding training session.

Remember that although ATP/CP is restored very quickly, the exhausted liver glycogen takes approximately 46 to 48 hours to replenish. It is logical, therefore, that heavy hypertrophy workouts to complete exhaustion be performed no more than three times per microcycle—preferably in the second, and especially in the third, step of the four-step loading pattern.

Constant exhaustive training depletes the body's energy stores and accelerates the breakdown of contractile protein (myosin). The undesirable outcome of such overloading can be that the muscles involved no longer increase in size. Maybe we should change the old adage to "too much pain, no gain!" If you already use the overload technique, do your body a favor and try the step-type approach to loading, and watch your body evolve. In addition, be sure to alternate intensities

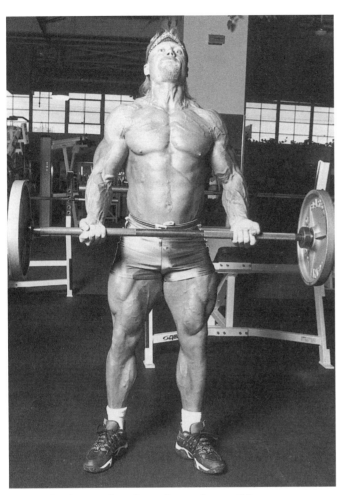

Trevor Butler performing cheated repetitions.

within each microcycle. Your body will respond well to proper sequences of loading and regeneration.

The Isokinetic Method

The term isokinetic means "equal motion" or "same velocity of motion throughout the range of motion." Isokinetic training is performed on specially designed equipment that provides muscles with the same resistance for both the concentric and eccentric parts of the contraction. This provides maximum activation of the muscles involved. Training velocity is very important in this type of training. Training at slower speeds seems to increase contractile strength, but *only* at slow speeds, and the major gains tend to be in muscle hypertrophy. On the other hand, training at higher speeds may increase the contractile strength at all speeds of contraction, either at or below the training speed, with major benefits being reaped for maximum strength (MxS). The more advanced computerized equipment allows athletes to select and set the desired training velocity. These machines are often used as strength-measuring devices.

Isokinetic equipment provides several key benefits:

- It offers a safe way to train, and is therefore suitable for entry-level athletes during their early years.
- It is well suited for the AA phase, when overall strength development and muscle attachment adaptation are the main purposes of training.
- It is useful for rehabilitation of injured athletes.
- It can be used for gains in muscle hypertrophy, if the load and number of repetitions are performed as suggested by this training method.
- With a higher velocity, it can result in gains in MxS.

Slow or Superslow Training

Although bodybuilders have successfully used the slow training system for years, proof of its effectiveness is mostly anecdotal. It is presumed that slow contraction works for the simple reason that it creates a high level of muscle tension, resulting in increased muscle hypertrophy and strength.

The proponents of slow or superslow contraction, whether using drop sets or any other variants, recommend that the duration of concentric contraction be half the length of the eccentric phase. For example: at 95 percent of 1RM, use four seconds for eccentric and only two seconds for concentric. The same ratio is suggested for lower loads: at 70 percent of 1RM, use six seconds for eccentric and only three for concentric. Some "experts," especially some self-proclaimed Internet gurus, suggest almost the opposite: 10 seconds to lift (concentric) and 5 to 10 seconds to lower the weight (eccentric).

The important thing is that the tension is high and prolonged for both the concentric and eccentric contractions. There is no magic secret regarding how many seconds one lowers or lifts the barbell, as long as the tension is consistently high and long. Note, however, that the eccentric phase creates lower tension than the concentric phase (using the same load), because the muscle needs to contract a reduced number of fibers to lower the barbell. Therefore, in order to have similar tension, the eccentric phase must be *either* longer (up to twice the length of the concentric contraction), *or* you have to increase the load to generate equal tension (i.e., add about 20 percent more weight).

Common Misconceptions

Many Internet publications, bodybuilding books, and especially some magazines, are full of misconceptions. They often refer to methods that promise miracles! Take care to recognize the fine line separating reality from fantasy. Here are some of the common misconceptions:

• *Slow movement reduces force, being the number one cause of injuries.* In reality, slow contraction increases muscle tension, keeping the myosin-actin coupling in longer contraction and leading to increased force and muscle size. Furthermore, since exercise form, or technique, is more easily controlled during slow contraction movements, they are safer than dynamic actions. The exception to this rule is when the muscles reach a state of exhaustion. In this instance, technical control is more difficult and athletes require a spotter's assistance to avoid problems.

• *The greater a muscle is fatigued in a limited time frame, the greater the exercise intensity.* In sport science, intensity refers to the load employed in training, which is calculated from 1RM, or 100 percent. The higher the load, the higher the intensity (both physiological and mental). Clearly, some of the Internet writers are confusing intensity with training demand.

• *No rest intervals between sets.* This might be accepted, with great reservation, in the "drop sets" method where the load decreases without rest. For example: two sets of two or three reps at 95 percent RM, then two sets of three or four reps at 90 percent RM, then two sets of 8 to 10 reps at 80 percent RM, and finally two sets of 12 to 15 reps at 70 percent RM. Considering the above statement, it is easy to understand why many bodybuilders are in a constant state of overtraining. The followers of such a theory will be physically and mentally exhausted.

• *Advanced trainees often require as many as seven or more rest days between workouts.* First, 48 hours is sufficient to complete protein synthesis, meaning that the muscles are ready for another workout. Second, targeting a muscle group every seven days may hamper some elements of muscle adaptation and will result in muscle damage and soreness when training is resumed.

High-Intensity Training

High-intensity training (HIT) systems follow traditional bodybuilding training principles, such as progression, overload (i.e., progressive increase of load in

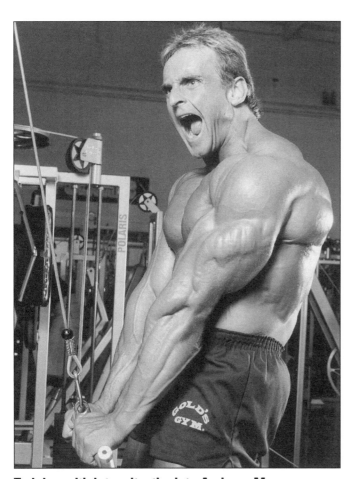

Training with intensity: the late Andreas Munzer.

steps), proper technique, multijoint exercises, superslow, pre-exhaust, drop sets, using full range of motion (ROM), 8 to 12 repetitions, and no split routines. But proponents of HIT promote some misconceptions about training. For example, they suggest that training should be brief (less than one hour). This is fine for those who cannot afford a longer time, such as recreational bodybuilders or strength fitness fans, but questionable for elite athletes who often perform many sets. It is simply impossible for them to do a complete workout in less than an hour. Some other misconceptions put forth by the HIT system are the following:

• *As you get stronger, you can tolerate less high intensity.* This claim strongly contradicts sport science, which has demonstrated that highly trained athletes are well adapted to tolerate high intensity. Many bodybuilders and athletes from various other sports train daily, often two or three times, without problems. This is possible for the simple reason that they are well adapted to both high intensity and volume (quantity) of training. In some programs, especially the Periodization system, training intensity is consistently alternated during the week, yet high intensity is the prevailing training standard. Consider the program followed by many Olympic weightlifters and throwers in track and field: they often train more than twice a day, six days a week, mostly at a high intensity.

• *Beginners should do 16 to 20 sets per workout, while advanced individuals should do only 8 to 12.* The reality is exactly the opposite. Beginners do not have the capacity and are not adapted to tolerate as much work and high intensity as advanced trained athletes. Therefore, beginners should start out performing less but progressively work toward more repetitions with a higher intensity.

• *Beginners should train three times a week, advanced bodybuilders just once.* This is another fallacy. This theory has been briefly discussed above in the section describing superslow contraction training. Some HIT advocates feel that the Periodization system doesn't work; yet when you read their publications you will realize they have never comprehended what Periodization actually is.

Manual Resistance

Manual resistance, generally shortened simply to *manuals,* refers to use of resistance provided by a partner. This method may be advisable for children who are not yet ready for intensive training. Note, however, that the only group of muscles for which the resistance provided by a partner can match or be slightly higher than that of the performer is the deltoids. All the other muscle groups of the body will easily overcome the resistance provided by a partner. Therefore, since resistance is low, strength increases can only be minor. The manuals method was tried in Eastern Europe in the 1950s for a very short time; the conclusion was that it is most advisable for young people and entry-level bodybuilders.

Program Design for the H Phase

As with any new training phase, H training should start with a test for 1RM. The test must be performed in the second part of the first week, because this is the lowest-intensity week in the step-type loading pattern. If it is performed in the early part of the week, the athlete is slightly fatigued from the previous high-intensity week. The brief delay ensures that fatigue does not affect the accuracy of the measurement.

One of the main objectives of H training is to consistently train all of the muscle groups in order to achieve the ultimate symmetrical shape. There are two muscle groups, however, to which additional reference should be made: hamstrings and calves.

Hamstrings

The hamstrings are often neglected and in many instances are not developed proportionately to the quads. When planning your own program, please keep this in mind. Furthermore, power loading is too often used for the hams in the same way it is for other muscles, despite the fact that most muscle strains and injuries occur in the hamstrings. In sprinting, the hams are called "nervous" muscles since they have more nerve end plates per square inch than the quads and many other muscles. The programs we suggest often propose a 10 to 20 percent lower load for the hams than for the quads. Work slowly and carefully on the hams!!

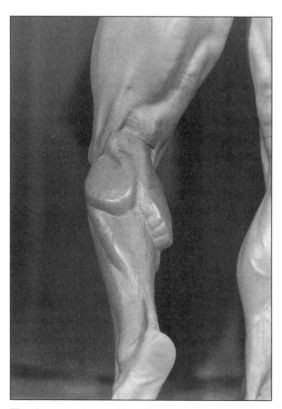

The impressive calf of Roger Stewart.

Calves

These muscles, along with the quads, support the human form in the standing or walking positions. Due to incessant low-level stimulation, they have biologically adapted by developing a higher proportion of slow twitch (76 percent) fibers than fast twitch (24 percent) fibers. As a result, it is difficult to stimulate the same growth in the calves as most of the other muscle groups. The special physiological composition of the calves prevents them from responding well to traditional bodybuilding and strength training programs, in which the same loading and RI are used for the calves as for other muscles.

Because the calves have a higher proportion of capillaries than other muscles, they are able to re-supply their energy needs (ATP/CP stores) more quickly than others. To offset the energy balance of the calves, their training must be slightly different. The RI should be no longer than 30 to 45 seconds, in order to inhibit immediate ATP and CP restoration. This forces the body to increase its energy transport capacity, thereby increasing the CP content of the cells and activating protein metabolism. The hypertrophy of the calves is therefore better stimulated, allowing athletes to build their calves in proportion with the rest of their bodies. Table 11.1 suggests training guidelines for the hypertrophy phase.

Table 11.1	Training Guidelines for the H Phase			
	Bodybuilder's classification			
	Entry-level	**Recreational**	**Advanced**	**Professional**
Duration of H phase (weeks)	6	3-6	3-6	12
Number of reps/set	6-12	9-12	9-12	9-12
Number of sets/exercise	2-3	4-5	4-5	3-7
RI between sets (seconds)	60-120	45-60	45-60	30-45
Workouts/week	2-3	3-5	4-5	5-6
Aerobic training sessions/week	1	1	1-2	2-3

Program Examples

Tables 11.2 to 11.5 on pages 216 to 219 present suggested H-phase programs for four different classifications of bodybuilders and strength trainers. Look at table 11.2 as an example.

- The top row of the chart is for the date. In our example, we simply numbered the six weeks of the program; but when making your individual program, use this space to indicate the dates of the week (e.g., September 1-7).

- The second row is the step row, which contains information about the load intensity, as per the step-type loading method. The first step is "low," indicating a low intensity and volume of training. Programs for the second step are of "medium" intensity. Finally, programs for the third step are of "high" intensity. The same pattern is repeated for weeks 4, 5, and 6.

- The third row shows the day of training. For example, days 1 and 4 will consist of the top program, while days 2 and 5 will consist of the bottom program. Days 3, 6, and 7 are for rest.

- The exercise prescriptions are in the form 40/15 + 3, meaning load/# of repetitions × sets (in this example, 3 sets of 15 repetitions, using a load equal to 40 percent of 1RM).

As you can see, this is an example of a two-day split routine, in which there are two groups of exercises, each performed twice a week. This simple split routine is superior to the traditional routines, because the muscles receive more stimulation when trained twice a week than only once a week. The obvious outcome is a more dramatic increase in muscle size.

All of the exercises numbered from weeks 1 to 6 are listed. If you look at prescriptions for one exercise for all six weeks, you can see the difference in the amount of work between the low-, medium-, and high-intensity training days, as well as the progression of expected strength gains. Changes in loading are made mostly by altering the load and number of sets.

HYPERTROPHY CUES

- Test for 1RM during week 1, during the second part of week 4, and during the first week of the next program.
- A few spaces are left open at the end of the lists so the athlete can add a preferred or needed exercise.
- The number of exercises can be slightly increased or decreased according to one's needs.
- Regardless of any of the above changes that might be made, always apply the suggested loading pattern.
- Decrease the load if it is too high, but maintain the same number of reps.
- The number of sets can be increased or decreased in response to the particular potential and needs of an individual.
- Do not forget to do 5 to 10 minutes of aerobic work before your weight session.
- During the hypertrophy phase, perform all of the sets per exercise before moving on to the next exercise (this is different from the AA phase).

Nutrition for the Hypertrophy Phase

This phase is similar to the "bulking up" phase most bodybuilders are familiar with. As usual, you'll be increasing your calorie intake. On the Metabolic Diet, your goal should be to *allow your body weight to increase to 15 percent above your ideal weight.*

By "ideal weight," we mean what you consider to be your optimum contest weight—and you must be practical about it. If you have been competing at 200 pounds for four or five years and then say your ideal weight is 315 pounds, that's not practical. More reasonable would be to define your ideal weight in this phase as 215 pounds or so and to increase your weight to 15 percent above that— or about 250 pounds.

If you go hog wild, eat like crazy, and end up going 30 percent above your ideal weight, your body will end up being 15 percent body fat or more. That's not what you want. The Metabolic Diet is designed to get you more muscle and limit body fat. Even though you will experience an increase in lean mass and put on less fat than you would on another diet, you still must exercise some discipline.

The specifics of the diet are the same in this phase as in the others—continue to eat a high-protein, high-fat diet on weekdays, and load up on carbohydrates on weekends. The only change will be in the number of calories you consume. If you want to get to a level 15 percent above your ideal weight, you obviously will have to eat more.

In this phase, bodybuilders should daily consume *25 calories per pound of the body weight they want to attain.* In the example above, the bodybuilder wants to get to 250 pounds, so he will take in $25 \times 250 = 6,250$ calories a day. When you consider that he's probably been on a 3,600 calorie diet before that, you can see the tremendous increase in calories he's going to experience.

Such an increase in calorie consumption can present a big problem for athletes who have trouble gaining weight. They're not used to eating and don't have big appetites. They may think they're eating huge amounts but they're not. They'll find themselves at 6,000 calories one day and down at 1,500 a few days later. When asked what happened, all they say is, "I wasn't hungry."

You can't do that on this diet. You have to be consistent. If you want, you can multiply that 6,250 daily calories times 7 and make your goal 43,750 for the week. That way you can vary some from day to day—for example, eat 7,500 calories one day and 5,000 the next—but by the end of the week you must be at the 43,750 calorie level. Keep a written record of calories eaten to make sure that you're reaching the desired levels.

KEYS TO SUCCESS IN THE HYPERTROPHY PHASE

- Increase bodyweight to 15 percent above your current "ideal" contest weight.
- Eat 25 calories per pound of your *new* ideal weight daily.
- If you have trouble eating enough, make calories a weekly rather than daily goal.
- Body fat should not rise above the 10 percent level.
- End the "mass phase" when you reach your new ideal weight *or* rise to the 10 percent body fat level, whichever comes first.
- Whether or not you have reached your new ideal weight, the mass phase must end 12 weeks before a contest.
- A gain of 2 pounds per week is best.

Controlling Body Fat

Body fat is of critical importance. Some athletes gain more body fat than others at similar calorie levels. Depending on personal goals, moreover, some individuals won't mind gaining a little more fat if it means more muscle and strength. While the 10 percent rule is best for competitive bodybuilders (and for any athlete who competes in a specific weight class), other athletes may be willing to go higher and find that even up to 15 percent is acceptable if it means more hypertrophy and strength. Just keep in mind that if your body fat levels get too high, it will be that much harder to get the fat off.

Since most athletes want to maximize muscle mass and strength and to minimize body fat, we will use the competitive bodybuilding model to discuss reaching ideal gains in weight and muscle mass during the mass phase.

We have found that most bodybuilders can maintain a 10 percent body fat level relatively easily if they properly use the Metabolic Diet. This is also a good level for keeping fat in check to prepare for competitive bodybuilding. That is why we advise those on the Metabolic Diet to keep close track of their body fat level and to not let it go above 10 percent.

The goal in the mass phase, then, is to continue eating and gaining weight until you either reach a level 15 percent above your ideal weight or hit 10 percent body fat, whichever comes first. Chances are, no matter which comes first, you will get the mass you want on this anabolically supercharged diet. It's not like the old days

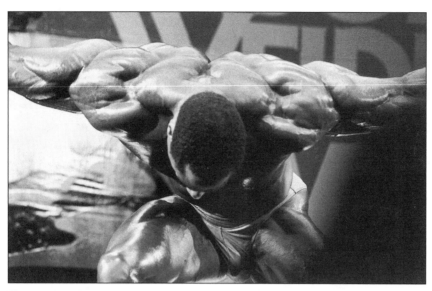

The recipe for muscles that look this big: (1) Start with hypertrophy training; (2) add just enough protein; and (3) stack the proper supplements.

with the high-carbohydrate diet on which you had to gain so much weight and fat to get mass.

You have to use your head here, though. If you find yourself still gaining weight but haven't reached your new ideal weight and your contest is in 12 weeks, it's time to stop the mass phase—regardless of your weight, you must begin the muscle definition phase of training to properly prepare yourself for the contest. Thus the amount of time before a contest joins body fat and weight as a determinant in how long you will stay in this phase.

While most bodybuilders generally believe they should not gain mass quickly, we disagree. Two pounds a week is good. If you can gain two pounds, you won't gain a lot of fat during the week on the Metabolic Diet. It will be mostly muscle. Though you may vary this goal plus or minus one pound given your individual metabolism, we think two pounds a week is the best benchmark for bulking up.

Hypertrophy Phase Duration Can Vary

By always maintaining about 10 percent body fat, you can quickly get into contest shape. We have seen people go through a 20-week cycle in which they bulked up for 8 weeks (three pounds a week) and then spent 12 weeks losing one to two pounds per week in the "cutting phase" (i.e., muscle definition phase—"cut" is jargon that means having highly defined muscles). Though they bulked for only 8 weeks and cut for 12, their weight for the contest was still above its previous level. And they were as cut if not more so.

The goal is to come into a contest a little better than before you were on the diet. This may mean a net gain of only 3 or 4 pounds. Or, in more long-term training, it could be 25 pounds. The important point is that *everybody makes progress with this diet*. For those people who have been the same for 15 years, here is a way to break out!

Some bodybuilders prefer to aim for a big contest, such as Mr. Olympia, and take the whole year to do it. That can easily be done on this diet. You may want to mass for 30 weeks and cut for 20, gaining 60 pounds and losing 40 over the course of a year. You'll come in 20 pounds ahead of where you were last year and be looking great.

Keep in mind that you may also want to use the start-up or maintenance phase described above as you go from mass to cutting phases. Assume you have a contest in 30 weeks. You have gained all the body mass you want in 10 weeks but you don't want to go yet to the cutting phase. You can maintain your gains by

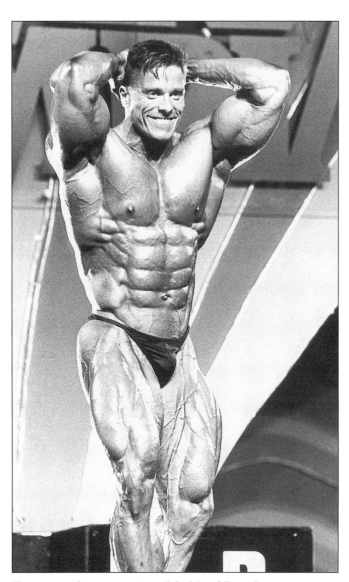

The muscular symmetry of Achim Albrecht.

staying on the maintenance phase for six to eight weeks. Then, when you're ready, you can go into the cutting phase in preparation for the contest.

Weekly Weight Gains

You may see big fluctuations in weight, especially at the beginning of the diet, as a result of your weekly carbohydrate loads. All the extra carbohydrates and water can make for a gain of 5 to 10 pounds between Friday and Monday.

If this happens, don't stress out. It's natural. When you go back on the Metabolic Diet on Monday, you'll immediately begin shedding those pounds (which are mostly water). On Monday through Wednesday you'll be cleaning out much of what you put into your body on the weekend. By Wednesday you should be pretty well flushed out and feeling good again. Depending on what phase of the diet you are on, you can manipulate calories so that by Friday you can reach either the weekly weight gain or loss you are looking for.

Supplements for the Hypertrophy Phase

In the hypertrophy phase, food counts more than supplements. Getting your quota of low-carbohydrate calories will supply you with much of what you need to pack on size and muscle. However, you should use several of the more general supplements on a regular basis, including one or more of MVM, Antiox, and EFA+; use others as needed—for example, ReNew, Regulate, JointSupport, LoCarb MRP, and sports bars. If you are running into training problems, joint pain, injuries, or overtraining, we recommend JointSupport and/or ReNew. LoCarb MRP and LoCarb Sports Bars can be extremely useful for snacks or after meals to help you reach your calorie goals in a healthy, low-carb way. Also, if you reach a plateau in this phase, especially in your training, you might want to use Exersol to maximize your training efforts.

For more information on these supplements, see "Supplements for the Muscle Definition Phase" in chapter 14; for complete information, log on to **www.MetabolicDiet.com**.

Table 11.2 A Suggested Training Program for the H Phase for an Entry-Level Bodybuilder or Strength Trainer

WEEK	1		2		3		4		5		6	
STEP	LOW		MEDIUM		HIGH		LOW		MEDIUM		HIGH	
EX. NO. / DAY	1	4	1	4	1	4	1	4	1	4	1	4
1 Leg press	40/10 × 2	40/12 × 2	40/15 × 2	40/15 × 2	50/12 × 2	50/10 × 3	40/12 × 2	40/12 × 3	50/12 × 3	50/12 × 3	60/10 × 2	60/10 × 3
2 Seated leg curl	40/8 × 2	40/10 × 2	40/10 × 2	40/8 × 3	50/10 × 2	50/8 × 3	40/10 × 3	40/10 × 3	50/10 × 3	50/10 × 3	50/10 × 3	50/10 × 3
3 Front dumbbell press	40/8 × 2	40/10 × 2	40/12 × 2	40/15 × 2	50/10 × 3	50/10 × 3	40/12 × 2	40/10 × 3	50/12 × 3	50/12 × 3	60/10 × 3	60/10 × 3
4 Incline side lateral	40/8 × 2	40/8 × 2	40/10 × 2	40/8 × 3	50/10 × 2	50/8 × 3	40/10 × 2	40/10 × 3	50/10 × 3	50/10 × 3	50/10 × 3	50/10 × 3
5 Back extension	2 × 10	2 × 12	2 × 15	2 × 15	3 × 10	3 × 10	2 × 15	3 × 10	3 × 12	3 × 15	3 × 15	3 × 15
6 Diagonal curl-up	2 × 12	2 × 12	2 × 15	2 × 15	3 × 10	3 × 10	2 × 12	3 × 10	3 × 12	3 × 15	3 × 15	3 × 15

EX. NO. / DAY	2	5	2	5	2	5	2	5	2	5	2	5
1 Shrug	40/10 × 2	40/10 × 2	40/12 × 2	40/15 × 2	50/10 × 2	50/10 × 3	40/12 × 2	40/10 × 3	50/12 × 3	50/12 × 3	60/10 × 3	60/10 × 3
2 Incline bench press	40/10 × 2	40/10 × 2	40/12 × 2	40/15 × 2	50/10 × 2	50/10 × 3	40/12 × 2	40/10 × 3	50/12 × 3	50/12 × 3	60/10 × 3	60/10 × 3
3 Seated pulley row	40/10 × 2	40/10 × 2	40/12 × 2	40/15 × 2	50/10 × 2	50/10 × 3	40/12 × 2	40/10 × 3	50/12 × 3	50/12 × 3	60/10 × 3	60/10 × 3
4 Triceps push-down	40/10 × 2	40/10 × 2	40/12 × 2	40/15 × 2	50/10 × 2	50/10 × 3	40/12 × 2	40/10 × 3	50/12 × 3	50/12 × 3	60/10 × 3	60/10 × 3
5 Standing calf raise	40/10 × 2	40/12 × 2	40/15 × 2	40/15 × 2	50/12 × 2	50/10 × 3	40/10 × 2	40/10 × 3	50/12 × 3	50/12 × 3	60/10 × 3	60/10 × 3
6 Seated calf raise	40/12 × 2	40/12 × 2	40/15 × 2	40/15 × 2	50/12 × 2	50/12 × 3	40/12 × 2	40/12 × 3	50/12 × 3	50/12 × 3	60/10 × 2	60/10 × 3

Note: RI between sets = 1–2 minutes; 40/10 × 2 means load/# of repetitions × sets (in this example, 2 sets of 10 repetitions using weight equal to 40 percent of 1RM).

Table 11.3 Suggested Training Program for the H Phase for a Recreational Bodybuilder or Strength Trainer

WEEK		1		2		3		4		5		6	
STEP		LOW		MEDIUM		HIGH		LOW		MEDIUM		HIGH	
EX. NO.	DAY	1	4	1	4	1	4	1	4	1	4	1	4
1	Hack squat	50/12 × 3	50/12 × 3	60/12 × 3	60/12 × 3	60/15 × 3	60/12 × 4	50/12 × 3	50/12 × 3	60/12 × 4	60/12 × 4	70/10 × 4	70/10 × 4
2	Standing leg curl	50/10 × 3	50/10 × 3	50/12 × 3	50/12 × 3	50/10 × 4	50/10 × 4	50/10 × 3	50/10 × 3	60/10 × 3	60/10 × 3	60/8 × 4	60/8 × 4
3	Lunge	50/12 × 3	50/12 × 3	60/12 × 3	60/12 × 3	60/15 × 3	60/12 × 4	50/12 × 3	50/12 × 3	60/12 × 4	60/12 × 4	70/10 × 4	70/10 × 4
4	Back extension	3 × 12	3 × 12	3 × 15	3 × 15	4 × 12	4 × 15	3 × 15	3 × 15	4 × 15	4 × 15	4 × 15	4 × 15
5	Diagonal curl-up	3 × 12	3 × 12	3 × 15	3 × 15	4 × 12	4 × 15	3 × 15	3 × 15	4 × 15	4 × 15	4 × 15	4 × 15
6	Biceps preacher curl	50/12 × 3	50/12 × 3	60/12 × 3	60/12 × 3	60/15 × 3	60/12 × 4	50/12 × 3	50/12 × 3	60/12 × 4	60/12 × 4	70/10 × 4	70/10 × 4
7	Triceps push-down	50/12 × 3	50/12 × 3	60/12 × 3	60/12 × 3	60/15 × 3	60/12 × 4	50/12 × 3	50/12 × 3	60/12 × 4	60/10 × 3	60/8 × 4	70/10 × 4
	DAY	2	5	2	5	2	5	2	5	2	5	2	5
1	Flat bench press	50/12 × 3	50/12 × 3	60/12 × 3	60/12 × 3	60/15 × 3	60/12 × 4	50/12 × 3	50/12 × 3	60/12 × 4	60/10 × 3	60/8 × 4	70/10 × 4
2	Incline dumbbell bench press	50/12 × 3	50/12 × 3	60/12 × 3	60/12 × 3	60/15 × 3	60/12 × 4	50/12 × 3	50/12 × 3	60/12 × 4	60/10 × 3	60/8 × 4	70/10 × 4
3	Front dumbbell press	50/12 × 3	50/12 × 3	60/12 × 3	60/12 × 3	60/15 × 3	60/12 × 4	50/12 × 3	50/12 × 3	60/12 × 4	60/12 × 4	70/10 × 4	70/10 × 4
4	Standing dumbbell side lateral	50/10 × 3	50/10 × 3	50/12 × 3	50/12 × 3	50/10 × 4	50/10 × 4	50/10 × 3	50/10 × 3	60/10 × 3	60/10 × 3	60/8 × 4	60/8 × 4
5	Shrug	50/12 × 3	50/12 × 3	60/12 × 3	60/12 × 3	60/15 × 3	60/12 × 4	50/12 × 3	50/12 × 3	60/12 × 4	60/12 × 4	70/10 × 4	70/10 × 4
6	Seated pulley row	50/12 × 3	50/12 × 3	60/12 × 3	60/12 × 3	60/15 × 3	60/12 × 4	50/12 × 3	50/12 × 3	60/12 × 4	60/10 × 3	60/8 × 4	70/10 × 4
7	Seated calf raise	50/12 × 3	50/12 × 3	60/12 × 3	60/12 × 3	60/15 × 3	60/12 × 4	50/12 × 3	50/12 × 3	60/12 × 4	60/12 × 4	70/10 × 4	70/10 × 4
8	Standing calf raise	50/12 × 3	50/12 × 3	60/12 × 3	60/12 × 3	60/15 × 3	60/12 × 4	50/12 × 3	50/12 × 3	60/12 × 4	60/12 × 4	70/10 × 4	70/10 × 4

Note: RI between sets = 1-2 minutes; 40/10 × 2 means load/# of repetitions × sets (in this example, 2 sets of 10 repetitions using weight equal to 40 percent of 1RM).

Table 11.4 An H Training Program for an Advanced Bodybuilder or Strength Trainer With Five Workouts Per Week

EX. NO.		WEEK 1 (LOW)			WEEK 2 (MEDIUM)			WEEK 3 (HIGH)			WEEK 4 (LOW)			WEEK 5 (MEDIUM)			WEEK 6 (HIGH)		
	DAY	1	3	5	1	3	5	1	3	5	1	3	5	1	3	5	1	3	5
1	Safety squat	60/12×4	OFF	60/15×4	60/15×4	70/10×4	70/10×4	75/10×4	OFF	75/10×4	60/12×4	70/10×4	70/10×4	75/10×4	OFF	80/8×4	80/8×5	80/8×5	85/5×5
2	Standing leg curl	60/8×3	OFF	60/8×3	60/8×4	60/8×4	60/8×4	65/7×4	OFF	65/7×4	60/10×3	60/10×3	60/10×4	65/10×4	OFF	65/10×4	70/8×4	70/8×4	70/8×4
3	Lunge	60/12×4	OFF	60/15×4	60/15×4	70/10×4	70/10×4	75/10×4	OFF	75/10×4	60/12×4	70/10×4	70/10×4	75/10×4	OFF	80/8×4	80/8×5	80/8×5	85/5×5
4	Bent-over barbell row	60/12×4	OFF	60/15×4	60/15×4	70/10×4	70/10×4	75/10×4	OFF	75/10×4	60/12×4	60/12×4	70/10×4	75/10×4	OFF	80/8×4	80/8×5	85/5×5	85/5×5
5	Back extension	3 × 15	OFF	4 × 15	4 × 12	4 × 12	4 × 12	4 × 15	OFF	4 × 15	3 × 15	3 × 15	4 × 12	4 × 15	OFF	4 × 15	5 × 15	5 × 15	5 × 15
6	Diagonal curl-up	3 × 15	OFF	4 × 15	4 × 12	4 × 12	4 × 12	4 × 15	OFF	4 × 15	3 × 15	3 × 15	4 × 12	4 × 15	OFF	4 × 15	5 × 15	5 × 15	5 × 15
7	Decline triceps extension	60/12×4	OFF	60/15×4	60/15×4	70/10×4	70/10×4	75/10×4	OFF	75/10×4	60/12×4	60/12×4	70/10×4	75/10×4	OFF	80/8×4	85/5×5	85/5×5	85/5×5
	DAY	2	4	6	2	4	6	2	4	6	2	4	6	2	4	6	2	4	6
1	Flat bench press	60/12×4	60/12×4	75/10×4	60/15×4	OFF	70/10×4	75/10×4	75/10×4	75/10×4	60/12×4	OFF	70/10×4	75/10×4	75/10×4	80/8×4	80/8×5	OFF	85/5×5
2	Incline flys	60/12×4	60/12×4	75/10×4	60/15×4	OFF	70/10×4	75/10×4	75/10×4	75/10×4	60/12×4	OFF	70/10×4	75/10×4	75/10×4	80/8×5	80/8×5	OFF	85/5×5
3	Front dumbbell press	60/12×4	60/12×4	75/10×4	60/15×4	OFF	70/10×4	75/10×4	75/10×4	75/10×4	60/12×4	OFF	70/10×4	75/10×4	75/10×4	80/8×5	80/8×5	OFF	85/5×5
4	Incline side lateral	60/10×3	70/8×4	65/8×4	65/8×4	OFF	60/10×4	70/8×4	70/8×4	70/8×4	60/10×3	OFF	60/10×4	70/8×4	75/6×4	75/6×4	75/6×4	OFF	75/6×4
5	Shrug	60/12×4	60/12×4	75/10×4	60/15×4	OFF	70/10×4	75/10×4	75/10×4	75/10×4	60/12×4	OFF	70/10×4	75/10×4	75/10×4	80/8×4	80/8×5	OFF	85/5×5
6	Biceps preacher curl	60/12×4	60/12×4	75/10×4	60/15×4	OFF	70/10×4	75/10×4	75/10×4	75/10×4	60/12×4	OFF	70/10×4	75/10×4	75/10×4	80/8×4	80/8×5	OFF	85/5×5
7	Donkey calf raise	60/12×4	60/12×4	75/10×4	60/15×4	OFF	70/10×4	75/10×4	75/10×4	75/10×4	60/12×4	OFF	70/10×4	75/10×4	75/10×4	80/8×4	80/8×5	OFF	85/5×5

Note: You could decrease the number of workouts to 4, but maintain same loading. If the number of workouts is reduced to 4, an aerobic training session should replace the 5th workout. RI between sets = 45 seconds; 60/12 × 4 means load/# of repetitions × sets (in this example, 4 sets of 12 repetitions using weight equal to 60 percent of 1RM).

Table 11.5 Suggested Three-Week H Training Program for a Professional Bodybuilder

EX. NO.		WEEK 1 — LOW			WEEK 2 — MEDIUM			WEEK 3 — HIGH		
	DAY	**1**	**3**	**5**	**1**	**3**	**5**	**1**	**3**	**5**
1	Safety squat	70/12 × 4	70/15 × 4	70/15 × 5	70/10 × 5	75/8 × 3	80/7 × 3	80/7 × 6	80/6 × 4	85/4 × 7
2	Standing leg curl	70/8 × 4	70/15 × 4	70/10 × 5	70/10 × 5	80/7 × 5	80/7 × 2	80/6 × 5	80/6 × 4	85/4 × 6
3	Lunge	70/12 × 3	70/15 × 3	70/10 × 3	70/10 × 3	75/8 × 1	80/7 × 2	80/6 × 3	80/6 × 3	85/4 × 3
4	Back extension	4 × 15	4 × 15	4 × 18	4 × 18	4 × 12	4 × 12	4 × 15	4 × 15	4 × 15
5	Biceps preacher curl	70/12 × 4	70/15 × 4	70/10 × 5	70/10 × 5	75/8 × 3	80/7 × 3	80/7 × 4	80/7 × 3	85/4 × 6
6	Decline triceps extension	70/12 × 4	70/15 × 4	70/10 × 5	70/10 × 5	75/8 × 3	80/7 × 3	80/7 × 4	80/7 × 3	85/4 × 6
	DAY	**2**	**4**	**6**	**2**	**4**	**6**	**2**	**4**	**6**
1	Flat bench press	70/12 × 4	70/15 × 4	75/10 × 5	75/10 × 5	75/8 × 1	80/7 × 2	80/7 × 6	80/7 × 4	85/4 × 6
2	Incline flys	70/12 × 3	70/15 × 3	75/10 × 3	75/10 × 3	75/8 × 1	80/7 × 2	80/7 × 3	80/7 × 3	85/4 × 3
3	One-arm dumbbell row	70/12 × 4	70/15 × 4	75/10 × 4	75/10 × 4	75/8 × 1	80/7 × 2	80/7 × 4	80/7 × 3	85/4 × 4
4	Incline side lateral	70/12 × 4	70/15 × 4	75/10 × 4	75/10 × 4	75/7 × 4	80/6 × 4	80/6 × 4	80/6 × 4	80/4 × 4
5	Front dumbbell press	70/12 × 3	70/15 × 3	75/10 × 3	75/10 × 4	75/8 × 1	80/7 × 2	80/7 × 3	80/7 × 3	85/4 × 3
6	Shrug	70/12 × 3	70/15 × 3	75/10 × 3	75/10 × 3	75/8 × 1	80/7 × 2	80/7 × 3	80/7 × 3	85/4 × 3
7	Two abdominal exercises	4 × 15	4 × 15	6 × 18	6 × 18	6 × 12	6 × 12	6 × 15	6 × 15	6 × 15
8	Donkey calf raise	70/12 × 4	70/15 × 4	75/10 × 5	75/15 × 5	75/8 × 3	80/7 × 3	80/7 × 4	80/6 × 4	85/4 × 4

Note: RI between sets = 30-45 seconds; 70/12 × 4 means load/# of repetitions × sets (in this example, 4 sets of 12 repetitions using weight equal to 70 percent of 1RM).

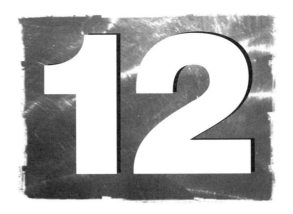

MIXED
TRAINING (M)

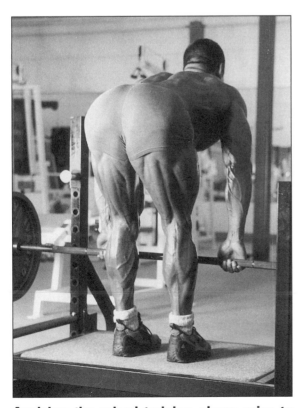

Applying the mixed-training phase prior to maximum-strength training has helped Erik Alstrup develop champion hamstrings.

Before entering the maximum-strength (MxS) phase, athletes must gradually introduce some specific training elements for the development of MxS. As the name implies, *mixed training* incorporates some workouts specific to H training and applies MxS methods for other sessions.

Duration of M Training— The Progressive Transition

In some instances, the strength of bodybuilders' muscles are not commensurate with their size. In other words, some bodybuilding training programs are more conducive to size than to maximum strength and its benefit of increased muscle tone. The main reason: for traditional bodybuilding programs, the load is only 60 to 80 percent of 1RM. But the load necessary to increase maximum strength is much higher,

Scope of M Training

- Continues to improve muscle hypertrophy.
- Introduces MxS methods in order to increase chronic hypertrophy, or long-term muscle tone and density.
- Uses desired proportions between the two types of training, depending on the needs of the athlete. For example:

  40% H and 60% MxS

  50% H and 50% MxS

  60% H and 40% MxS

often up to 95 to 100 percent. Therefore, one of the goals of M training is a better progression from H to MxS training. This progression is insured by employing in training a given proportion between the H and MxS phases.

Regardless of the proportions used, M training ensures a more progressive transition into the maximum-strength phase, where extremely heavy loads might challenge the athlete's ability to cope with the stress and strains of high-intensity workouts.

Program Design for the M Phase

Table 12.1 presents the proportions of an H and MxS mixed-training program for four classifications of bodybuilders. The program can be repeated as many times as necessary, depending on the length of the M phase. As the chart shows, MxS training is consistently recommended for the first workout of the week, or after a rest day. Since MxS training employs loads that come close to maximum potential, planning for these sessions must take into account the athlete's ability to reach maximum concentration before and during training.

The Fatigue Factor

It is well known that fatigue affects one's ability to lift heavy loads, such as those used in MxS. If, for example, athletes perform an MxS workout after an H workout, they will have decreased lifting efficiency for the heavy loads. On the other hand, starting H

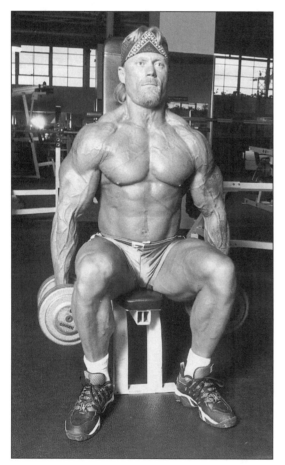

Intensity personified.

Table 12.1	Suggested Proportion Between MxS and H Training for the M Phase							
No.	Classification	Mon	Tues	Wed	Thurs	Fri	Sat	Sun
1	Entry-level	H	H	Off	MxS	Off	H	Off
2	Recreational	MxS	H	Off	MxS	Off	H	Off
3	Advanced	MxS	H	MxS	H	Off	H	Off
4	Professional	MxS	H	H	Off	MxS	H	Off

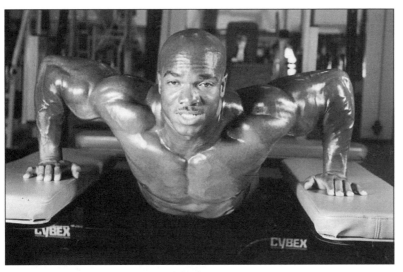

Fatigue seems to exhaust ATP/CP stores more quickly, which appears to stimulate muscle growth.

training with slight residual fatigue tends to have a stimulating effect on the development of muscle. A slightly fatigued muscle seems to exhaust the ATP/CP stores more quickly, thereby stimulating muscle growth. In the case of mixed training, therefore, always plan MxS workouts before H workouts.

In this chapter we offer M training programs for entry-level, recreational, advanced, and professional athletes (see tables 12.2-12.9 on pages 226-231). To follow the same sequence of H and MxS training days shown in table 12.1, an athlete must split the plan for each level into two parts—one for the hypertrophy portion and one for the Mx portion. The suggested training programs in table 12.2 (page 226) show the H portion of the M program for entry-level athletes, with three days planned for the development of H—days 1, 2, and 6. Table 12.3 on page 227 shows the MxS portion of the M program for entry-level athletes, with only one day planned for MxS training. Day 6 consists of a selection of exercises from both programs. Please perform only those exercises you have chosen and *not* both complete programs.

MIXED TRAINING CUES

- The exercises that we have recommended may be substituted with similar exercises according to one's needs and preferences.
- The recommended programs for the M phase are all three weeks in duration; if a longer M phase is needed, the entire program can be repeated.

Achieve Optimum Recovery

Unlike the exercise pattern for H training, where all the planned sets for one exercise are performed before moving on to the next exercise, MxS training requires that the athlete always reach optimum recovery between sets. The MxS exercise pattern is to perform one set for the first exercise, then to perform one set for the next exercise. Always work the exercises in series of twos from the top down. The rest interval should be about 5 to 6 minutes, before going back to the original exercise. In order to enhance the recovery process further, the exercises are planned in such a way that the muscle groups are constantly being alternated.

It is extremely important to religiously observe the proposed rest intervals! Do not make the mistake of performing your sets too soon. Regardless of whether you feel ready before the RI is up, your body needs the time to recover from this type of training. Your last set should be as good as your first set.

MIXED TRAINING CUES

- Test for 1RM as suggested for the other training phases.

- You may select exercises other than those suggested above, but apply the same loading pattern.

- The suggested loading is not carved in stone. If a given load is too high for you, reduce it slightly until you can perform the recommended number of reps.

- The number of sets can be increased or decreased according to your own potential.

- Do your aerobic training.

Nutrition for the Mixed Phase

This phase, and the maximum-strength phase, are intermediate phases between the classical hypertrophy, or bulk, phase and the definition phase. The nutrition goals in the mixed phase are at the very least to maintain the weight and muscle mass gained during the hypertrophy phase and ideally to increase both marginally, while at the same time developing the strength that would normally go along with the increased weight and muscle mass. During this phase, athletes begin the process of solidifying and marginally adding to the muscle mass gains of the hypertrophy phase; they also begin increasing their strength.

During this phase, bodybuilders should daily consume between 17 and 25 calories per pound of the top bodyweight they attained during the hypertrophy phase. Using the example from chapter 11, the 250-pound bodybuilder will now cut back roughly 2 calories per pound per week. That means that the first week of the mixed phase he will take in 23 calories per pound of bodyweight, or $23 \times 250 = 5,750$ calories per day. The following week he will take in 21 calories per pound of bodyweight, or 5,250 calories per day. The third week, 19 calories per pound of bodyweight, or 4,750 calories per day. The fourth week, 17 calories per pound of bodyweight, or 4,250 calories per day, and so on. Once the weight stabilizes so that the individual is no longer gaining weight, he or she should keep the calories at that level until beginning the definition phase.

KEYS TO SUCCESS IN THE MIXED PHASE

- Stabilize your body weight at or slightly above your weight in the hypertrophy phase.

- Body fat should not rise above the levels of the hypertrophy phase.

- Consume 17 to 25 calories per pound of your top hypertrophy-phase weight daily.

- Cut back 2 calories per pound of bodyweight every week.

- End the calorie cutting when your weight stabilizes.

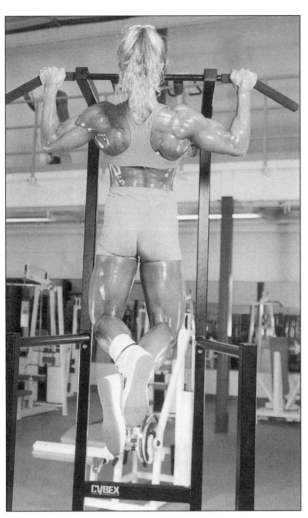

MVM, Antiox, and EFA should be used on a regular basis by bodybuilders who are training hard.

Supplements for the Mixed Phase

In the mixed phase, as in the hypertrophy phase, the food counts more than the supplements. Getting your quota of low-carb calories will supply you with much of what you need to solidify your increased muscle mass and start getting ready to decrease your body fat. However, as you drop your calories, nutritional supplements gain in importance.

You will need more than just your basic daily vitamin and mineral tablet. You should use MVM (my complete vitamin, mineral, and nutrient supplement), Antiox (my antioxidant mix), and EFA+ (my essential fatty acid formula that contains much more than just the essential fatty acids) on a regular basis. As in the hypertrophy phase, other supplements—such as Exersol (made up of Resolve, Power Drink, and Amino), ReNew, Regulate, JointSupport, LoCarb MRP, and LoCarb Sports Bars—can be used as needed.

Table 12.2   Mixed Phase: H Training Portion for an Entry-Level Bodybuilder or Strength Trainer

EX. NO.		WEEK 1 — LOW			WEEK 2 — MEDIUM			WEEK 3 — HIGH		
	DAY	1	3	6	1	3	6	1	3	6
1	Leg extension	40/15 × 3	Off		50/12 × 3	Off		60/12 × 3	Off	
2	Leg press	40/12 × 3	Off	40/12 × 3	50/12 × 3	Off	50/12 × 3	60/10 × 3	Off	60/10 × 3
3	Lunge	40/12 × 3	Off	40/12 × 3	50/12 × 3	Off	50/12 × 3	60/10 × 3	Off	60/10 × 3
4	Standing leg curl	40/10 × 3	Off	40/10 × 3	50/10 × 3	Off	50/12 × 3	50/10 × 3	Off	50/10 × 3
5	T-Bar row	40/12 × 3	Off		50/12 × 3	Off		60/10 × 3	Off	
6	Back extension	3 × 10	Off		3 × 12	Off		3 × 15	Off	
7	Seated calf raise	40/12 × 3	Off		50/12 × 3	Off		60/10 × 3	Off	
8	Flat flies	40/12 × 3	Off	40/12 × 3	50/12 × 3	Off	50/12 × 3	60/10 × 3	Off	60/10 × 3
	DAY	2	5	6	2	5	6	2	5	6
1	Front dumbbell press	40/12 × 3	Off		50/12 × 3	Off		60/10 × 3	Off	
2	Incline side lateral	40/12 × 3	Off	40/12 × 3	50/12 × 3	Off	50/12 × 3	60/10 × 3	Off	60/10 × 3
3	Upright row	40/12 × 3	Off	40/12 × 3	50/12 × 3	Off	50/12 × 3	60/10 × 3	Off	60/10 × 3
4	Shrug	40/12 × 3	Off	40/12 × 3	50/12 × 3	Off	50/12 × 3	60/10 × 3	Off	60/10 × 3
5	Decline triceps extension	40/12 × 3	Off	40/12 × 3	50/12 × 3	Off	50/12 × 3	60/10 × 3	Off	60/10 × 3
6	Diagonal curl-up	3 × 10	Off	3 × 10	3 × 12	Off	3 × 12	3 × 15	Off	3 × 15

Note: RI between sets: 1-2 minutes; 40/15 × 3 means load/# of repetitions × sets (in this example, 3 sets of 15 repetitions using weight equal to 40 percent of 1RM).

	WEEK	1	2		3
EX.	**STEP**	**LOW**	**MEDIUM**		**HIGH**
NO.	**DAY**	**4**	**4**		**5**
1	**Leg press**	70/7 × 3	70/8 × 1	80/6 × 2	80/6 × 3
2	**Flat bench press**	70/7 × 3	70/8 × 1	80/6 × 2	80/6 × 3
3	**Supine leg curl**	50/10 × 3	60/10 × 3		70/7 × 3
4	**T-Bar row**	50/10 × 3	60/10 × 3		70/8 × 3
5	**Seated calf raise**	70/7 × 3	70/8 × 1	80/6 × 2	80/6 × 3

Table 12.3 — Mixed Phase, MxS Training Portion for Entry-Level Bodybuilders or Strength Trainers

Note: 70/7 × 3 means load/# of repetitions × sets (in this example, 3 sets of 7 repetitions using weight equal to 70 percent of 1RM).

	WEEK	1	2	3
EX.	**STEP**	**LOW**	**MEDIUM**	**HIGH**
NO.	**DAY**	**2**	**2**	**2**
1	**Front dumbbell press**	50/12 × 3	60/12 × 3	70/8 × 4
2	**Incline side lateral**	50/12 × 3	60/12 × 3	70/8 × 4
3	**Biceps preacher curl**	50/12 × 3	60/12 × 3	70/8 × 4
4	**Shrug**	50/12 × 3	60/12 × 3	70/8 × 4
5	**Seated calf raise**	50/12 × 3	60/12 × 3	70/8 × 4
	DAY	**6**	**6**	**6**
1	**Hack squat**	50/12 × 3	60/12 × 3	70/8 × 4
2	**Supine leg curl**	50/12 × 3	60/12 × 3	70/8 × 4
3	**Seated pulley row**	50/12 × 3	60/12 × 3	70/8 × 4
4	**Incline fly**	50/10 × 3	60/10 × 3	60/8 × 4
5	**Triceps push-down**	50/12 × 3	60/12 × 3	70/8 × 4
6	**Crunch**	3 × 10	3 × 12	4 × 15

Table 12.4 — Mixed-Phase H Training Portion for Recreational Bodybuilders and Strength Trainers

Note: 50/12 × 3 means load/# of repetitions × sets (in this example, 3 sets of 12 repetitions using weight equal to 50 percent of 1RM).

Table 12.5 — Mixed Phase, MxS Training Portion for Recreational Bodybuilders and Strength Trainers

EX. NO.		WEEK 1 — STEP LOW		WEEK 2 — STEP MEDIUM		WEEK 3 — STEP HIGH	
		DAY 1	DAY 4	DAY 1	DAY 4	DAY 1	DAY 4
1	Leg press	70/8 × 3	70/8 × 2, 80/6 × 1	70/8 × 1, 80/7 × 2	80/7 × 3	80/8 × 4	80/8 × 4
2	Flat bench press	70/8 × 3	70/8 × 2, 80/6 × 1	70/8 × 1, 80/7 × 2	80/7 × 3	80/8 × 4	80/8 × 4
3	Supine leg curl	60/10 × 3	60/10 × 3	70/8 × 3	70/8 × 3	70/8 × 4	70/8 × 4
4	Lat pull-downs	70/8 × 3	70/8 × 2, 80/6 × 1	70/8 × 1, 80/7 × 2	80/7 × 3	80/8 × 4	80/8 × 4

Note: 70/8 × 3 means load/# of repetitions × sets (in this example, 3 sets of 8 repetitions using weight equal to 70 percent of 1RM); RI between sets = 3 minutes.

Table 12.6 — Mixed Phase, MxS Training Portion for Advanced Bodybuilders and Strength Trainers

EX. NO.		WEEK 1 — STEP LOW		WEEK 2 — STEP MEDIUM		WEEK 3 — STEP HIGH	
		DAY 1	DAY 3	DAY 1	DAY 3	DAY 1	DAY 3
1	Safety squat	70/8 × 4	80/7 × 5	90/3 × 3	85/4 × 2	90/3 × 5	90/2 × 5
2	Standing leg curl	60/8 × 5	60/8 × 5		70/7 × 5	80/6 × 5	80/6 × 5
3	Flat bench press	70/8 × 4	80/7 × 5	90/3 × 3	85/4 × 2	90/3 × 5	90/2 × 5
4	Bent-over barbell row	70/8 × 4	80/7 × 5	90/3 × 3	85/4 × 2	90/3 × 5	90/2 × 5
5	Front dumbbell press	70/8 × 4	80/7 × 5	90/3 × 3	85/4 × 2	90/3 × 5	90/2 × 5
6	Donkey calf raise	60/8 × 5	60/8 × 5		70/7 × 5	80/6 × 5	80/6 × 5

Note: 70/8 × 4 means load/# of repetitions × sets (in this example, 4 sets of 8 repetitions, using weight equal to 70 percent of 1RM); RI between sets = 3-4 minutes.

Table 12.7 Example of H Training Program for the M Phase for Advanced Bodybuilders and Strength Trainers

WEEK		1	2	3
STEP		LOW	MEDIUM	HIGH
DAY		6	6	6
EX. NO.				
1	Lunge	70/8 × 4	80/9 × 5	85/5 × 5
2	Diagonal curl-up	4 × 12	5 × 15	5 × 15
3	Biceps preacher curl	70/8 × 4	80/7 × 5	85/5 × 5

WEEK		1		2		3	
STEP		LOW		MEDIUM		HIGH	
DAY		2/4	6	2/4	6	2/4	6
EX. NO.							
1	Decline triceps extension	70/8 × 4	70/8 × 4	80/7 × 5	80/7 × 5	85/5 × 3	80/7 × 2
2	Pull-down behind neck	70/8 × 4	70/8 × 4	80/7 × 5	80/7 × 5	85/5 × 3	80/7 × 2
3	Standing dumbbell bent lateral	60/10 × 4	70/8 × 4	70/7 × 5	80/7 × 5	75/6 × 5	
4	Shrug	70/8 × 4		80/7 × 5	80/7 × 2	85/5 × 3	85/5 × 3
5	Back extension	4 × 12		4 × 15		5 × 15	

Note: 70/8 × 4 means load/# of repetitions × sets (in this example, 4 sets of 8 repetitions using weight equal to 70 percent of 1RM); RI between sets = 30-45 seconds.

Table 12.8 Suggested H Training Program for the M Phase for Professional Bodybuilders and Strength Trainers

	WEEK	1		2		3	
EX.	STEP	LOW		MEDIUM		HIGH	
NO.	DAY	2	6	2	6	2	6
1	Front dumbbell press	60/12 × 3	60/12 × 3	70/10 × 3	75/8 × 3	80/7 × 2	80/7 × 2
2	Incline side lateral	60/12 × 4	60/12 × 4	70/10 × 4	75/8 × 4	80/7 × 3	80/7 × 3
3	Shrug	60/12 × 6	60/12 × 6	70/10 × 6	75/8 × 6	80/7 × 6	80/7 × 6
4	Decline triceps extension	60/12 × 4	60/12 × 4	70/10 × 6	75/8 × 6	80/7 × 6	80/7 × 6
5	Biceps preacher curl	60/12 × 3	60/12 × 3	70/10 × 3	70/10 × 3	80/7 × 3	80/7 × 3
	DAY	3		3		3	
1	Safety squat	60/12 × 6		70/10 × 7		80/7 × 3	
2	Standing leg curl	60/12 × 6		70/10 × 7		70/7 × 3	
3	Flat bench press	60/12 × 6		70/10 × 7		80/7 × 3	
4	Barbell bent-over row	60/12 × 6		70/10 × 7		80/7 × 3	
5	Back extension	60/12 × 3		70/10 × 3		80/7 × 3	
6	Nautilus crunch	60/12 × 3		70/10 × 3		80/7 × 3	
7	Donkey calf raise	60/12 × 6		70/10 × 7		80/7 × 3	

Note: 60/12 × 3 means load/# of repetitions × sets (in this example, 3 sets of 12 repetitions using weight equal to 60 percent of 1RM); RI between sets = 30-45 seconds.

Table 12.9 — Mixed Phase, MxS Training Portion for Professional Bodybuilders and Strength Trainers

EX. NO.	Exercise	WEEK 1 — LOW		WEEK 2 — MEDIUM		WEEK 3 — HIGH	
		DAY 1	DAY 5	DAY 1	DAY 5	DAY 1	DAY 5
1	Safety squat	80/7 × 6	80/7 × 6	85/4 × 3	90/3 × 3	90/3 × 2	95/2 × 4
2	Standing leg curl	70/6 × 5	70/6 × 5	80/6 × 5	80/6 × 5	80/6 × 5	80/6 × 5
3	Barbell bent-over row	80/7 × 6	80/7 × 6	85/4 × 3	90/3 × 3	90/3 × 2	95/2 × 4
4	Flat bench press	80/7 × 6	80/7 × 6	85/4 × 3	90/3 × 3	90/3 × 2	95/2 × 4

Note: 80/7 × 6 means load/# of repetitions × sets (in this example, 6 sets of 7 repetitions using weight equal to 80 percent of 1RM).

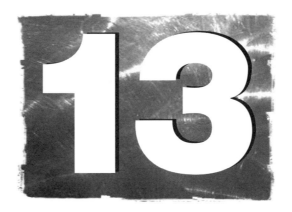

13

MAXIMUM STRENGTH (MXS)

Maximum strength is developed by increasing the training load and in the process increasing the contractile capability of the muscles. Training loads higher than 80 percent increase the tension in the muscle and recruit the powerful fast twitch motor units. The result is higher protein content in the muscle via increased thickness of myosin filaments. Since motor units are recruited by size, beginning with slow twitch followed by fast twitch, loads greater than 80 percent are required to recruit the powerful fast twitch motor units.

We recommend that this phase last six weeks, although other variations are possible.

The Physiology Behind MxS Training

An athlete's ability to develop maximum strength depends to a high degree on the following factors:

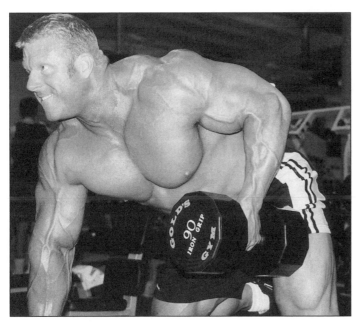

Scott Milnes, 25-year-old bodybuilding sensation, understands the importance of strength training.

• **The diameter, or cross-sectional area, of the muscle involved.** More specifically, this means the diameter of the myosin filaments, including their cross bridges. Although muscle size depends largely on the duration of the H phase, the diameter of the myosin filaments depends specifically on the volume and duration of the MxS phase. This is because MxS training is responsible for increasing the protein content of the muscles.

• **The capacity to recruit FT muscle fibers.** This ability depends largely on training content. Use of maximum loads, with high application of force against resistance, is the only type of training that completely involves the powerful fast twitch motor units.

• **The ability to successfully synchronize all of the muscles involved in the action.** This develops over time as a function of learning, which is based on performing many repetitions of the same exercise, with heavy loads. Most North American bodybuilders use only bodybuilding (i.e., H) methods to increase muscle size. They tend to neglect training approaches that stimulate recruitment of FT muscle fibers to build high-density muscle, tight muscle tone, impressive muscle separation, and more visible muscle striations. While North American bodybuilders do increase their muscle size, the increases are usually not chronic: the growth is largely due to fluid displacement within the muscles rather than a thickening of the muscle fibers. The MxS phase in the Periodization program can correct this deficiency. Maximum strength improves as a result of creating high tension in the muscle—and this tension can be achieved only by using loads that result in higher FT muscle fiber recruitment (loads over 80 to 85 percent of 1RM).

Scope of MxS Training

- Increases protein content of muscle, thereby inducing chronic hypertrophy and increasing muscle tone and density.
- Increases thickness of the cross bridges and myosin filaments (this is the only way to induce chronic hypertrophy).
- Conditions muscles to recruit as many fast twitch muscle fibers as possible, through the application of heavy loads; this develops maximum strength and improves muscle tone and density.

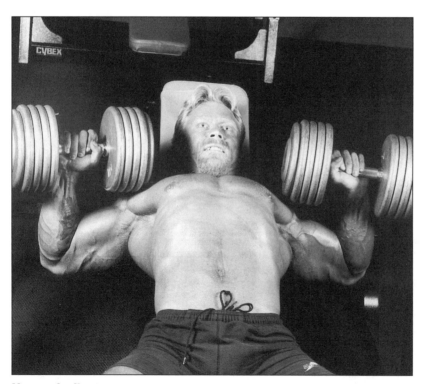

Heart of a lion.

Training Methods and Duration for MxS

Exercises for the development of MxS must not be carried out under the conditions of exhaustion as in the H phase. During MxS training, the muscles should be allowed to recover maximally between sets. Due to its maximum activation of the central nervous system, and the high levels of concentration and motivation it requires, MxS training improves the links with the CNS that lead to improved muscle coordination and synchronization. Strength depends not only on the size of the muscle and the total number of cross bridges, but also on the CNS' capacity to "drive" that muscle.

High activation of the CNS (i.e., muscle synchronization) also results in inhibition of the antagonistic muscles. When maximum force is applied, therefore, the antagonistic muscles are coordinated in such a way that they do not contract to oppose the movement—allowing the athlete to lift even heavier weights.

Most changes in strength are said to occur at the level of muscle tissue. Little is said, however, about the involvement of the nervous system during MxS training. In fact, very little research has been conducted on the subject. The research that has been done suggests that the CNS acts as a stimulus for gains in strength. The CNS normally acts as an inhibitor of motor units during contraction. Under extreme circumstances, such as a life-and-death situation, this inhibition is removed and all the motor units are activated, providing what seems to be superhuman strength. One of the main objectives of MxS training is to teach the body to eliminate CNS inhibition, which results in a huge improvement of strength potential.

The Maximum Load Method (MLM)

MxS improvement occurs almost solely through the *maximum load method* (MLM). This method should only be performed after a minimum of two or three years of general bodybuilding or strength training, because of the strain of training and the utilization of maximum loads. The gains are largely due to motor learning, whereby athletes learn to use and coordinate the muscles involved in training more efficiently.

Benefits of MLM

- Increases motor unit activation, resulting in high recruitment and firing frequency of FT muscle fibers.
- Increases secretion of growth hormones and raises levels of catecholamines (compounds—primarily epinephrine and norepinephrine—that increase the strong physiological response to this type of training).
- Improves coordination and synchronization of muscle groups during performance. The better the coordination and synchronization of the muscles involved in contraction and the more they learn to recruit FT muscles, the better will be the performance.
- Increases diameter of the muscle's contractile elements.
- Raises the body's testosterone level.

The gains obtained through MLM are predominantly gains in MxS, with muscle hypertrophy as a secondary benefit. Large gains in muscle size through MLM are possible, but generally only in athletes who are just beginning to use MLM. For athletes with a more solid background, gains in muscle size will not be as noticeable as the gains made in MxS. The MxS phase sets the stage for future growth explosions through better synchronization and increased recruitment of FT fibers. Highly trained athletes, with three or four years of MLM training, are so well adapted to such training that they are able to recruit approximately 85 percent of their FT fibers. The remaining 15 percent represent a "latent reserve" that is not easily tapped through training.

Once athletes have reached such an advanced level, they may find it very difficult to further increase MxS. In order to avoid stagnating and to further improve muscle density and separation, they must use alternative methods to provide greater stimulation to the muscles. One such method is to increase the eccentric component of contractions—the increased tension helps the body to continue developing MxS despite an already high level of adaptation.

The most important elements to be considered in MLM training are the load used in training, the loading pattern, the RI, and the speed of performing the contraction. A brief explanation of these factors will help clarify the above statement.

Load

As already mentioned, MxS develops only when maximum tension is created in the muscle. While lower loads stimulate the ST muscle fibers, loads exceeding 85 percent RM are necessary if most muscle fibers, and especially FT fibers, are to be recruited in contraction. Maximum loads with low repetitions result in significant nervous system adaptation, better synchronization of the muscles involved, and increased capacity to recruit FT muscle fibers.

A suggestion by Goldberg et al. (1975), that the tension developed within myofilaments is the stimulus for protein synthesis, further illustrates why training for MxS should be performed only with maximum loads. It is because the load for the MLM is maximum that the number of repetitions per set is low—only from one to four (or at most up to six).

Rest Interval

The RI between sets depends partially on the athlete's fitness level and should be carefully calculated to ensure adequate recovery of the neuromuscular system. For MLM, a three- to five-minute RI is necessary because maximum loads involve the CNS (which recovers more slowly than the skeletal system). If the RI is too short, the nervous system participation—in the form of maximum concentration, motivation, and the power of the nerve impulses sent to the contracting muscle—could be less than optimal. In addition, complete restoration of the required fuel for contraction (ATP/CP) can also be jeopardized if the RI is too brief.

Speed

The speed of execution plays an important role in MLM. Even when using typical maximum loads, the athlete's force against resistance must be exerted as quickly as possible. Although the magnitude of the load restricts the speed of contraction, the athlete must concentrate on activating the muscles as briskly as possible.

The Eccentric Method

Strength exercises, using either free weights or most isokinetic apparatuses, involve both concentric and eccentric types of contraction. During the concentric phase, force is produced while the muscle shortens; during the eccentric segment, force is produced while the muscle lengthens, or returns to the resting position.

Everyone knows that the eccentric phase is easier than the concentric phase. For example, when performing the bench press, the lowering of the barbell to the chest (eccentric part of the lift) is easier than pressing the bar upwards. Because eccentric work is easier, it allows athletes to work with heavier loads than if they

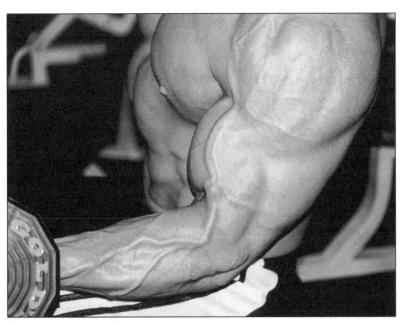

Eccentric contractions.

were performing only concentric work, and heavier loads translate into greater strength gains. Strength training specialists and researchers have arrived at the same conclusion, which is that eccentric training creates a higher tension in the muscles than isometric or isotonic contractions. And since higher muscle tension is normally equated with greater strength development, eccentric training is a superior training method.

Training specialists from the former East Germany claim that the eccentric strength-training method results in a 10 to 35 percent higher strength gain than that of other methods.

The load in eccentric training is much higher than the athlete's 1RM, so the speed of performance is quite slow. Such a slow rate of contraction produces a larger stimulus for protein synthesis, and therefore normally results in muscle hypertrophy and greater strength development.

During the first few days of using the eccentric method, athletes may experience muscle soreness, because higher tensions provoke some minor muscle damage. As athletes adapt, the muscle soreness disappears in about 7 to 10 days. Athletes can avoid this short-term discomfort by increasing the load progressively, using the step-type approach.

There are a number of differences in mechanical, metabolic, and neural stimuli between concentric and eccentric contractions. While maximum concentric contractions lead to maximum muscle activation, maximum eccentric contractions do not appear to elicit complete muscle activation. In other words, a bodybuilder and strength athlete must work with heavier loads during the eccentric phase in order to develop a positive adaptation in strength. The neural command for eccentric contractions is unique in that it decides (1) which motor units should be activated, (2) how much they have to be activated, (3) when they should be activated, and (4) how the activity should be distributed within a group of muscles.

Program Design for the MxS Phase

Since the eccentric method employs the heaviest loads in strength training (110 to 160 percent), only athletes with a solid strength-training background (i.e., two to four years of strength training or bodybuilding experience) should use it. Moreover, they should use it only after they are experiencing no further gains with the maximum load method (MLM).

The eccentric method can be used alone, or in combination with MLM but for only a short period of time. Eccentric training should not be abused. When overused it has limitations and can lead to a plateau that might be difficult to break. In addition, because eccentric training requires such intense mental concentration, every time maximum or supermaximum loads are used there is a great deal of psychological stress.

For maximum training benefits, athletes should use MLM for as long as practically possible. When they reach a plateau in which they are achieving little or no improvement, then they should begin using the eccentric method. This training approach will break through the ceiling of adaptation created by the plateau and permit achievement of new levels of strength.

During eccentric training, which is usually performed with free weights, the assistance of two spotters is always necessary because the weights are always greater than the athletes can lift concentrically by themselves. The spotters' job is to help lift the weight during the concentric portion and to watch the lifters carefully during the eccentric portion to ensure that they can handle the huge load.

Training parameters for the eccentric method are presented in table 13.1. The load is expressed as a percentage of 1RM for the concentric contraction, and is recommended to be between 110 to 160 percent. The most effective load for athletes of high caliber is around 130 to 140 percent. Less experienced athletes should use lower loads. These loads are to be used after at least two phases of MxS training in which the eccentric contraction is included. Eccentric contractions should not be used under any circumstances in the first few months of training.

The number of sets per exercise and training session recommended in table 13.1 are a guideline only for experienced bodybuilders. Entry-level and recreational athletes need a lower number of sets depending on their training potential.

The RI is an important element in the capacity to perform highly demanding work. If, after a set, athletes do not recover sufficiently to perform the next set at the same level, they should slightly increase the RI.

As eccentric contractions use extremely heavy loads, athletes must be highly motivated and have maximum concentration before performing each set. Only under such mental conditions will they be capable of performing eccentric contraction effectively.

The eccentric method is rarely performed in isolation from the other MxS methods. Even during the MxS phase, the eccentric method is used together with MLM. We recommend only one eccentric training session. The frequency may eventually be increased for high-caliber athletes during the third step of the step-type approach to load patterning.

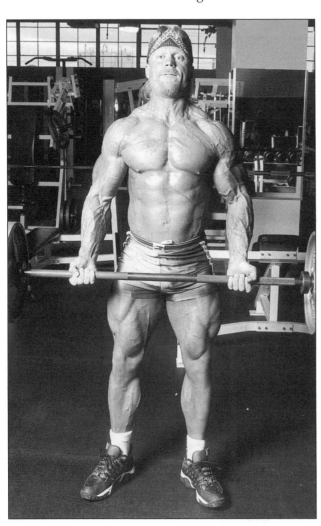

Trevor Butler used maximum-strength training to his benefit.

Table 13.1	Training Guidelines for the MxS Phase			
	Bodybuilder's classification			
	Entry-level	**Recreational**	**Advanced**	**Professional**
Reps/set	1-4	3-8	3-8	2-8
Sets/session	10-15	15-20	20-32	25-40
RI between sets (minutes)	4-5	3-5	3-5	3-5
Frequency/week:				
MLM	None	2-3	2-3	2-3
Eccentric	None	None	1	1-2
Rhythm/speed of contraction	Slow	Slow	Active	Active

MAXIMUM STRENGTH CUES

- Test for 1RM during the second part of the first week and during the first week of the next phase.
- Since MxS training is very taxing for the neuromuscular system, reduce the number of exercises to the lowest realistic level. As much as possible, use multijoint exercises that involve several muscle groups; however, this does not exclude the use of single-joint exercises.
- Because of the physiological and psychological stress of MxS training, the RI between sets must be 3 to 5 minutes long. Throughout the RI, relax the muscles, keep them warm with dry clothing, and do mild stretching exercises.
- If the suggested load is too high, lower it, and maintain the recommended number of repetitions.
- Adjust the program/exercises to meet your own needs and training potential.
- Remember to do 20 to 25 minutes of aerobic training for most training sessions.
- Advanced and professional bodybuilders and strength trainers may use more complex exercises such as dead lifts or power lifts, which involve up to six joints.

Tables 13.2 to 13.4 on pages 242 and 243 provide MxS programs for recreational, advanced, and professional bodybuilders and strength trainers. The load differs quite visibly among the three groups, as it must match ability and training potential.

Nutrition for the Maximum-Strength Phase

This phase, like the mixed phase, is intermediate between the classical hypertrophy (bulk) phase and the definition phase. The nutrition goals in the maximum-strength phase are to maintain much of the weight and solidify all of the muscle mass gained during the hypertrophy phase—and ideally to increase muscle mass marginally, while maximizing the strength that would normally go along with the increased weight and muscle mass.

During this phase, continue to consume the same number of calories as in the mixed phase—that is, the daily caloric intake that resulted in your weight being stabilized. Keep the calories at about that level until you go into the definition phase.

KEYS TO SUCCESS IN THE MXS PHASE

- Stabilize your muscle mass gained through the hypertrophy phase.
- Body fat should not rise above the levels of the hypertrophy phase.
- Stay at the same daily calorie intake that you reached during the mixed phase.
- Dietary protein intake should be at the same level, and dietary fat at a lower level as compared to intakes in the hypertrophy phase.
- For maximum results, use of nutritional supplements is a must.

Supplements for the Maximum-Strength Phase

In the maximum-strength phase, supplements are more important than in the previous three phases. It is still important to get your quota of low-carbohydrate calories and dietary protein to supply you with much of what you need to solidify your increased muscle mass (by increasing muscle protein content and fiber density) and to start getting yourself ready to shed body fat. However, because the daily calories have decreased substantially over the hypertrophy phase, and your training intensity is increasing, supplementing your diet with some targeted supplements will allow you to make better progress.

You will need more than just your basic daily vitamin or mineral tablet. Use MVM, Antiox, and EFA+ on a regular basis. As in the hypertrophy phase, use other supplements—such as Exersol, ReNew, Regulate, JointSupport, LoCarb MRP, and LoCarb Sports Bars—as needed.

For more information on these supplements, see the supplement sections in the chapters describing the hypertrophy (chapter 11) and muscle definition (chapter 14) phases.

In addition to the supplements detailed above, the MxS phase demands a more sophisticated array. At this time it's usually necessary to supplement the diet with additional "lean" protein and to make up the added protein calories by decreasing dietary fat. You also need to use three or four new formulations to maximize the anaerobic energy systems and the anabolic drive.

1. **Myosin Protein** allows you to keep protein levels up at a time when it might be difficult to take in enough protein from foods while at the same time cutting calories. It is an advanced synergistic blend of high-quality protein powders, including a specially developed source of glutamine peptides. Myosin Protein

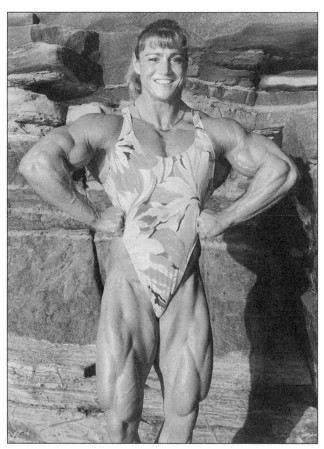

The sensational Laura Binetti has always believed that stacking, cycling, and proper timing of nutritional supplements, along with a sound MxS training program, have played an enormous role in her success.

Complex, containing both fast- and slow-absorbed proteins, is engineered to increase protein synthesis and decrease muscle breakdown. It does this by increasing the anabolic and decreasing the catabolic hormones and by providing the body with an increased immune response to combat overtraining and maximize the anabolic and fat-burning effects of exercise. Because of the gentle processes used to isolate the various proteins, the formula maintains the beneficial immune and other effects of undenatured whey, casein, and soy proteins.

2. **Creatine Advantage** keeps the energy system in high gear despite the decreased caloric intake. By increasing endogenous levels of phosphocreatine, Creatine Advantage increases the immediately available energy that is necessary to fuel the MxS phase's increased exercise intensity. Added amino acids and dipeptides allow a natural increase in the absorption and utilization of creatine and increase the volumizing, anticatabolic, and anabolic effects of the formula.

3. **TestoBoost** contains several natural ingredients; it is designed to improve natural testosterone formation and to decrease any potential side effects from the conversion of testosterone to estrogens and dihydrotestosterone. By boosting the body's natural testosterone levels, TestoBoost lowers body fat while increasing muscle mass.

4. **GHboost** is formulated to increase muscle mass and decrease body fat by enhancing the body's natural production of growth hormone (GH) and insulin-like growth factor-1 (IGF-1). The natural physiological increase in both GH and IGF-1, up to a level consistent with an individual's genetic potential, will enhance muscle development, strength, and size, while decreasing body fat.

Used together, TestoBoost and GHboost maximize endogenous production of and the anabolic and fat-burning effects of testosterone, growth hormone, and IGF-1.

Table 13.2 — Suggested Training Program for the MxS Phase for Recreational Bodybuilders or Strength Trainers

EX. NO.		WEEK 1 — LOW			WEEK 2 — MEDIUM			WEEK 3 — HIGH		
	DAY	1	3	5	1	3	5	1	3	5
1	Leg press	70/8 × 3	75/8 × 4	75/8 × 4	80/6 × 4	80/6 × 3	90/3 × 1	90/3 × 4	90/3 × 4	90/3 × 4
2	Supine leg curl	60/10 × 3	60/10 × 3	70/7 × 4	70/7 × 4	70/7 × 4	70/7 × 4	70/7 × 4	70/7 × 4	70/7 × 4
3	Lat pull-down	70/8 × 3	75/8 × 4	75/8 × 4	80/6 × 4	80/6 × 3	90/3 × 1	90/3 × 4	90/3 × 4	90/3 × 4
4	Front dumbbell press	70/8 × 3	75/8 × 4	75/8 × 4	80/6 × 4	80/6 × 3	90/3 × 1	90/3 × 4	90/3 × 4	90/3 × 4
5	Donkey calf raise	70/8 × 3	75/8 × 4	75/8 × 4	80/6 × 4	80/6 × 3	90/3 × 1	90/3 × 4	90/3 × 4	90/3 × 4

Note: 70/8 × 3 means load/# of repetitions × sets (in this example, 3 sets of 8 repetitions using weight equal to 70 percent of 1RM); combinations of programs are possible, such as 4 MxS, 3 MxS plus 1 H training, etc.

Table 13.3 — An Illustration of an MxS Training Program for Advanced Bodybuilders or Strength Trainers

EX. NO.		WEEK 1 — LOW				WEEK 2 — MEDIUM				WEEK 3 — HIGH				
	DAY	1	3	5	7	1	3	5	7	1	3	5	7	7
1	Safety squat	75/8 × 4	75/8 × 4	75/8 × 4	75/8 × 4	80/6 × 5	85/5 × 5	90/3 × 5	90/3 × 5	90/3 × 5	95/2 × 5	95/2 × 3	100/1 × 2	120/3 × 5
2	Standing leg curl	60/10 × 4	60/10 × 4	65/10 × 4	65/10 × 4	70/7 × 5	85/5 × 5	90/3 × 5	90/3 × 5	80/6 × 5	80/6 × 5	80/6 × 5		80/6 × 5
3	Incline bench press	75/8 × 4	75/8 × 4	75/8 × 4	75/8 × 4	80/6 × 5	85/5 × 5	90/3 × 5	90/3 × 5	90/3 × 5	95/2 × 5	95/2 × 3	100/1 × 2	120/3 × 5
4	Barbell bent-over row	75/8 × 4	75/8 × 4	75/8 × 4	75/8 × 4	80/6 × 5	85/5 × 5	90/3 × 5	90/3 × 5	90/3 × 5	95/2 × 5	95/2 × 3	100/1 × 2	120/3 × 5
5	Donkey calf raise	75/8 × 4	75/8 × 4	75/8 × 4	75/8 × 4	80/6 × 5	85/5 × 5	90/3 × 5	90/3 × 5	90/3 × 5	95/2 × 5	95/2 × 3	100/1 × 2	120/3 × 5
6	Nautilus crunch	60/10 × 4	60/10 × 4	65/10 × 4	65/10 × 4	70/7 × 5	85/5 × 5	90/3 × 5	90/3 × 5	80/6 × 5	80/6 × 5	80/6 × 5		80/6 × 5

Note: In the last workout of the 3rd week there is a session entirely dedicated to eccentric exercises; 75/8 × 4 means load/# of repetitions × sets (in this example, 4 sets of 8 repetitions using weight equal to 75 percent of 1RM).

Table 13.4 Suggested MxS Program for a Professional Bodybuilder, With a Mixture of MLM and Eccentric Method

EX. NO.		WEEK	1						2						3					
	STEP	LOW						MEDIUM						HIGH					
	DAY	1	2	3	4	5	6	1	2	3	4	5	6	1	2	3	4	5	6
1	Safety squat	70/8×6	70/8×6	Off	75/8×3	80/6×5	Off	80/6×6	85/4×6	120/4×6	Off	90/3×7	120/3×7	90/3×6	95/2×3	130/3×7	Off	95/2×7	130/3×7
2	Standing leg curl	70/8×5	70/8×5	Off	75/8×6	75/8×6	Off	75/8×6	75/8×6	80/6×5	Off	80/6×6	80/6×6	80/6×6	80/6×6	85/4×5	Off	85/4×5	85/4×5
3	T-bar row	70/8×6	70/8×6	Off	75/8×3	80/6×5	Off	80/6×6	85/4×6	85/4×6	Off	90/3×7	90/3×7	90/3×6	95/2×3	100/1×3	Off	95/2×7	95/2×7
4	Flat bench press	70/8×6	70/8×6	Off	75/8×3	80/6×5	Off	80/6×6	85/4×6	120/4×6	Off	90/3×7	120/3×7	90/3×6	95/2×3	130/3×7	Off	95/2×7	130/3×7
5	Donkey calf raise	70/8×5	70/8×5	Off	75/8×3	80/6×5	Off	80/6×6	85/4×6	120/4×6	Off	90/3×7	120/3×7	90/3×6	95/2×3	130/3×7	Off	95/2×7	130/3×7
6	Nautilus crunch	70/8×5	70/8×5	Off	75/8×6	75/8×6	Off	75/8×6	75/8×6	80/6×5	Off	80/6×6	80/6×6	80/6×6	80/6×6	85/4×5	Off	85/4×5	85/4×5

Note: Where the load is over 100 percent, it is performed eccentrically; for exercises 2, 3, and 6, where the load is lower, use only MLM, since these exercises are inappropriate for eccentric training; 75/8×4 means load/# of repetitions×sets (in this example, 4 sets of 8 repetitions using weight equal to 75 percent of 1RM).

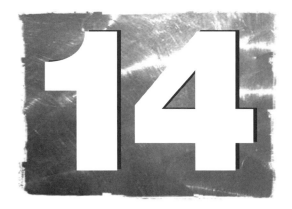

MUSCLE DEFINITION (MD)

During the muscle definition training phase, athletes strive to develop the most refined, polished, and visible muscles possible—known as "getting ripped." Specific high-repetition training methods stimulate the body to use fatty acids as a fuel source, thus helping to burn the subcutaneous fat that is responsible for hiding those precious "cuts."

The duration of the MD phase depends on the needs of the individual. The phase can be three weeks or six weeks; or, as in our model (figure 2.1, page 23), it can comprise two six-week portions. Since the latter choice ensures better achievement of MD, a bodybuilder preparing for a contest would probably opt for it.

Scope of MD Training

- Burns off subcutaneous fat and increases the visibility of muscle striations.
- Increases the protein content of muscles through performance of long, high-rep sets. In addition to better muscle definition, in some instances these exercises also increase muscle strength.
- Clearly increases capillary density within the muscle through increased adaptation to aerobic work, which may result in a slight increase in muscle size.

Training Methods for MD

The vast majority of today's bodybuilders and strength trainers are convinced that the highest number of repetitions they ever need to perform is 12 to 15. These traditionalists believe that in order to increase muscle size a larger number of repetitions are not necessary, and this is certainly true.

The difference is that we are breaking away from the traditional approach to bodybuilding and strength training and believe that the overall body package is more important than plain mass. We want to promote better-looking bodies with higher muscle density, perfect symmetry, and increased muscle separation and striations. The type of training we promote will revolutionize the training philosophy of many bodybuilders and strength trainers. Those who use the Periodization technique will never want to go back to traditional methods. The MD phase plays a very important role in sculpting the ideal body.

Burn Off Fat

In order to maximize muscle separation, striation, and definition, one must burn off as much fat as possible. To accomplish this, the duration of nonstop muscular contraction must be increased. Bodybuilders traditionally have tried to burn off fat through aerobic work, such as running, or by using rowing machines, stationary bikes, or stair climbers. This type of work, however, does not and should not satisfy most bodybuilders who want to become extremely lean. These activities do not entirely achieve their goal of burning off most of the body's subcutaneous fat.

The training methods we promote will result in elimination of fat from the overall body—and, more importantly, from the local muscle groups involved in the activity. The number of repetitions per muscle group and per workout must be drastically but progressively increased. It is equally important to perform the program in a nonstop fashion—to perform hundreds of repetitions per muscle group per workout. Since it is impossible to do work of such long duration nonstop for only one muscle group, the exercises must be continually alternated during the workout. Please refer to the suggested training programs.

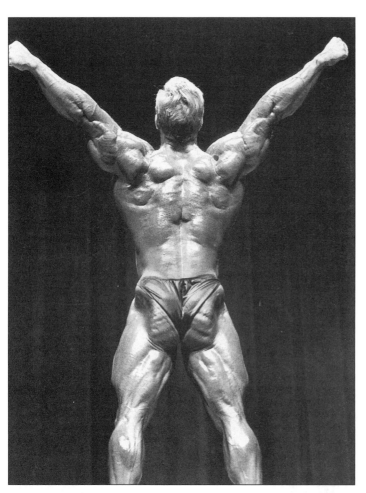

Dave Fisher's signature pose showcases his deeply striated glutes.

Decrease Load With More Reps

In order to perform extremely high repetitions per muscle group, one must decrease the load to 30 to 50 percent of 1RM. At the beginning of a high-rep, low-load set, only a limited number of muscle fibers are active. The other fibers are at rest, but they become activated as the contracting fibers become fatigued. This progressively increasing recruitment of muscle fibers allows a person to perform work for a prolonged period of time. Prolonged work exhausts the ATP/CP and glycogen energy supplies, leaving fatty acids as the only fuel available to sustain this activity. Use of this fuel source burns fat from the body, and especially the subcutaneous fat. The burning off of this type of fat increases muscle striations and muscle definition.

Program Design for the MD Phase

In order to use fatty acids as fuel, an athlete must perform a high number of repetitions per set nonstop. Short RIs will prevent ATP/CP and glycogen from being restored, thus forcing the body to tap its fatty acid reserves. The MD program must be carefully designed. *It is necessary to select exercises and work stations so that it takes no more than two or three seconds to move from one station to another.*

Exercises are often paired together, so it is advisable to select an even number of exercises for each session, as illustrated in our sample programs. Tables 14.1 and 14.2 on page 256 present MD programs both for recreational and for advanced or professional athletes. The suggested exercises are for reference only, and the user has the choice of employing other exercises if needed. In the first three weeks, the purpose of training is to increase the number of reps to 50 or higher for each exercise. When this is accomplished, the exercises are grouped into two, then four, and so on, until eventually all eight exercises can be performed together without stopping. For maximum MD benefits, the ideal program is the one containing two six-week MD phases. The longer the time spent on MD, the greater the amount of fat burned, and the better the muscles will show their striations.

MUSCLE DEFINITION CUES

- MD training requires that muscle groups be constantly alternated.
- The same exercise may be performed twice per set, especially one targeting a desired muscle group.
- The number of reps may not be exactly the same for each exercise. The decision depends on individual strengths and weaknesses for given muscle groups or on an individual's choice in targeting specific muscle(s).
- Speed should be moderate throughout the set. A fast lifting rhythm may produce a high level of lactic acid, which can hamper ability to finish the entire set.
- In order to avoid wasting time between exercises, athletes should (if this is possible) set up all the equipment needed before the training session begins.
- Since the physiological demand of MD training can be quite severe, entry-level athletes should not use it.
- The total number of MD workouts per week can be from 2 to 4, depending on an athlete's experience—lower for recreational, and higher for advanced or professional athletes. The additional 1 to 2 workouts can be divided between aerobic, H, or MxS training.
- The number of reps per exercise should not be restricted to 50, as shown in our example. A very well-trained athlete may go as high as 60 to 75.

Nutrition for the Muscle Definition Phase

The mechanics of the Metabolic Diet remain constant in all phases in terms of carbohydrate intake. The regimen always includes five high-protein days followed by 36 to 48 hours of carbohydrate loading. The only thing that changes is the number of calories consumed—and since it is important to keep protein levels high, and since carbohydrates are already low, athletes must decrease the amount of fat they eat during the low-carb phase and to a lesser extent through the higher-carb phase.

In the muscle definition phase, commonly called the "cutting phase" by bodybuilders, athletes cut calories as a way of trimming fat off the body. The reason for this practice is simple: after athletes have trained their bodies to burn fat as the primary fuel, lowering intake of both calories and fat primes the body to use body fat as fuel—while sparing muscle tissues.

As a rule of thumb, you should cut 500 calories per day from your diet the first week. If you were at 4,000 during the MxS phase, cut intake to 3,500 per day during the first week of your MD phase. The next week you should drop another 200 to 500 calories from the daily diet, depending on how many calories you're taking in. Someone consuming only 2,000 calories, for example, would cut down by only 200 calories. During this time you must measure body fat weekly. What you want to do is *lose 1.5 to 2.0 pounds of body fat each week*—that way you will not lose appreciable lean mass as you cut.

If you find at the end of the second week that you have lost less than 1.5 pounds during the week, cut another 200 to 500 calories the next week and continue cutting calories (anywhere from 100 to 500) in subsequent weeks until you are losing 1.5 pounds a week. If you are losing more than 2 pounds of body fat during the week, you have cut too many calories and will need to adjust them upward.

You don't have to make the cuts in 500-calorie increments. You can fine-tune how many calories you add or subtract. The usual progression is to make the changes 500 calories at a time at first, then perhaps 100 to 500 calories the next few weeks, and then 100 to 200 calories at a time as you get closer to your goal.

The important thing to remember is that it is not calories that you are really after—it's body fat. You must allow for individual variations in calorie count to get that optimum 1.5 to 2.0 pounds of fat loss per week.

You will do plenty of experimentation in this phase to find the right caloric intake for you. Though 500-calorie drops seem to be a good general starting point, especially for people with higher calorie intakes, you must find what works best for you. The calorie levels to which you eventually drop will vary according to your initial caloric intake and your individual metabolism. I have dropped some bodybuilders from 5,000 to 3,000 calories per day in the cutting phase. I have taken others as low as 1,500 to see what happens. If they are losing a fair amount of body fat (remember the 1.5 to 2 pound per

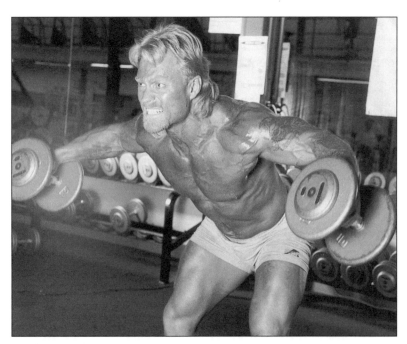

Working hard.

week guideline), and they are getting leaner and not losing significant lean body mass, I leave them at that level until they "lean out." At that point, I increase calories to the point that they maintain or possibly even lose body fat while increasing lean mass again.

Bodybuilders who just want to cut up and are starting at a higher body fat level can go directly into the definition phase. They should start at a reasonable daily calorie value, usually *15 calories per pound of body weight*. Someone weighing 200 pounds at 17 percent body fat should start at around 3,000 calories a day and then follow the instructions above on calorie adjustments needed to maintain the optimum weekly fat loss and minimal loss of muscle mass. Don't start too low—you will have plenty of time to lose body fat in the correct way. If you start too low, the lack of food may be more of a problem than the lack of carbohydrates, and may sabotage your efforts to stick to the diet through the all-important first week.

KEYS TO SUCCESS IN THE MUSCLE DEFINITION PHASE

- Measure body fat weekly.
- Lose 1.5 to 2.0 pounds per week.
- Experiment with caloric intake. Cutting 1,000 calories per day the first week and 500 per day in subsequent weeks is a rough guideline.
- Refine your contest preparation.
- Experiment with foods.

Experimenting With Foods

The Metabolic Diet's five-day, two-day week is almost like getting a person in shape for a contest every week. In the weekend carbohydrate-loading part of the diet, you will find out exactly how many hours you can load up on carbs before you begin to smooth out and lose your contest look.

When you get to your precontest phase, you won't have to make many changes: you will be doing the same thing you have been doing for the previous several weeks in the cutting phase. You will go off the higher-fat, high-protein diet and carb up to dramatically increase the glycogen and water inside the muscle cells. You want the cells swollen and big, but you want to cut off the carbohydrates before you begin to reservoir extracellular water or fat and smooth out.

During the muscle definition phase, you should be refining contest preparation. Play with the kinds of foods you eat on the weekends to see what gives you maximum muscle size. You will know on Monday morning if what you've been eating is right for you. If it is, you will look good—your muscles will be huge and you will be cut up with a nice, pronounced vascularity. If you don't look good, you'll know you did something wrong. Modify your diet the next weekend to see if you can get some improvement. That's the beauty of this diet—by the time a contest approaches, you have already perfected your contest diet by practicing it during the muscle definition phase.

On the old carbohydrate diet, you did this only once. On the Metabolic Diet you do it every week during the cutting phase and you become an expert in how to manipulate your body for a contest.

Experiment with high- and low-sugar foods and with percentages of fat intake on these weekends. See what they do for you. Treat each weekend as if your contest were imminent. That way you will know what it takes to come into a contest looking your best. Your confidence will also grow because you will know what to expect from your body and how to get it contest ready.

The Precontest Phase

One of the many advantages of this diet is that, if you want to enter a lot of contests, you can manipulate your diet so you never get much above the eight percent body fat level. You don't have huge gains in body fat here. At eight percent, you can drop to contest level in just two or three weeks.

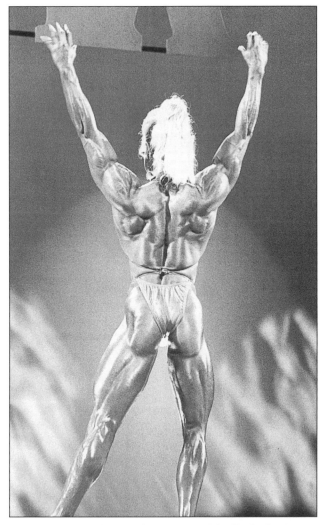

Not an ounce of body fat on this chiselled physique.

You generally will want to go into the precontest phase of diet and training about 16 weeks before a major contest. Because you already know what you need to do from previous weekends on the diet, you will only be doing some fine tuning by lowering and increasing calories a bit as needed. You shouldn't be doing anything much out of the ordinary.

By the final 6 to 8 weeks before the contest, you should look fairly close to how you want to appear on stage. With this diet you can control exactly where you're at each week. After the weekend carb-loading portion of your diet, you should be looking great on Monday—ready to hit the gym hard with the high glycogen levels, muscle swelling, and other benefits derived from a well-honed weekend diet strategy.

You can go through the precontest phase in preparation for several contests a year as long as you keep your fat levels low; yet we suggest that you go through the precontest phase no more than four times a year. That means, obviously, a maximum of four contests a year. More than this will probably prevent you from going back into the mass phase and using it properly.

You must build up lean body mass to some extent between contests, which means that you will gain a bit of fat. You will still be bulking up and cutting down—but it won't be like on other diets with which you gain so much body fat that by the time you lose it you're no better off than when you started.

Being Consistent Before Competition

Two things bodybuilders do to sabotage themselves before contests is to panic or try something new. Both of these scenarios can be disastrous.

Bodybuilders who find themselves too fat may begin doing aerobics, thinking it will get the extra body fat off. Doing about half an hour of aerobics certainly will not harm you—you will burn up more free fatty acids than you would burn doing too little work, and you will take off some body fat. But people sometimes begin to panic and overdo it. They start doing three to four hours a day of aerobics to burn off the fat; but all they do is exhaust energy stores so that their bodies start using muscle tissue for energy.

Some people start pigging out to build mass as they go into super aerobic mode, thinking that aerobics will make up for the fat buildup. It doesn't work. Increasing calories and aerobics will most probably just increase catabolic activity in your body. Aerobics, while burning fat, can also destroy muscle. Even if it doesn't do appreciable damage, it will still limit to some degree the amount of muscle you can put on. As a rule, the fewer calories you take in and the more time you allow yourself to lose the body fat, the less aerobics you will need to do and the more lean body mass you will retain. Allow yourself time to lose extra body fat and gauge yourself effectively as you move toward a contest.

The Metabolic Diet is particularly effective in helping you fine-tune your levels of body fat. With the weekend portion of the diet, you learn what foods to eat, and how much, in order to make yourself successful. You are better able to track your progress and to know precisely what you need to do before the contest.

Other bodybuilders decide to try something new just before a contest, looking to get that final edge. But this is a mistake. They may start with the sodium-depletion or sodium-loading trick. They try all sorts of things they've never tried before, and all of a sudden they end up wondering how it was that they were looking so great and now look so bad. Don't shock your system before a contest. Make a smooth landing into it. Don't throw everything away by trying to get the extra edge through a crazy stunt. Do nothing out of the ordinary, and certainly do not panic.

Fluid Retention

If you tend to retain fluid, begin to restrict yourself to distilled water and low levels of sodium 24 hours before the competition. Also increase your potassium, magnesium, and calcium intake. Since most people tend to retain some fluid, all bodybuilders should consider these suggestions. You want as little extracellular fluid as possible to avoid smoothing out. On the other hand, intracellular fluid will increase cell size so you'll be bigger. It also aids vascularity.

Distilled water and low sodium levels lower the extracellular fluid. Potassium increases the amount of fluid inside the cell. Higher potassium levels are also better for muscle contractions, though you should not create potassium levels that are too high. Calcium and magnesium help you to avoid cramping.

One to Two Weeks Out

Stop training one to two weeks before the contest. That's pretty standard wherever you go. Our advice is to do your last heavy training session 10 days before the contest, to give your muscles maximum time to recuperate and achieve maximum growth. Don't worry about maintaining muscle mass and tone. Your posing will take care of that and also give you some aerobic activity. Posing should, of course, be continued throughout this entire period, with the exception of the day before the contest.

But though you shut down heavy training 10 days or so before a contest, this is the *only* time you should back off. Some people think that just because they're on the Metabolic Diet, they don't have to work as hard. That's simply not true. All you do by cutting back in training is limit the effectiveness of the diet and your ultimate growth.

Diet and training work hand-in-hand. Exercise complements the Metabolic Diet. Hormonal changes caused by exercise result in increased activity of the enzyme lipoprotein lipase (LPL) in the muscle, which in turn increases breakdown of free fatty acids and decreases fat buildup.

Countdown to Contest

During the weekend carbohydrate loading part of your diet, note how many hours into it that you look your very best. Further refine that time, by experimenting with the types of food you eat, to precisely dial in that time when you're at your best. Then use this information when the contest arrives.

Identify Your Best Day

What you eventually will find is that there is a day in the week when you look your very best. All the water you have gained during your carb load is gone, and you have just the right balance between muscle glycogen and water to look your best. You also feel great. Everyone's system works differently, and there are wide differences among individuals. The goal is to find the right day *for you*, that day each week—Monday, Tuesday, Wednesday, whatever—when you are consistently at your best.

Most contests occur on Saturday. Suppose you have found that you look your best on Wednesday of each week. Your goal then is to basically make the Saturday of your contest like a Wednesday. Because you look your best three days after your carbohydrate load, you should complete a carb loading three days—in this case, on Tuesday and Wednesday—before the contest. Three days later, on Saturday, you will look your best.

Note that the weekend before the contest, you won't carb up as usual. To carb up on the weekend and repeat the process two or three days later may well spill you back over to a carb-burning metabolism and

Laura Binetti displays the results of dedicated contest preparation.

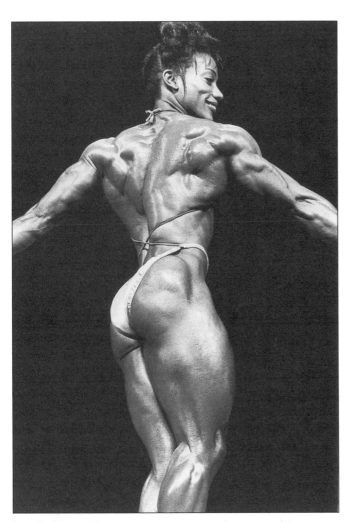

Lenda Murray's precontest preparation was always one of the best in the sport.

smooth you out for that Saturday contest. Rather, skip your carbohydrate load the weekend before a contest. That way you will be on the high-protein, higher-fat part of the Metabolic Diet for eight straight days, from the Monday two weeks before the contest to the Tuesday before the contest. Then begin your precontest carbohydrate load so you will hit the contest just right.

This is one area where the Metabolic Diet has a big advantage over the competition. Because you are basically *always* loading up on carbohydrates when you're on the high-carb diet, it's difficult to manipulate the diet so that the body responds well to your carb loading before the contest.

What often happens on high-carbohydrate diets is that you get off your high-carb diet for three days at the beginning of the week before a competition and go low-carb for 72 hours; then you again load up on carbohydrates in an attempt to hit the contest right. The problem is, you really don't know how your body is going to react. Everything could work out well, or you could experience a complete disaster. It's Russian roulette. You have perhaps a 50 percent chance of hitting the mark: you've had maybe a year to prepare for the contest, you've been disciplined and dedicated, yet you miss the mark when you hit the stage because of the uncertainty of the high-carb diet.

With the Metabolic Diet, you know the exact hour when you look your best. Because your body goes through the cycle every week, it has become predictable and consistent. You know precisely what to expect, since you won't be doing anything different from what you have done in the preceding months.

KEYS TO SUCCESS IN THE PRECONTEST PHASE

- Begin this phase 16 weeks before contest.
- By 6 to 8 weeks out, you should be close to your contest look.
- Don't panic or make rash decisions.
- Stick with the program.
- Don't overdo aerobics.
- Stop training 1 to 2 weeks out.
- Skip your carbohydrate load the weekend before the contest.
- Time your carbohydrate load so you'll look your best at prejudging.

- Allow a 4-hour "fail-safe" period.
- Begin to drink distilled water, increase potassium, magnesium, and calcium, and reduce sodium 24 hours before contest.
- Be careful with diet after prejudging.

Prejudging

You want that exact hour when you look your best to coincide with prejudging; this is where most decisions are made. But the body is not a perfectly predictable instrument. To be certain that you don't smooth out, therefore, give yourself four hours of extra time as a kind of fail-safe mechanism for prejudging. That is, if you are at your best 48 hours after carbohydrate loading, and prejudging will take place at 2 o'clock on Saturday, count back 48 hours. This puts you at 2 o'clock Thursday. Giving yourself the extra four hours mentioned above, you should complete your carb loading at 6 P.M. on Thursday.

You also will want to look good at the evening show, especially if judging is close and will be ultimately decided in the evening. Fortunately, you usually have a several-hour window during which you look good; and that window usually will overlap the evening session.

Yet you still need to be careful. Some competitors look great for prejudging, then go out and eat, thinking it's all over. They come in bloated and retaining water for the evening show and in a close competition will lose because of it. You must stay tight all day. Keep diet minimal and in the higher-fat mode. Even having food in your stomach will create a slight bulge. You want to keep everything nice and flat; so keep your regimen going through the evening contest.

The above, of course, is just an example. You have to work with the diet to find the best approach for you. The big difference between this diet and whatever you've been on before is the precision with which you can plan your contest regimen. Not only does the Metabolic Diet build muscle and burn fat, it also gives you a weekly opportunity to practice and prepare for a contest so that you can manipulate your diet to the very best effect.

Supplements for the Muscle Definition Phase

Cycling nutritional supplements means using those supplements that are phase-specific so that a different set of supplements is used in each phase. Always use supplements at the right times and for the right reasons. For example, there are vast differences in dietary needs and in the effects of various supplements between the mass and definition phases. The nutritional supplements you need on days when you train differ from what you need on rest days. Manipulating the diet and nutritional supplement use in and around training increases the anabolic and fat-burning effects of the training, and it can decrease recuperation time and enhance your abilities to perform at the next training session.

Other variables that affect diet and use of nutritional supplements include bodybuilders' training backgrounds and the levels that they have reached. Novice bodybuilders—in which gains come relatively easy even with simple training routines and a diet high in calories and protein—don't need the sophisticated dietary modifications and cutting-edge nutritional supplements that are necessary to improve more advanced bodybuilders.

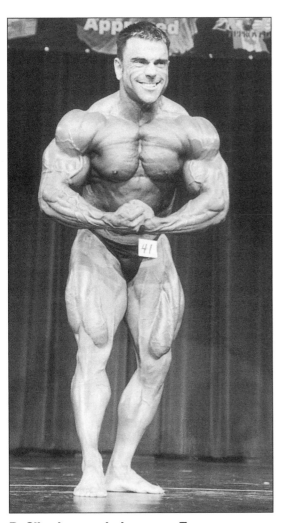

DaSilva has got it down to a T.

Supplements come into their own in the muscle definition phase, in which they are extremely useful in maintaining and raising the anabolic and fat-burning response to the Metabolic Diet and training. In this phase you consistently cut calories so that your body effectively uses your body fat as fuel; yet in so doing, your system tends to change its hormones and metabolism to a survivalist mode that is counter-productive to your goals. The Metabolic Diet is a big help here, but the supplements are also important. The following supplements work well in this phase:

- Exersol
- LoCarb MRP and Bars
- TestoBoost
- GHboost
- Creatine Advantage*Myosin Protein
- Metabolic

There is little difference between supplements used in the cutting and precontest phases. The only thing to watch out for is the effect some of the supplements may have on your definition. For example, some bodybuilders discontinue creatine a few weeks before a competition because they retain more water and are less defined if they stay on it. Also the use of certain supplements—such as Myosin Protein, Metabolic, ReNew, and JointSupport—usually should increase as the competition gets closer.

Training Programs for Muscle Definition

We will use the eight exercises suggested in tables 14.1 and 14.2 to illustrate how to apply the muscle definition training method.

In the first week, the load is dropped to 30 to 50 percent 1RM, with lower loads for recreational athletes and higher loads for advanced and professional athletes. Using table 14.1 as an example, the actual program is as follows:

1. Perform 30 reps with the appropriate load on the leg press machine. Without any rest, perform 30 reps of the front barbell press.
2. Place a bar with the appropriate load on the preacher curl bench and then perform 30 crunches followed immediately by 30 preacher curls.
3. Next, lie down on a bench and perform 30 bench presses followed by 30 leg extensions, 30 supine leg curls, and finally 30 lat pull-downs.

For the MD program, a set is the performance of all eight exercises. The suggested number of sets is not a standard or a limitation. Depending on your working potential and motivation, the number of sets can be slightly increased. You may perform a higher number of sets if the number of exercises and work stations is lower, or fewer sets if you are using 8 to 12 exercises.

Table 14.1 An MD Training Program for Recreational Bodybuilders and Strength Trainers

No.	Exercise	Week 1	Week 2	Week 3	Week 4	Week 5	Week 6
1	Leg press	Increase number of reps to 30 for each exercise. RI between exercises = 1 minute.	Perform 40 reps per exercise. RI between exercises = 1 minute.	Perform 50 reps per exercise. RI between exercises = 1 minute.	Perform 2 exercises together nonstop, or 100 reps (e.g., 50 leg presses and 50 upright rows). Do the same for the other 3 pairs. RI between exercises = 1 minute.	Perform 4 exercises together nonstop, or 200 reps. Same for the other 4. RI between set of 4 exercises = 1 minute.	Perform all 8 exercises together nonstop, or 400 reps. RI between set of 8 exercises = 1 minute.
2	Front barbell press						
3	Crunch						
4	Biceps preacher curl						
5	Flat bench press						
6	Leg extension						
7	Supine leg curl						
8	Lat pull-down						

Duration = 6 weeks; load = 30 percent; number of sets = 2-3.

Table 14.2 An MD Training Program for Advanced or Professional Bodybuilders and Strength Trainers

Week	1-4	5-6	7	8-9	10-12
Training program	First 4 weeks as per table 14.1.	Perform 4 exercises together nonstop, or 200 reps. Same for the other 4.	A light week of training for regeneration.	Perform 4 exercises together nonstop, or 200 reps. Same for the other 4.	Perform 8 exercises together nonstop, or 400 reps.

Duration = 6 + 6 weeks = total of 12 weeks; load = 40-50 percent depending on individual's ability and work tolerance; number of sets = 3-5; RI between sets = 1 minute (if too short, increase slightly and reduce to 1 minute at a later date); RI between exercises: none.

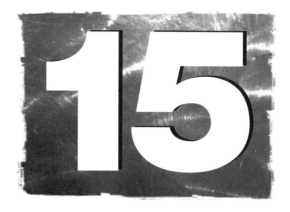

TRANSITION (T)

An annual plan, as suggested in our examples, should finish with a transition phase. Following many months of intensive training, athletes must give their bodies a respite to allow recovery and regeneration to occur before beginning a new year of training.

In addition to a year-end transition phase, we recommend employing a brief transition period between each different training phase.

Scope of T Training

- Decreases the volume and intensity of training and facilitates removal of the fatigue acquired during the previous phase or annual plan.
- Replenishes exhausted energy stores.
- Relaxes the body and the mind.

Duration of T Training

If the year-end T phase exceeds four to six weeks, the hard-sought training benefits will fade away and the athlete will experience a detraining effect. Also, the athlete who adheres to the four- to six-week time frame but does no strength training during the T phase may experience a decrease in muscle size together with a considerable loss in power (Wilmore and Costill 1999).

During transition, physical activity is reduced by 60 to 70 percent. It is advisable, however, to lightly train those muscles that are or may become asymmetrically developed during a period of low-intensity training.

Program Design for T Phase: Detraining

Improvement or maintenance of muscle size and strength is possible only if the body is constantly exposed to an adequate training stimulus. When training decreases or stops, as it does during a long transition phase, there is a disturbance in the biological state of the muscle cell and of bodily organs. Consequently, there is a marked decrease in the athlete's physiological well-being and work output (Fry et al. 1991; Kuipers and Keizer 1988).

This state of diminished training can leave athletes vulnerable to the *detraining syndrome* (Israel 1972) or *exercise-dependency syndrome* (Kuipers and Keizer 1988), the extent of which depends on the length of time away from training.

Effects of Detraining

A decrease in the cross-sectional area of the muscle fibers becomes visible after only a couple of weeks of inactivity. These changes result from higher rates of protein degradation (catabolism) that reverse the muscle gains made during training. Greater levels of sodium and chloride ions in the muscles also play a role in the breakdown of muscle fibers (Appell 1990).

Strength loss occurs during the first week of inactivity at a rate of roughly 3 to 4 percent per day (Appell 1990), largely due to the degeneration of motor units. Slow twitch fibers are usually the first to lose their force-producing capabilities, while fast twitch fibers generally take longer to be affected by inactivity. During the state of detraining the body cannot recruit the same number of motor units that it once could, resulting in a net decrease in the amount of force that can be generated within the muscle (Hainaut and Duchatteau 1989; Houmard 1991).

Detraining causes the body's natural testosterone levels to fall. And since the presence of testosterone is crucial for gains in size and strength, protein synthesis within the muscles diminishes as these levels fall (Houmard 1991). Headaches, insomnia, feelings of exhaustion, loss of appetite, increased tension, mood disturbances, and depression are among the usual symptoms associated with total abstinence from training. An athlete may develop any number of these symptoms, all of which appear to be associated with the lowered levels of testosterone and beta-endorphin (a neuroendocrine compound that is the main forerunner to euphoric postexercise feelings) (Houmard 1991).

Nutrition for the T Phase

I usually suggest going off the strict part of the Metabolic Diet and reintroducing a moderate amount of carbohydrates (20-50 percent of total caloric intake), cutting back on protein, and consuming only moderate amounts of fat—in other words, almost the normal North American diet. Don't worry about having problems getting strict with the Metabolic Diet when it is time to back onto it. Your body will "remember" and it will be much easier to get back into the groove.

Nutritional Supplements for the T Phase

During the T phase, back off all your supplements except maybe MVM, the vitamin and mineral supplement. The one other supplement you may want to use during this phase is ReNew, since this supplement is meant to get your system, especially your immune system, back to normal.

ReNew is formulated not only to enhance the immune system, but also to normalize the metabolism and to naturally support thyroid, testosterone, GH, insulin, and adrenergic function. It is the perfect nutritional supplement to deal with workout fatigue at the end of a long Periodization session.

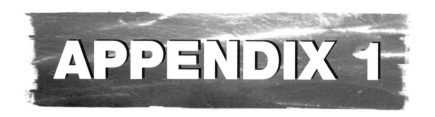

APPENDIX 1

Training Log

Enter exercise, load, and number of repetitions per set (i.e., 180 × 6).

No.	Exercise	SETS									
		1	2	3	4	5	6	7	8	9	10

Reprinted from Bompa 1996.

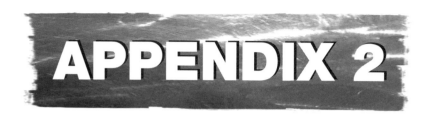

APPENDIX 2

Maximum Lift Based on Repetitions

% of 1RM REPS	100 1	95 2	90 4	85 6	80 8	75 10
Pounds lifted	700.00	665.00	630.00	595.00	560.00	525.00
	695.00	660.25	625.50	590.75	556.00	521.25
	690.00	655.50	621.00	586.50	552.00	517.50
	685.00	650.75	616.50	582.25	548.00	513.75
	680.00	646.00	612.00	578.00	544.00	510.00
	675.00	641.25	607.50	573.75	540.00	507.00
	670.00	636.50	603.00	569.50	536.00	502.50
	665.00	631.75	598.50	565.25	532.00	498.75
	660.00	627.00	594.00	561.00	528.00	495.00
	655.00	622.25	589.50	556.75	524.00	491.25
	650.00	617.50	585.00	552.50	520.00	487.50
	645.00	612.76	580.50	548.25	516.00	483.75
	640.00	608.00	576.00	544.00	512.00	480.00
	635.00	603.25	571.50	539.75	508.00	476.25
	630.00	598.50	567.00	535.50	504.00	472.50
	625.00	593.75	562.50	531.25	500.00	468.75
	620.00	589.00	558.00	527.00	496.00	465.00
	615.00	584.25	553.50	522.75	492.00	461.25
	610.00	579.50	549.00	518.50	488.00	457.50
	605.00	574.75	544.50	514.25	484.00	453.75
	600.00	570.00	540.00	510.00	480.00	450.00
	595.00	565.25	535.50	505.75	476.00	446.25
	590.00	560.50	531.00	501.50	472.00	442.50
	585.00	555.75	526.50	497.25	468.00	438.75
	580.00	551.00	522.00	493.00	464.00	435.00
	575.00	546.25	517.50	488.75	460.00	431.25
	570.00	541.50	513.00	484.50	456.00	427.50
	565.00	536.75	508.50	480.25	452.00	423.75
	560.00	532.00	504.00	476.00	448.00	420.00
	555.00	527.50	499.50	471.75	444.00	416.25
	550.00	522.50	495.00	467.50	440.00	412.50
	545.00	517.75	490.50	463.25	436.00	408.75
	540.00	513.00	486.00	459.00	432.00	405.00
	535.00	508.25	481.50	454.75	428.00	401.25
	530.00	503.50	477.00	450.50	424.00	397.50
	525.00	498.75	472.50	446.25	420.00	393.75

(continued)

Maximum Lift Based on Repetitions *(continued)*

% of 1RM REPS	100 1	95 2	90 4	85 6	80 8	75 10
Pounds lifted	520.00	494.00	468.00	442.00	416.00	390.00
	515.00	489.25	463.50	437.75	412.00	386.25
	510.00	484.50	459.00	433.50	408.00	382.50
	505.00	479.75	454.50	429.25	404.00	378.75
	500.00	475.00	450.00	425.00	400.00	375.00
	495.00	470.25	445.50	420.75	396.00	371.25
	490.00	465.50	441.00	416.50	392.00	367.50
	485.00	460.75	436.50	412.25	388.00	363.75
	480.00	456.00	432.00	408.50	384.00	360.00
	475.00	451.25	427.50	403.75	380.00	356.25
	470.00	446.50	423.00	399.50	376.00	352.50
	465.00	441.75	418.50	395.25	372.00	348.75
	460.00	437.00	414.00	391.00	368.00	345.00
	455.00	432.75	409.50	386.75	364.00	341.25
	450.00	427.50	405.00	382.50	360.00	337.50
	445.00	422.75	400.50	378.25	356.00	333.75
	440.00	418.00	396.00	374.00	352.00	330.00
	435.00	413.25	391.50	369.75	348.00	326.25
	430.00	408.50	387.00	365.50	344.00	322.50
	425.00	403.75	382.00	361.25	340.00	318.75
	420.00	399.00	378.00	357.00	336.00	315.00
	415.00	394.25	373.50	352.75	332.00	311.25
	410.00	389.50	369.00	348.50	328.00	307.50
	405.00	384.75	364.50	344.25	324.00	303.75
	400.00	380.00	360.00	340.00	320.00	300.00
	395.00	375.25	355.50	335.75	316.00	296.25
	390.00	370.50	351.00	331.50	312.00	292.50
	385.00	365.76	346.50	327.25	308.00	288.75
	380.00	361.00	342.00	323.00	304.00	285.00
	375.00	356.25	337.50	318.75	300.00	281.25
	370.00	351.50	330.00	314.50	296.00	277.50
	365.00	346.75	328.50	310.25	292.00	273.75
	360.00	342.00	324.00	306.00	288.00	270.00
	355.00	337.25	319.50	301.75	284.00	266.25
	350.00	332.50	315.00	297.50	280.00	262.50
	345.00	327.75	310.50	293.25	276.00	258.75
	340.00	323.00	306.00	289.00	272.00	255.00
	335.00	318.25	301.50	284.75	268.00	251.25
	330.00	313.50	297.00	280.50	264.00	247.50
	325.00	308.75	292.50	276.25	260.00	243.75
	320.00	304.00	288.00	272.00	256.00	240.00
	315.00	299.25	283.50	267.75	252.00	236.25
	310.00	294.50	279.00	263.50	248.00	232.50
	305.00	289.75	274.50	259.25	244.00	228.75
	300.00	285.00	270.00	255.00	240.00	225.00
	295.00	280.25	265.50	250.75	236.00	221.25

Maximum Lift Based on Repetitions

% of 1RM REPS	100 1	95 2	90 4	85 6	80 8	75 10
Pounds lifted	290.00	275.50	261.00	246.50	232.00	217.50
	285.00	270.75	256.50	242.25	228.00	213.75
	280.00	266.00	252.00	238.00	224.00	210.00
	275.00	261.25	247.50	233.75	220.00	206.25
	270.00	256.50	243.00	229.50	216.00	202.50
	265.00	251.75	238.50	225.25	212.00	198.75
	260.00	247.00	234.00	221.00	208.00	195.00
	255.00	242.25	229.50	216.75	204.00	191.25
	250.00	237.50	225.00	212.50	200.00	187.50
	245.00	232.75	220.50	208.25	196.00	183.75
	240.00	228.00	216.00	204.00	192.00	180.00
	235.00	223.25	211.50	199.75	188.00	176.25
	230.00	218.50	207.00	195.50	184.00	172.50
	225.00	213.75	202.50	191.25	180.00	168.75
	220.00	209.00	198.00	187.00	176.00	165.00
	215.00	204.25	193.50	182.75	172.00	161.25
	210.00	199.50	189.00	178.50	168.00	157.50
	205.00	194.75	184.50	174.25	164.00	153.75
	200.00	190.00	180.00	170.00	160.00	150.00
	195.00	185.25	175.50	165.75	156.00	146.25
	190.00	180.50	171.00	161.50	152.00	142.50
	185.00	175.75	166.50	157.25	148.00	138.75
	180.00	171.00	162.00	153.00	144.00	135.00
	175.00	166.25	157.50	148.75	140.00	131.25
	170.00	161.50	153.00	144.50	136.00	127.50
	165.00	156.75	148.50	140.25	132.00	123.75
	160.00	152.00	144.00	136.00	128.00	120.00
	155.00	147.25	139.50	131.75	124.00	116.25
	150.00	142.50	135.00	127.50	120.00	112.50
	145.00	137.75	130.50	123.24	116.00	108.75
	140.00	133.00	126.00	119.00	112.00	105.00
	135.00	128.25	121.50	114.75	108.00	101.25
	130.00	123.50	117.00	110.50	104.00	97.50
	125.00	118.75	112.50	106.25	100.00	93.75
	120.00	114.00	108.00	102.00	96.00	90.00
	115.00	109.25	103.50	97.75	92.00	86.25
	110.00	104.50	99.00	93.50	88.00	82.50
	105.00	99.75	94.50	89.25	84.00	78.75

Reprinted from Bompa 1996.

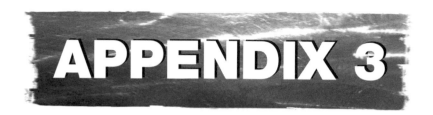

APPENDIX 3

Maximum Weight Chart

If for any reason, (i.e., equipment) an athlete cannot lift the load necessary to calculate 1RM, but only 3, 4, or 5RM and so on, one can still figure out his or her 1RM by using the chart below. In order to calculate 1RM, perform the maximum number of repetitions with the load available (say 4 repetitions with 250 pounds), and then do the following:

1. Choose from the top of the chart the column headed "4"—the number of repetitions you did.
2. Find the row for 250 pounds—the maximum load you had available.
3. Find the number where column (4) and row 250 meet.
4. This number is your 1RM at that given time.

Maximum Weight Chart

Pounds	10	9	8	7	6	5	4	3	2
5	7	6	6	6	6	6	6	5	5
10	13	13	13	12	12	11	11	11	11
15	20	19	19	18	18	17	17	16	16
20	27	26	25	24	24	23	22	22	21
25	33	32	31	30	29	29	28	27	26
30	40	39	38	36	35	34	33	32	32
35	47	45	44	42	41	40	39	38	37
40	53	52	50	48	47	46	44	43	42
45	60	58	56	55	53	51	50	49	47
50	67	65	63	61	59	57	56	54	53
55	73	71	69	67	65	63	61	59	58
60	80	77	75	73	71	69	67	65	63
65	87	84	81	79	76	74	72	70	68
70	93	90	88	85	82	80	78	76	74
75	100	97	94	91	88	86	83	81	79
80	107	103	100	97	94	91	89	86	84
85	113	110	106	103	100	97	94	92	89
90	120	116	113	109	106	103	100	97	95
95	127	123	119	115	112	109	106	103	100
100	133	129	125	121	118	114	111	108	105
105	140	135	131	127	124	120	117	114	111
110	147	142	138	133	129	126	122	119	116
115	153	148	144	139	135	131	128	124	121
120	160	155	150	145	141	137	133	130	126
125	167	161	156	152	147	143	139	135	132
130	173	168	163	158	153	149	144	141	137

(continued)

Maximum Weight Chart *(continued)*

Pounds	10	9	8	7	6	5	4	3	2
135	180	174	169	164	159	154	150	146	142
140	187	181	175	170	165	160	156	151	147
145	193	187	181	176	171	166	161	157	153
150	200	194	188	182	176	171	167	162	158
155	207	200	194	188	182	177	172	168	163
160	213	206	200	194	188	183	178	173	168
165	220	213	206	200	194	189	183	178	174
170	227	219	213	206	200	194	189	184	179
175	233	226	219	212	206	200	194	189	184
180	240	232	225	218	212	206	200	195	189
185	247	239	231	224	218	211	206	200	195
190	253	245	238	230	224	217	211	205	200
195	260	252	244	236	229	223	217	211	205
200	267	258	250	242	235	229	222	216	211
205	273	265	256	248	241	234	228	222	216
210	280	271	263	255	247	240	233	227	221
215	287	277	269	261	253	246	239	232	226
220	293	284	275	267	259	251	244	238	232
225	300	290	281	273	265	257	250	243	237
230	307	297	288	279	271	263	256	249	242
235	313	303	294	285	276	269	261	254	247
240	320	310	300	291	282	274	267	259	253
245	327	316	306	297	288	280	272	265	258
250	333	323	313	303	294	286	278	270	263
255	340	329	319	309	300	291	283	276	268
260	347	335	325	315	306	297	289	281	274
265	353	342	331	321	312	303	294	286	279
270	360	348	338	327	318	309	300	292	284
275	367	355	344	333	324	314	306	297	289
280	373	361	350	339	329	320	311	303	295
285	380	368	356	345	335	326	317	308	300
290	387	374	363	352	341	331	322	314	305
295	393	381	369	358	347	337	328	319	311
300	400	387	375	364	353	343	333	324	316
305	407	394	381	370	359	349	339	330	321
310	413	400	388	376	365	354	344	335	326
315	420	406	394	382	371	360	350	341	332
320	427	413	400	388	376	366	356	346	337
325	433	419	406	394	382	371	361	351	342
330	440	426	413	400	388	377	367	357	347
335	447	432	419	406	394	383	372	362	353
340	453	439	425	412	400	389	378	368	358
345	460	445	431	418	406	394	383	373	363
350	467	452	438	424	412	400	389	378	368
355	473	458	444	430	418	406	394	384	374
360	480	465	450	436	424	411	400	389	379
365	487	471	456	442	429	417	406	395	384
370	493	477	463	448	435	423	411	400	389

Maximum Weight Chart

Pounds	10	9	8	7	6	5	4	3	2
375	500	484	469	455	441	429	417	405	395
380	507	490	475	461	447	434	422	411	400
385	513	497	481	467	453	440	428	416	405
390	520	503	488	473	459	446	433	422	411
395	527	510	494	479	465	451	439	427	416
400	533	516	500	485	471	457	444	432	421
405	540	523	506	491	476	463	450	438	426
410	547	529	513	497	482	469	456	443	432
415	553	535	519	503	488	474	461	449	437
420		542	525	509	494	480	467	454	442
425		548	531	515	500	486	472	459	447
430		555	538	521	506	491	478	465	453
435		561	544	527	512	497	483	470	458
440		568	550	533	518	503	489	476	463
445		574	556	539	524	509	494	481	468
450		581	563	545	529	514	500	486	474
455		587	569	552	535	520	506	492	479
460		594	575	558	541	526	511	497	484
465		600	581	564	547	531	517	503	489
470		606	588	570	553	537	522	508	495
475		613	594	576	559	543	528	514	500
480		619	600	582	565	549	532	519	505
485		626	606	588	571	554	539	524	511
490		632	613	594	576	560	544	530	516
495		639	619	600	582	566	550	535	521
500		645	625	606	588	571	556	541	526
505		652	631	612	594	577	561	546	532
510		658	638	618	600	583	567	551	537
515		665	644	624	606	589	572	557	542
520		671	650	630	612	594	578	562	547
525		677	656	636	618	600	583	569	553
530		684	663	642	624	606	589	573	558
535		690	669	648	629	611	594	578	563
540		697	675	655	635	617	600	584	568
545		703	681	661	641	623	606	589	574
550		710	688	667	647	629	611	595	579
555		716	694	673	653	634	617	600	584
560		723	700	679	659	640	622	605	589
565		729	706	685	665	646	628	611	595
570		735	713	691	671	651	633	616	600
575		742	719	697	676	657	639	622	605
580		748	725	703	682	663	644	627	611
585		755	731	709	688	669	650	632	616
590		761	738	715	694	674	656	638	621
595		768	744	721	700	680	661	643	626
600		774	750	727	706	686	667	649	632
605		781	756	733	712	691	672	654	637
610		787	763	739	718	697	678	659	642

(continued)

Maximum Weight Chart *(continued)*

Pounds	10	9	8	7	6	5	4	3	2
615		794	769	745	724	703	683	665	647
620		800	775	752	729	709	689	670	653
625		806	781	758	735	714	694	676	658
630		813	788	764	741	720	700	681	663
635		819	794	770	747	726	706	686	668
640		826	800	776	753	731	711	692	674
645		832	806	782	759	737	717	697	679
650		839	813	788	765	743	722	703	684
655		845	819	794	771	749	728	708	689
660		852	825	800	776	754	733	714	695
665		858	831	806	782	760	739	719	700
670		865	838	812	788	766	644	724	705
675		871	844	818	794	771	750	730	711
680		877	850	824	800	777	756	735	716
685		884	856	830	806	783	761	741	721
690		890	863	836	812	789	767	746	726
695		897	869	842	818	794	772	751	732
700		903	875	848	824	800	778	757	737
705		910	881	855	829	806	783	762	742
710		916	888	861	835	811	789	768	747
715		923	894	768	841	817	794	773	753
720		929	900	873	847	823	800	778	758
725		935	906	879	853	829	806	784	763
730		942	913	885	859	834	811	789	768
735		948	919	891	865	840	817	795	774
740		955	925	897	871	846	822	800	779
745		961	931	903	876	851	828	805	784
750		968	938	909	882	857	833	811	789
755		974	944	915	888	863	839	816	795
760		981	950	921	894	869	844	822	800
765		987	956	927	900	874	850	827	805
770		994	963	933	906	880	856	832	811
775		1,000	969	939	912	886	861	838	816
780		1,006	975	945	918	891	867	843	821
785		1,013	981	952	924	897	872	849	826
790		1,019	988	958	929	903	878	854	832
795		1,026	994	964	935	908	883	859	837
800		1,032	1,000	970	941	914	889	865	842
820		1,058	1,025	994	965	937	911	886	863
840		1,084	1,050	1,018	988	960	933	908	884
860		1,110	1,075	1,042	1,012	983	956	930	905
880		1,135	1,100	1,067	1,035	1,006	978	951	926
900		1,161	1,125	1,091	1,059	1,029	1,000	973	947
920		1,187	1,150	1,115	1,082	1,051	1,022	995	968

Reprinted from Bompa 1996.

GLOSSARY

actin—A protein involved in muscle activity.

adaptation threshold—The level of adaptation an individual reaches in a given training phase. To surpass the threshold, one has to increase the stimulation (loading) level.

adaptation—Persistent changes in structure or function of a muscle as a direct response to progressively increased training loads.

agonist—A muscle directly engaged in a muscle contraction and working in opposition to the action of other muscles.

all-or-none law—A stimulated muscle or nerve fiber contracts or propagates a nerve impulse either completely or not at all (i.e., a minimal stimulus causes a maximum response).

amino acid—Basic unit of structure in proteins.

anabolic—Protein building.

androgenic—Possessing masculinizing properties.

antagonist—A muscle that has the opposite effect of an agonistic muscle, opposing its contraction.

ATP deficiency theory—The theory that constant taxation of ATP (i.e., disturbance in the equilibrium between consumption and manufacturing of ATP) results in increased muscle hypertrophy.

atrophy—A gradual shrinking of muscle tissue as a result of disuse or disease.

ballistic—Dynamic muscular movements.

beta-endorphin—A naturally occurring chemical substance (a peptide) produced in the brain. Endorphins produce a natural analgesic effect by binding to certain receptor sites in the body (the same sites that bind morphine). Endorphins are believed to be released during prolonged exercise.

beta-lipotropin—A trophic hormone secreted by the anterior lobe of the pituitary gland. Its physiological function is unclear, but its amino acid sequence is similar to that of endorphins and enkephalins (endogenous morphine-like substances) and hence it is also believed to produce analgesia.

bioelectrical impedance analysis—A method of measuring body fat. An electrical current is transmitted through the body, and the resistance or impedance to the current is measured. Because the body's fat-free mass contains much of the body's water and electrolytes and is therefore a better conductor of electrical current, impedance to the current gives information about the person's percentage of body fat.

biological value—Describes how efficiently body tissue can be created from food proteins.

calorie cycling—The practice of alternating low-, medium-, and high-calorie days to prevent the body from adapting to any particular amount of food intake. Helps to keep the metabolism from slowing down during periods of dieting.

carbohydrate—Any of a group of chemical compounds, including sugars, starches, and cellulose, containing only carbon, hydrogen, and oxygen. One of the basic food stuffs.

cardiac stroke volume (or stroke volume)—The amount of blood pumped out of the left ventricle per beat. The average amount is approximately 70 ml/beat in a resting man of average size tested in a supine position.

catabolic—Increases the degradation of protein.

ceiling of adaptation—A certain level of adaptation an individual has reached during training. The goal of training is to break through the ceiling of adaptation in order to raise it, and as a result, to improve performance.

central nervous system (CNS)—The spinal cord and the brain.

cheat day—A planned day used during periods of dieting to help prevent the body from adapting to specific caloric intakes.

chronic hypertrophy—Long-lasting hypertrophy resulting from structural changes at the muscle level after the employment of heavy loads (over 80 percent 1RM).

complete protein—Protein that contains all of the nine essential amino acids. Found in animal protein sources.

complex carbohydrates—Also known as polysaccharides or starches. They are composed of many glucose units and are found in vegetables, fruits, and grains.

creatine kinase—A soluble muscle protein that when found in the circulatory system is indicative of muscle damage. Specific isomers of creatine kinase are used to differentiate between damage to skeletal muscle and damage to cardiac muscle.

creatine phosphate (CP)—A high-energy compound stored in muscles; it supplies energy for high-intensity activities that last less than 30 seconds.

cross bridge—Extensions of myosin, a contractile protein. Cross bridges play a major role in muscle contraction.

detraining—Reversal of adaptation to exercise. Effects of detraining occur more rapidly than training gains, with significant reduction of strength (and work) capacity only two weeks after training stops.

disaccharide—Simple sugar composed of two monosaccharides. The most common are sucrose (table sugar) and lactose (found in milk).

double pyramid load pattern—Pertaining to increasing the load from the bottom up, and decreasing it again to the initial level.

dynamic flexibility—The performance of a motion requiring flexible muscles in an active manner (as opposed to static). Often called ballistic flexibility.

eccentric contraction—A muscle action that lengthens muscle fibers as it develops tension.

edema—Swelling. A local or generalized condition in which the body tissues contain an excessive amount of tissue fluid. Acute swelling, or edema, refers to the rapid build-up of tissue fluid in an area that lasts for only a short time (i.e., not chronic).

electromyography (EMG)—Measurement of the electrical activity of the excitable membranes of a muscle or muscle group.

endorphin—Powerful opioid peptide manufactured in the brain that regulates pain perception. Responsible for the euphoric sensations experienced during vigorous exercise, such as the runner's high, second wind, and so on. A member of the morphine family.

essential amino acid—Amino acid that cannot by synthesized by the body, and therefore must be supplied by the diet.

excitation—Ability to react to a stimulus.

fasciculus (pl. fasciculi)—A group or bundle of skeletal muscle fibers held together by a connective tissue called the perimysium.

fast twitch fiber (FT)—A muscle fiber characterized by fast contraction time, high anaerobic capacity, and low aerobic capacity, all making the fiber suited for high-power output activities.

fat—A compound containing glycerol and fatty acids. One of the major basic foods.

fat-free mass—Weight of the body minus the fat.

fixators—Muscles that are stimulated to act in order to stabilize the position of a bone to perform a motion. Also know as stabilizers.

flat pyramid load pattern—A loading pattern that after the warm-up lift stabilizes the load for the entire duration of strength training.

flexibility—Range of motion about a joint (static flexibility); opposition or resistance of a joint to motion (dynamic flexibility).

glycemic index—A measure of how quickly a food is digested as compared with the speed of glucose digestion. Indicates whether or not a food may cause harmful insulin fluctuations. Bodybuilders have found this to be a useful tool for dieting purposes.

glycogen—The form in which carbohydrates (glucose) are stored in the muscles and liver.

glycolysis—The metabolism of glucose into pyruvic acid or lactic acid to produce ATP for energy.

growth hormone—A hormone, secreted by the anterior lobe of the pituitary gland, that stimulates growth and development.

heavy load—A load using a percentage over 80 to 85 percent of the maximum.

homeostasis—Maintenance of a relatively stable internal physiological condition. As the stress of exercise causes changes in the internal environment, the body is constantly working to restore balance, or achieve homeostasis.

hydrostatic weighing—An accurate technique used to measure body fat, whereby the subject is submerged in a water tank and weighed. This value, along with the dry weight, residual volume, and water temperature, are used to calculate percentage of body fat.

hyperemia—Increase in the quantity of blood flowing through any part of the body. This is often experienced as a "pump" or the feeling of blood-engorged muscles after weight training.

hyperplasia—Increase in the number of cells in a tissue or organ.

hypertrophy—Increase in the size of a tissue or organ due to increased cell size rather than increased cell number.

incomplete protein—Protein that does not contain all of the nine essential amino acids. Found in plant proteins.

inhibition—To repress, or slow down, the stimulating (excitation) effect of the CNS (by decreasing the electrical activity).

intensity—Refers to the qualitative element of training. In bodybuilding training, intensity is expressed as a percentage of 1RM.

isokinetic contraction—Contraction in which tension is developed but there is no change in the length of the muscle.

isotonic contraction—Contraction in which the muscle shortens while lifting a constant load. Also know as a concentric, or dynamic, contraction.

joint—Junction of two or more bones in the human body in which the bones are joined in a functional relationship.

lactic acid system—An anaerobic energy system in which ATP is manufactured through the breakdown of glucose, in the absence of oxygen, to lactic acid. The energy is used in high-intensity work over a short duration (less than 2 minutes).

lactic acid—Fatiguing metabolite of the glycolytic (anaerobic, or lactic acid) system resulting from the incomplete breakdown of glucose.

ligament—Strong band of fibrous tissue that connects bones to each other.

limiting amino acid—The essential amino acid that is in shortest supply in the body and that is consequently responsible for the stop of protein synthesis.

line of pull—The line of action of the tension developed by a muscle.

low load—Pertaining to loads between 0 and 79 percent of one's maximum.

macrocycle—A phase of training of two to six weeks in duration.

maximum load—Refers to a load of 90 to 100 percent of one's maximum.

medium load—Pertaining to loads between 50 to 89 percent of one's maximum.

membrane—A structural barrier composed of lipids and proteins.

microcycle—A phase of training of approximately one week in duration.

microtear—Small tear found in muscle, ligaments, or tendons.

monosaccharide—Simple sugar. The two most common are glucose (blood sugar) and fructose (found in fruit).

motor unit—Individual motor nerve and all the muscle fibers it innervates.

motor neuron—A nerve cell that when stimulated effects muscular contraction. Most motor neurons innervate skeletal muscle.

myofibril—The part of a muscle fiber containing two protein filaments—myosin and actin.

myosin—A protein involved in muscular contraction.

negative calorie balance—A state in which the body is burning more calories than it is consuming. This is necessary if weight loss is to occur.

neural adaptation—Increased nervous coordination of a group of muscles involved in contraction. Gains in strength before puberty often result from improved neural adaptation.

neuromuscular junction—The union of a muscle and its nerve.

neuron—A nerve cell specialized to initiate, integrate, and conduct electric signals.

nonessential amino acid—An amino acid that can be synthesized by the body and therefore does not need to be supplied by the diet.

one-repetition maximum (1RM)—The maximum amount of weight that a person can lift once; 100 percent of one's lifting capacity.

overcompensation—Often called supercompensation, refers to the relationship between work and regeneration as a biological base for physical and psychological arousal before a heavy workout.

overloading—An increase of work in training with the goal of improving strength.

Periodization of nutrition—The structure of using nutritional and training supplements in order to match training phases.

Periodization of bodybuilding—The methodological structure of training phases intended to bring about the best improvements in muscle size, tone, and definition.

phase-specific—Pertaining to a particular training phase, for example, hypertrophy phase, muscle definition phase, and so on.

plantar flexion—Movement of the foot forward and downward.

plateau—Period during training when no observable progress is made.

PNF (proprioceptive neuromuscular facilitation)—Flexibility technique designed to enhance the relaxation and contraction of a body part, based on neurophysiological principles.

polysaccharide—See complex carbohydrates.

prime movers—Muscles primarily responsible for performance of a technical movement.

protein—Substance composed of amino acid chains. It is used for tissue growth and repair, as opposed to fuel for the body.

pump—The thick, full feeling during weight training that results from blood engorging the muscles being trained.

pyramid load pattern—Method of load patterning whereby the load for an exercise starts low, gradually increases with each set, hits a high point, and then decreases.

RDA (recommended dietary allowance)—A guideline of food intake for the general population. RDA values may not be appropriate for serious bodybuilders, because of the heightened demands placed on their bodies.

receptor—Specific protein-binding site in plasma membrane or interior of target cell.

sensory neuron—A nerve cell that conveys impulses from a receptor to the CNS. Examples of sensory neurons are those excited by sound, pain, light, and taste.

skewed pyramid load pattern—A pattern in which the load is constantly increased throughout the session, with exception being made for the last set, when the load is lowered.

slow twitch fiber (ST)—A muscle fiber characterized by slow contraction time, low anaerobic capacity, and high aerobic capacity, all making the fiber suited for low-power output activities.

specificity training—Principle underlying construction of a training program for a specific activity or skill.

spotter—Individual who watches and/or assists a lifter while a set is being performed.

stabilizers (fixators)—Muscles that are stimulated to act, to anchor, or to stabilize the position of a limb.

standard loading—A load that remains at the same level for a certain period of time.

static flexibility—Passively stretching an antagonistic muscle by placing it in a maximal stretch position and holding it in place.

step-loading principle—Pertaining to increasing the load from week to week, normally for three weeks, followed by a week of unloading so that the body can regenerate before a new increase.

stretch, or myostatic, reflex—Reflex that responds to the rate of muscle stretch. This reflex has the fastest known response to a stimulus (in this case, the rate of muscle stretch). The stretch reflex elicits a contraction of the muscle being stretched and the synergistic muscles, while inhibiting the antagonistic muscles, when it senses that a stretch is being performed too quickly or rigorously.

supermaximum load—A load that exceeds 100 percent of one's 1RM (1-repetition maximum). These weights should only be used by experienced lifters, especially in the maximum-strength phase of training.

synergist—A muscle that actively provides an additive contribution to the agonist muscle during a muscle contraction.

tendon—Collagen fiber bundle that connects muscle to bone and transmits muscle contractile force to the bone.

testosterone—Male sex hormone produced in the testes; responsible for secondary male sexual characteristics.

transient hypertrophy—Temporary enlargement of muscles due to water accumulation, not to permanent tissue growth. Occurs during and shortly after an intense weight-training session and subsides after a short time when the body returns to its normal state (homeostasis).

twitch—A brief period of contraction followed by relaxation in the response of a motor unit to a stimulus (nerve impulse).

unloading—Decrease of load, often for the purpose of allowing the body and mind to regenerate and refresh itself before a new loading phase.

urea—Major body waste product formed from the breakdown of amino acids.

vasodilation—Expansion of the blood vessels, especially the arteries and their branches.

yo-yo dieting—The process of repeatedly gaining and losing large amounts of body weight.

REFERENCES

Alway, S.E. 1997. Anatomy and kinesiology of skeletal muscle: The framework for movement. *Muscle Development* 31(3):34-35, 180-81.

Ameredes, B.T., W.Z. Zhan, R. Vanderboom, Y.S. Prakash, and G.C. Sieck. 2000. Power fatigue of the rat diaphragm muscle. *J Appl Physiol* 89:2215-19.

Anderson, R.A. 1986. Chromium metabolism and its role in disease processes in man. *Clin Physiol Biochem* 4(1):31-41.

Anderson, R.A., M.M. Polansky, N.A. Bryden, et al. 1982. Effect of exercise (running) on serum glucose, insulin, glucagon, and chromium excretion. *Diabetes* 31(3):212-16.

Appell, H.J. 1990. Muscular atrophy following immobilization: A review. *Sports Med* 10(1): 42-58.

Armstrong, R.B. 1986. Muscle damage and endurance events. *Sports Med* 3:370-81.

Arnheim, D. 1989. *Modern principles of athletic training*, 7th ed. St. Louis: Times Mirror/Mosby College.

Asmussen, E., and K. Mazin. 1978. A central nervous component in local muscular fatigue. *Europ J Appl Physiol* 38:9-15.

Awad, A.B., and E.A. Zepp. 1979. Alteration of rat adipose tissue lipolytic response to norepinephrine by dietary fatty acid manipulation. *Biochem Biophys Res Comm* 86:138-44.

Babichev, V.N., T.A. Peryshkova, N.I. Aivazashvili, and I.V. Shishkin. 1989. Effect of alcohol on the content of sex steroid receptors in the hypothalamus and hypophysis of male rats. *Biull Eksp Biol Med* 107(2):204-7.

Barnett, G., C.W. Chiang, and V.J. Licko. 1983. Effects of marijuana on testosterone in male subjects. *Theor Biol* 104(4):685-92.

Baroga, L. 1978. Contemporary tendencies in the methodology of strength development. *Educatia Fizica si Sport* 6:22-36.

Behm, D.G. 1995. Neuromuscular implications and applications of resistance training. *J Strength Condit Res* 9:264-74.

Belzung, F., T. Raclot, and R. Groscolas. 1993. Fish oil n-3 fatty acids selectively limit the hypertrophy of abdominal fat depots in growing rats fed high-fat diets. *Am J Physiol* 264(6 Pt 2): R1111-18.

Bendich, A. 1989. Symposium conclusions: Biological actions of carotenoids. *J Nutr* 119(1):135-36.

Bhathena, S.J., E. Berlin, J.T. Judd, et al. 1989. Dietary fat and menstrual-cycle effects on the erythrocyte ghost insulin receptor in premenopausal women. *Am J Clin Nutr* 50(3):460-64.

Biolo, G., R.Y.D. Fleming, and R.R. Wolfe. 1995. Physiologic hyperinsulinemia stimulates protein synthesis and enhances transport of selected amino acids in human skeletal muscle. *J Clin Invest* 95:811-19.

Blankson, H., J.A. Stakkestad, H. Fagertun, E. Thom, J. Wadstein, and O. Gudmundsen. 2000. Conjugated linoleic acid reduces body fat mass in overweight and obese humans. *J Nutr* 130(12):2943-48.

Bompa, T.O. 1999. *Periodization: Theory and methodology of training.* Champaign, Illinois: Human Kinetics.

Bompa, T.O., and L.J. Cornacchia. 1998. *Serious strength training.* Champaign, IL: Human Kinetics.

Borer, K.T. 1994. Neurohumoral mediation of exercise-induced growth. *Med Sci Sport Exerc* 26(6): 741-54.

Brilla, L.R., and T.F. Haley. 1992. Effect of magnesium supplementation on strength training in humans. *J Am Coll Nutr* 11(3):326-29.

Bucci, L., J.F. Hickson Jr., J.M. Pivarnik, et al. 1990. Ornithine ingestion and growth hormone release in bodybuilders. *Nutr Res* 10(3):239-45.

Butterfield, G., and D.H. Calloway. 1984. Physical activity improves protein utilization in young men. *Br J Nutr* 51:171-84.

Chung, K.W. 1989. Effect of ethanol on androgen receptors in the anterior pituitary, hypothalamus and brain cortex in rats. *Life Sci* 44(4):2273-80.

Cook, M.E., C.C. Miller, Y. Park, and M. Pariza. 1993. Immune modulation by altered nutrient metabolism: Nutritional control of immune-induced growth depression. *Poultry Sci* 72(7):1301-5.

Cordova, A., and M. Alvarez-Mon. 1995. Behaviour of zinc in physical exercise: A special reference to immunity and fatigue. *Neurosci Biobehav Rev* 19(3):439-45.

Coronado, R., J. Morrissette, M. Sukhareva, and D.M. Vaughan. 1994. Structure and function of ryanodine receptors. *Am J Physiol Cell Physiol* 266:C1485-504.

DeLuca, C.J., R.S. LeFever, M.P. McCue, and A.P. Xenakis. 1982. Behaviour of human motor units in different muscles during lineally varying contractions. *J Physiol* (Lond) 329:113-28.

Denke, M.A., and S.M. Grundy. 1991. Effects of fats high in stearic acid on lipid and lipoprotein concentrations in men. *Am J Clin Nutr* 54(6):1036-40.

Diamond, F., L. Ringenberg, D. MacDonald, et al. 1986. Effects of drug and alcohol abuse upon pituitary-testicular function in adolescent males. *Adol Health Care* 7(1):28-33.

DiPasquale, M.G. 2001. *The Metabolic Diet*. Austin, TX: Allprotraining.com Books.

Dodd, S.L., R.A. Herb, and S.K. Powers. 1993. Caffeine and exercise performance. An update. *Sports Med* 15(1):14-23.

Dorup, I., A. Flyvbjerg, M.E. Everts, and T. Clausen. 1991. Role of insulin-like growth factor-1 and growth hormone in growth inhibition induced by magnesium and zinc deficiencies. *Brit J Nutr* 66(3):505-21.

Dragan, G.I., A. Vasiliu, and E. Georgescu. 1985. Research concerning the effects of Refit on elite weightlifters. *J Sports Med Physical Fitness* 25(4):246-50.

Dragan, G.I., W. Wagner, and E. Ploesteanu. 1988. Studies concerning the ergogenic value of protein supply and l-carnitine in elite junior cyclists. *Physiologie* 25(3):129-32.

Dray, F., B. Kouznetzova, D. Harris, and P. Brazeau. 1980. Role of prostaglandins on growth hormone secretion: PGE2 a physiological stimulator. *Adv Prostagl Thrombox Res* 8:1321-28.

Durnin, J.V. 1982. Muscle in sports medicine—Nutrition and muscular performance. *Int J Sports Med* 3(Suppl 1):52-57.

Ebbing, C., and P. Clarkson. 1989. Exercise-induced muscle damage and adaptation. *Sports Med* 7:207-34.

Enoka, R. 1996. Eccentric contractions require unique activation strategies by the nervous system. *J Appl Physiol* 81:2339-46.

Eritsland, J., H. Arnesen, I. Seljeflot, and A.T. Hostmark. 1995. Long-term metabolic effects of n-3 polyunsaturated fatty acids in patients with coronary artery disease. *Am J Clin Nutr* 61(4):831-36.

Evans, W.J. 1987. Exercise-induced skeletal muscle damage. *Phys Sports Med* 15(1):89-100.

Fahey, T.D. 1991. How to cope with muscle soreness. *Power Research*.

Fossati, P., and P. Fontaine. 1993. Endocrine and metabolic consequences of massive obesity. *Rev Praticien* 43(15):1935-39.

Fox, E.L., R.W. Bowes, and M.L. Foss. 1989. *The physiological basis of physical education and athletics*. Dubuque, Iowa: Wm. C. Brown.

Fry, R.W., R. Morton, and D. Keast. 1991. Overtraining in athletics. *Sports Med* 2(1):32-65.

Garg, M.L., A. Wierzbicki, M. Keelan, A.B. Thomson, and M.T. Clandinin. 1989. Fish oil prevents change in arachidonic acid and cholesterol content in rat caused by dietary cholesterol. *Lipids* 24(4):266-70.

Ghavami-Maibodi, S.Z., P.J. Collipp, M. Castro-Magana, C. Stewart, and S.Y. Chen. 1983. Effect of oral zinc supplements on growth, hormonal levels and zinc in healthy short children. *Ann Nutr Metab* 273:214-19.

Gohil, K., L. Rothfuss, J. Lang, and L. Packer. 1987. Effect of exercise training on tissue vitamin E and ubiquinone content. *J Appl Physiol* 63(4):1638-41.

Goldberg, A.L., J.D. Etlinger, D.F. Goldspink, and C. Jablecki. 1975. Mechanism of work-induced hypertrophy of skeletal muscles. *Med Sci Sports Exerc* 7:185-98.

Grandjean, A.C. 1983. Vitamins, diet, and the athlete. *Clin Sports Med* 2(1):105-14.

Grimby, G. 1992. *Strength and power in sport*, ed. P.V. Komi. Oxford: Blackwell Scientific.

Habito, R.C., J. Montalto, E. Leslie, and M.J. Ball. 2000. Effects of replacing meat with soybean in the diet on sex hormone concentrations in healthy adult males. *Br J Nutr* 84(4):557-63.

Hainaut, K., and J. Duchatteau. 1989. Muscle fatigue: Effects of training and disuse. *Muscle and Nerve* 12:660-69.

Han, Y.S., D.N. Proctor, P.C. Geiger, and G.C. Sieck. 2001. Reserve capacity for ATP consumption during isometric contraction in human skeletal muscle fibers. *J Appl Physiol* 90(2):657-64.

Harris, D.B., R.C. Harris, A.M. Wilson, and A. Goodship. 1997. ATP loss with exercise in muscle fibres of the gluteus medius of the thoroughbred horse. *Res Vet Sci* 63(3):231-37.

Hartman, J.H., and H. Tünneman 1988. *Fitness and strength training*. Berlin: Sportsverlag.

Hartoma, T.R., K. Nahoul, and A. Netter. 1977. Zinc, plasma androgens and male sterility. *Lancet* 2:1125-26.

Houmard, J.A. 1991. Impact of reduced training of performance in endurance athletes. *Sports Med* 12(6):380-393.

Hsu, J.M. 1977. Zinc deficiency and alterations of free amino acid levels in plasma, urine and skin extract. *Progr Clin Biol Res* 14:73-86.

Hunt, C.D., P.E. Johnson, J. Herbel, and L.K. Mullen. 1992. Effects of dietary zinc depletion on seminal volume of zinc loss, serum testosterone concentrations and sperm morphology in young men. *Am J Clin Nutr* 56(1):148-57.

Ip, C., J.A. Scimeca, and H.J. Thompson. 1994. Conjugated linoleic acid. A powerful anticarcinogen from animal fat sources. *Cancer* 74(3 Suppl):1050-54.

Ip, C., M. Singh, H.J. Thompson, and J.A. Scimeca. 1994. Conjugated linoleic acid suppresses mammary carcinogenesis and proliferative activity of the mammary gland in the rat. *Cancer Res* 54(5):1212-15.

Israel, S. 1972. The acute syndrome of detraining. *GDR National Olympic Committee* 2:30-35.

Iwasaki, K., K. Mano, M. Ishihara, et al. 1987. Effects of ornithine or arginine administration on serum amino acid levels. *Biochem Int* 14(5):971-76.

Jacobson, B.H., M.D. Weber, L. Claypool, and L.E. Hunt. 1992. Effect of caffeine on maximal strength and power in elite male athletes. *Br J Sports Med* 26(4):276-80.

Katan, M.B., P.L. Zock, and R.P. Mensink. 1994. Effects of fats and fatty acids on blood lipids in humans: An overview. *Am J Clin Nutr* 60(6 Suppl):1017-22S.

Kieffer, F. 1986. [Trace elements: Their importance for health and physical performance.] *Deut Zeit Sportmed* 37(4):118-23.

Kobayashi Matsui, H. 1983. Analysis of myoelectric signals during dynamic and isometric contraction. *Electromyog Clin Neurophysiol* 26:147-60.

Kuipers, H., and H.A. Keizer. 1988. Overtraining in elite athletes: Review and directions for the future. *Sports Med* 6:79-92.

Laricheva, K.A., N.I. Ialovaia, V.I. Shubin, P.V. Smirnov, and V.S. Beliaev. 1977. Use of the specialized protein product, SP-11, in the nutrition of highly trained sportsmen in heavy athletics. *Vopr Pitan* Jul-Aug(4):47-51.

Lavy, A., A. Ben-Amotz, and M. Aviram. 1993. Preferential inhibition of LDL oxidation by the all-trans isomer of beta-carotene in comparison with 9-cis beta-carotene. *Eur J Clin Chem Clin Biochem* 31(2):83-90.

Lefavi, R.G., R.A. Anderson, R.E. Keith, et al. 1992. Efficacy of chromium supplementation in athletes: Emphasis on anabolism. *Int J Sport Nutr* 2(2):111-22.

Lefebvre, P.J., and A.J. Scheen. 1995. Improving the action of insulin. *Clin Invest Med—Medecine Clinique et Experimentale* 18(4):340-47.

Lemon, P.W. 1998. Effects of exercise on dietary protein requirements. *Int J Sport Nutr* 8(4):426-47.

Lemon, P.W. 2000. Beyond the zone: Protein needs of active individuals. *J Am Coll Nutr* Oct19(5 Suppl):513-21S.

Lichtenstein, A.H., L.M. Ausman, W. Carrasco, et al. 1993. Effects of canola, corn, and olive oils on fasting and postprandial plasma lipoproteins in humans as part of a National Cholesterol Education Program Step 2 diet. *Arterioscl Thromb* 13(10):1533-42.

Malomsoki, J. 1983. [The improvement of sports performance by means of complementary nutrition]. *Sportorvosi szemle/Hungarian Review of Sports Medicine* 24(4):269-82.

Mariotti, F., S. Mahe, C. Luengo, R. Benamouzig, and D. Tome 2000. Postprandial modulation of dietary and whole-body nitrogen utilization by carbohydrates in humans. *Am J Clin Nutr* 72:954-62.

Marsden, C.D., J.C. Meadows, and P.A. Merton. 1971. Isolated single motor units in human muscle and their rate of discharge during maximum voluntary effort. *J Physiol (London)* 217:12P.

Matsuda, J.J., R.F. Zermocle, A.C. Vailus, V.A. Perrini, A. Pedrini-Mille, and J.A. Maynard. 1986. Structural and mechanical adaptation of immature bone to strenuous exercise. *J Appl Physiol* 60(6):2028-34.

May, M.E., and M.G. Buse. 1989. Effects of branched-chain amino acids on protein turnover. *Diab Metab Rev* 5(3):227-45.

Mcbride, J.M., W.J. Kraemer, T. Triplett-Mcbride, and W. Sebastianelli. 1998. Effect of resistance exercise on free radical production. *Med Sci Sports Exerc* l(3):67-72.

McCall, G.E., W.C. Byrnes, A. Dickinson, P.M. Pattany, and S.J. Fleck. 1996. Muscle fiber hypertrophy, hyperplasia and capillary density in college men after resistance training. *J Appl Physiol* 81:2004-12.

McNamara, D.J. 1992. Dietary fatty acids, lipoproteins, and cardiovascular disease. *Adv Food Nutr Res* 36:253-351.

McNaughton, L.R. 1986. The influence of caffeine ingestion on incremental treadmill running. *Br J Sports Med* 20(3):109-12.

Melo, G.L., and E. Cararelli. 1994-95. Exercise physiology laboratory manual, 25.

Mendelson, J.H., N.K. Mello, S.K. Teoh, J. Ellingboe, and J. Cochin. 1989. Cocaine effects on pulsatile secretion of anterior pituitary, gonadal and adrenal hormones. *J Clin Endocrinol Metab* 69(6): 1256-60.

Metges, C.C., and C.A. Barth. 2000. Metabolic consequences of a high dietary-protein intake in adulthood: Assessment of the available evidence. *J Nutr* 130:886-89.

Miller, C.C., Y. Park, M.W. Pariza, and M.E. Cook. 1994. Feeding conjugated linoleic acid to animals partially overcomes catabolic responses due to endotoxin injection. *Biochem Biophysic Res Comm* 198(3):1107-12.

Millward, D.J. 1999. Optimal intakes of protein in the human diet. *Proc Nutr Soc* 58(2):403-13.

Morgan, R.E., and G.T. Adamson. 1959. *Circuit weight training*. London: G. Bell and Sons.

Moritani, T., and H.A. deVries. 1987. Re-examination of the relationship between the surface integrated electromyogram (IEMG) and force of isometric contraction. *Am J Physiol Med* 57: 263-77.

Moritani, T., M. Muro, and A. Nagata. 1986. Intramuscular and surface electromyogram changes during muscle fatigue. *J Appl Physiol* 60:1179-85.

National Research Council. 1989. Protein and amino acids. In *Recommended dietary allowances*, 10th ed. Washington, DC: National Academy Press.

Nielsen, O.B., F. de Paoli, and K. Overgaard. 2001. Protective effects of lactic acid on force production in rat skeletal muscle. *J Physiol* 536(Pt 1):161-66.

Noth, R.H., and R.M. Walter. 1984. The effects of alcohol on the endocrine system. *Med Clin North Am* 68(1):133-46.

Nybo, L., and B. Nielsen. 2001. Hyperthermia and central fatigue during prolonged exercise in humans. *J Appl Physiol* 91:1055-60.

Opstad, P.K., and A. Asskvaag. 1983. The effect of sleep deprivation on the plasma levels of hormones during prolonged physical strain and calorie deficiency. *Eur J Appl Phys Occup Phys* 51(1):97-107.

Oteiza, P.I., K.L. Olin, C.G. Fraga, and C.L. Keen. 1995. Zinc deficiency causes oxidative damage to proteins, lipids and DNA in rat testes. *J Nutr* 125(4):823-29.

Packer, L. 1997. Oxidants, antioxidant nutrients and the athlete. *J Sports Sci* 15(3):353-63.

Packer, L., and S.I. Landvik. 1989. Vitamin E: Introduction to biochemistry and health benefits. *Ann NY Acad Sci* 570:1-6.

Paffenbarger, R.S. Jr., J.B. Kampert, I.M. Lee, et al. 1994. Changes in physical activity and other lifeway patterns influencing longevity. *Med Sci Sports Exerc* 26(7):857-65.

Pariza, M.W., Y.L. Ha, H. Benjamin, et al. 1991. Formation and action of anticarcinogenic fatty acids. *Adv Exper Med Biol* 289:269-72.

Parrish, C.C., D.A. Pathy, and A. Angel. 1990. Dietary fish oils limit adipose tissue hypertrophy in rats. *Metabolism: Clin Exp* 39(3):217-19.

Parrish, C.C., D.A. Pathy, J.G. Parkes, and A. Angel. 1991. Dietary fish oils modify adipocyte structure and function. *J Cell Phys* 148(3):493-502.

Philip, W., T. James, and A. Ralph. 1992. Dietary fats and cancer. *Nutr Res* 12(Suppl):S147-58.

Posterino, G.S., T.L. Dutka, and G.D. Lamb. 2001. L(+)-lactate does not affect twitch and tetanic responses in mechanically skinned mammalian muscle fibres. *Pflugers Arch* May 442(2):197-203.

Prasad, A.S. 1996. Zinc deficiency in women, infants and children. *J Am Coll Nutr* 15(2):113-20.

Prentice, W.J. 1990. *Rehabilitation techniques in sports medicine.* Toronto: Times Mirror/Mosby College.

Reid, M.B., K.E. Haack, K.M. Franchek, et al. 1992. Reactive oxygen in skeletal muscle. I. Intracellular oxidant kinetics and fatigue in vitro. *J Appl Physiol* 73(5):1797-1804.

Rennie, M.J., P.A. MacLennan, H.S. Hundal, et al. 1989. Skeletal muscle glutamine transport, intramuscular glutamine concentration, and muscle-protein turnover. *Metabolism* 38(8 Suppl 1):47-51.

Richardson, J.H., T. Palmerton, and M. Chenan. 1980. Effect of calcium on muscle fatigue. *J Sports Med Phys Fit* 20(2):149-51.

Sahlin, K. 1986. Metabolic changes limiting muscular performance. *Biochem Exerc* 16:22-31, 42-53.

Sanchez-Gomez, M., K. Malmlof, W. Mejia, A. Bermudez, M.T. Ochoa, S. Carrasco-Rodriguez, and A. Skottner. 1999. Insulin-like growth factor-I, but not growth hormone, is dependent on a high protein intake to increase nitrogen balance in the rat. *Br J Nutr* 81(2):145-52.

Schurch, P.M., A. Reinke, and W. Hollmann. 1979. Carbohydrate-reduced diet and metabolism: About the influence of a 4-week isocaloric, fat-rich, carbohydrate-reduced diet on body weight and metabolism. *Mediz Klinik-Muich* 74(36):1279-85.

Sherwood, L. 1993. *Human physiology from cells to systems,* 2nd ed. St. Paul, MN: West.

Shultz, T.D., B.P. Chew, W.R. Seaman, and L.O. Luedecke. 1992. Inhibitory effect of conjugated dienoic derivatives of linoleic acid and beta-carotene on the in vitro growth of human cancer cells. *Cancer Letters* 63(2):125-33.

Sidery, M.B., I.W. Gallen, and I.A. Macdonald. 1990. The initial physiological responses to glucose ingestion in normal subjects are modified by a 3 day high-fat diet. *Br J Nutr* 64(3):705-13.

Sies, H., W. Stahl, and A.R. Sundquist. 1992. Antioxidant functions of vitamins. Vitamins E and C, beta-carotene, and other carotenoids. *Ann N Y Acad Sci* 669:7-20.

Simopoulos, A.P. 1999. Essential fatty acids in health and chronic disease. *Amer J Clin Nutr* 70:560S-69S.

Soszynski, P.A., and L.A. Frohman. 1992. Inhibitory effects of ethanol on the growth hormone (GH)-releasing hormone-GH-insulin-like growth factor-I axis in the rat. *Endocrinology* 131(6):2603-8.

Starkey, D.B., M.L. Pollock, Y. Ishida, M.A. Welsh, W.F. Breshue, J.F. Graves, and M.S. Feigembaum. 1996. Effect of resistance training volume on strength and muscle thickness. *Med Sci Sports Exerc* 28:1311-20.

Staron, R.S., D.L. Karapondo, W.J. Kraemer, A.C. Fry, S.E. Gordon, J.E. Falkel, F.C. Hagerman, and R.S. Hikida. 1994. Skeletal muscle adaptations during early phase of heavy resistance training in men and women. *J Appl Physiol* 76:1247-55.

Terjung, R.L., and D.L. Hood. 1986. Biochemical adaptation in skeletal muscle induced by exercise training. *J Appl Physiol* 70:1021-28.

Tesch, P.A., E.G. Colliander, and P. Kaiser. 1986. Muscle metabolism during intense, heavy-resistance exercise. *Eur J Appl Physiol Occup Ther*.

Tipton, K.D., B.B. Rasmussen, S.L. Miller, S.E. Wolf, S.K. Owens-Stovall, B.E. Petrini, and R.R. Wolfe. 2001. Timing of amino acid-carbohydrate ingestion alters anabolic response of muscle to resistance exercise. *Am J Physiol Endocrinol Metab* Aug281(2):E197-206.

Wahrburg, U., H. Martin, M. Sandkamp, H. Schulte, and G. Assmann. 1992. Comparative effects of a recommended lipid-lowering diet vs a diet rich in monounsaturated fatty acids on serum lipid profiles in healthy young adults. *Am J Clin Nutr* 56(4):678-83.

Westerblad, H., D.G. Allen, J.D. Bruton, F.H. Andrade, and J. Lannergren. 1998. Mechanisms underlying the reduction of isometric force in skeletal muscle fatigue. *Acta Physiol Scand* 162:253-60.

Williams, J.H. 1991. Caffeine, neuromuscular function and high-intensity exercise performance. *J Sports Med Phys Fitness* 31(3):481-89.

Wilmore, J.H, and D.L Costill. 1999. *Physiology of sports and exercise*. Champaign, Illinois: Human Kinetics.

Wolfe, R.R. 2000. Protein supplements and exercise. *Am J Clin Nutr* 72:551-57S.

Yoshida, H., and G. Kajimoto. 1989. Effect of dietary vitamin E on the toxicity of autoxidized oil to rats. *Ann Nutr Metab* 33(3):153-61.

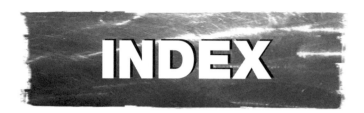
INDEX

Note: The italicized *f* and *t* following page numbers refer to figures and tables, respectively.

ABOUT THE AUTHORS

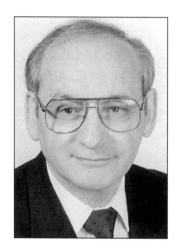

Tudor O. Bompa, PhD, revolutionized Western training methods when he introduced his groundbreaking theory of Periodization in Romania in 1963. After adopting his training system, the Eastern Bloc countries dominated international sports through the 1970s and 1980s. In 1988, Dr. Bompa applied his principle of periodization to the sport of bodybuilding. He has personally trained 11 Olympic Games medalists (including four gold medalists) and has served as a consultant to coaches and athletes worldwide.

Dr. Bompa's books on training methods, including *Theory and Methodology of Training: The Key to Athletic Performance* and *Periodization of Training for Sports,* have been translated into 17 languages and used in more than 130 countries for training athletes and educating and certifying coaches. Bompa has been invited to speak about training in more than 30 countries and has been awarded certificates of honor and appreciation from such prestigious organizations as the Argentinean Ministry of Culture, the Australian Sports Council, the Spanish Olympic Committee, and the International Olympic Committee.

A member of the Canadian Olympic Association and the Romanian National Council of Sports, Dr. Bompa is professor emeritus at York University, where he has taught training theories for 25 years. He and his wife, Tamara, live in Sharon, Ontario.

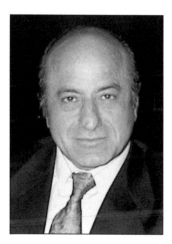

Mauro Di Pasquale, MD, a physician specializing in nutrition and sports medicine, spent 10 years at the University of Toronto teaching and researching nutritional supplements and drug use in sports. He wrote both *Bodybuilding Supplement Review* and *Amino Acids and Proteins for the Athlete* and has written hundreds of articles for *Muscle and Fitness, Flex, Men's Fitness, Shape, Muscle Media,* and *Ironman,* among many others. Di Pasquale was a powerlifter for over 20 years, winning the powerlifting world championships in 1976 and the World Games in 1981.

Di Pasquale received his medical degree from the University of Toronto and is a certified medical review officer. Currently the president of the International United Powerlifting Federation and the Pan American Powerlifting Federation, he lives in Ontario, Canada.

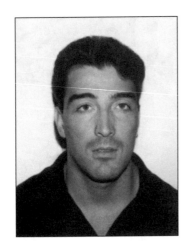

As a former bodybuilder, former professional wrestler for the National Wrestling Alliance (NWA), and kinesiologist, **Lorenzo J. Cornacchia** has conducted extensive electromyography (EMG) research to identify which exercises cause the greatest muscle stimulation and which could potentially cause harm. The Periodized Program that developed out of his research helped professional bodybuilder Laura Binetti win the World Championship in Detroit, Michigan, and go on to receive her highest ranking title ever in Ms.Olympia. Cornacchia is presently a contributing editor and author for *Ironman* magazine.

Cornacchia received his B.A. in physical education and health from York University. A member of the Association of Kinesiologists of Canada, he presently resides in Oak Ridges, Ontario.

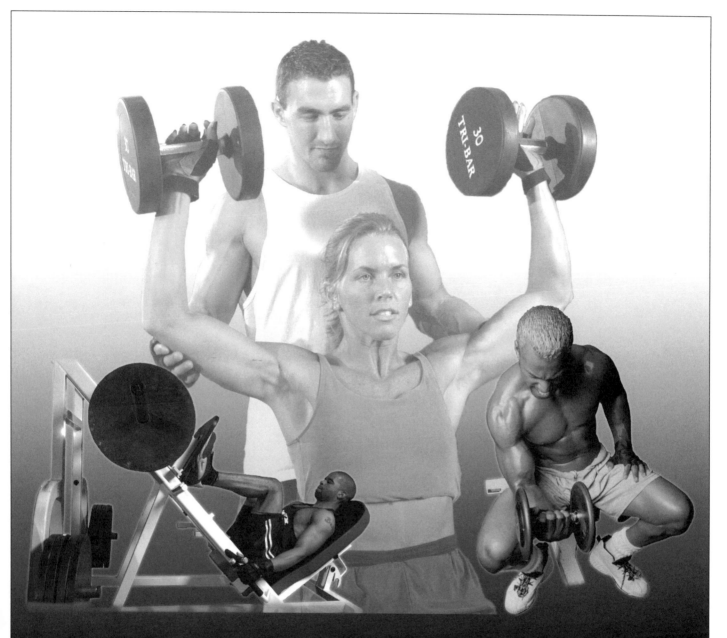

You'll find other outstanding strength training resources at

http://strengthtraining.humankinetics.com

In the U.S. call 1-800-747-4457

Australia 08 8372 0999 • Canada 1-800-465-7301
Europe +44 (0) 113 255 5665 • New Zealand 0064 9 448 1207

 HUMAN KINETICS
The Premier Publisher for Sports & Fitness
P.O. Box 5076 • Champaign, IL 61825-5076 USA